CRITICAL MASS

The Extremely Dangerous Life of an
Emergency Nurse

Ron Martin

PAGE PUBLISHING, INC.
Conneaut Lake, PA

First originally published by Page Publishing 2020

ISBN 978-1-6624-0465-8 (pbk)
ISBN 978-1-6624-0466-5 (digital)

Printed in the United States of America

Contents

PROLOGUE

First of all, if you are one of those avid bicyclists who participate in one of the phenomenal worldwide Critical Mass bicycle rides typically held on the last Friday of every month, and you thought this book might be a chronicling of these events, *do not* put this book down. Critical Mass bike tours originated over forty years ago in Stockholm, Sweden, in 1972, quickly spreading to over three hundred cities around the world, and finally gripped America on Friday, September 25, 1992, in San Francisco, soon to become a monthly social protest movement.

Rather, my book is more focused on the *phenomenon* of critical mass that got its origins in the early 1950s during an unknown scientist's research and observation of macaque monkeys (*Macaca fuscata*) on the remote island of Koshima, Japan. This very intelligent, omnivorous, mostly terrestrial, matrilineal Old World monkey species, aka the snow monkey, is the most north-living primate on earth, save for *Homo sapiens*. The major difference between us and them besides our opposing thumb is the fact that macaques have evolutionarily evolved to survive extremes of snow and cold, whereas *H. sapiens* learned to survive the weather extremes by covering themselves with the furs of other dead animals. It seems there was a serious drought and famine on Koshima, so the researchers provided sweet potatoes dipped in sand to the local simian population. The macaques loved the sweet potatoes but disliked the taste and feel of the sand, much like myself; eating clam chowder with sand and clam shell fragments can really ruin the soup appetizer on a typical Friday Night Fish Fry in Milwaukee, Wisconsin.

One day, an eighteen-month-old macaque picked up the sweet potato, carried it over to the nearby stream, and washed the sand off. He was instantly rewarded by having no sand in his meal, so he taught the lesson to his mom and playmates, who taught this new behavior to their mothers. News soon spread throughout the macaque colony over a six-year period. One day, when the one hundredth macaque, *as the story is told*, learned to wash his food before eating, an amazing phenomenon occurred. Suddenly, *all* the monkeys on Koshima began washing their food before eating. This added energy of the one hundredth monkey had created an extraordinary behavioral change. More importantly and even more mysteriously, this behavior of washing food before eating suddenly spread to monkeys on islands all around the Pacific, some as far as five hundred miles away.

The phenomenon of *critical mass* became a shared consciousness. When a limited number of people learn something in a new way, that knowledge remains in their conscious proprietary awareness. However, at some point, when that awareness permeates just *one more person*, it generates the critical-mass effect, and that consciousness and awareness is picked up by everyone. Our collective consciousness must be proactive in order to effect prompt positive changes.

If 999 people read my book, I will provide the thousandth copy, autographed and free of charge, to the next interested reader, hoping to duplicate the critical-mass effect it had nearly seventy years ago to the macaques on Koshima, Japan.

This biographical account of my life, and how it has truly already affected literally tens of thousands of people's lives firsthand, has not come without great cost and sacrifice to myself and my family. Many great things are in store for my future, even though my days of being one of the many great emergency nurses are now past tense. How the end of my illustrious career was finally determined will be disclosed in explicit detail in this saga's closing chapters. The *reasons* are what are most upsetting, not just for myself, but for those health care professionals (HCPs), nurses, doctors, PAs, EMTs, paramedics, and all EMS personnel that I have loved, adored, mentored, partied, and worked with for nearly four decades, that I leave behind to continue caring for the sick and infirm during the

"Reign of Obamacare" (Affordable Care Act) or "Obama Trauma" (my idiom). As much as I despise more legislation and government intervention into the private lives of Americans (and the rest of the world!), I feel my mission is to make more people aware—hence, the critical mass phenomenon—of what is happening inside the doors of our hospitals that *administrations so desperately try to hide* from the public. Once safe refuges of healing, hospitals and especially ERs have become soft targets, havens for the pharmaceutical opioid drug seeking (prescription drug overdose is now *the number 1 cause of accidental death in America*, surpassing automobile accidents), drop-off centers for society's rejects, shelters for the homeless, and places of *extreme* violence. The health care profession *leads the nation in all occupations* with the number of work-related violence and assaults resulting in lost days of work. Hospital administrations refuse to acknowledge the growing problem, and mostly (76 percent) fail to acknowledge when one of its own employees is assaulted, raped, or killed. Instead, they would like to portray hospitals as a hotel-like atmosphere with security guards dressed more like upscale hotel concierges rather than security guards, *and* with no defensive deterrents except their body as a shield. Hospital administrators rightfully go to great efforts to provide a safe environment for their "clients" (if you were sick or injured, you were my "patient," not my "client," and I was your "nurse," not your "mother") but have failed miserably to provide a safe working environment for their dedicated employees. Verbal abuse, physical abuse, assault, rape, and murder should *not* be considered "part of the job." Slapping, pinching, biting, hitting, kicking, punching, shoving, breaking bones, and being shot at, spit on, and urinated on have all occurred to me numerous times during my nursing career. I finally met my Waterloo almost three hundred years after Napoleon when my last assault caused permanent, irreparable damage. Legislative standards must be imposed to protect the hospital staff first and foremost so that we can continue to provide excellent nursing care to our patients into the twenty-first century.

The original intention of this book was to be a composite of my life as a helicopter flight nurse, my dream for many years, with flashbacks from my past and how they became relevant years later in forming the unique individual I am today. However, during the writing of my book, I became gravely ill from an unknown, undetected blood-borne (*and* work-related I might add) disease that I will hopefully die *with*, not *from*. I lost track of my manuscript for several years through several moves over the US, and after finally rediscovering my disk, I had to seek professional computer guidance to transfer my data from four-inch floppy disk to CD format. So much had transpired during those ten-plus years that were worthy of mention that I decided to extend my story to cover my life to present day. I have experienced and survived more bizarre, exotic, frightening, life-altering, life-threatening experiences in my nursing career than likely most anyone in the same profession. The proof is in the fact that I am alive to complete this account. The final insult that ended my inimitable, exceptional career as one of most experienced clinical emergency nurses to walk the halls of any hospital is one that I sincerely hope will raise questions for hospital administrators, managers, state and federal legislators, attorneys, and idealistic young men and women who dare enter the *most dangerous profession in the US*, the health care industry. I feel fortunate that I no longer have to experience the fallout from Obamacare as an emergency room nurse, but must endure the repercussions of increasingly socialized medicine as a patient. Thank dog one day soon I will utilize the VA as my primary medical care provider.

Over a career spanning four decades, I have been personally accountable for saving hundreds of lives and have given those individuals a second chance on life. I hope they have all realized their unique good fortune and have lived their new lives with a renewed sense of purpose. Unfortunately, during that same span, I have seen literally thousands of people die, most of them young and most of them tragic. This toll has weighed heavily on my conscience over the years; the demons still haunt me, and my heart mourns when I hear their silent screams in the still darkness of night, despite months of psychological counseling. It is part of who I am, and I feel blessed that I was able to save those I could and accept death for those I could not.

The greatest unselfish act on the planet is placing the life of another human being unequivocally above that of your own. John

15:13 states, "Greater love has no man than this; that a man lay down his life for his friends." I have toiled and struggled for over seventy years trying to discover the true meaning of life. I believe strong faith and morals, responsibly, honesty and integrity, facing life's challenges head-on, being accountable for one's actions, and walking proudly and honorably along life's course is the honorable path, but not the final destination. I offered my life as millions did for my country in the US Marines in Viet Nam but was somehow graciously and questioningly spared, only to serve a more dangerous mission in life, once again fighting an unseen deadly enemy. Unknowingly at that time, it unleashed its enigmatic lethal fury upon me at a time when my only thoughts were to save the life of a human being on the worst day of his life—*mine!* My lifespan on Mother Earth has been directly affected as a result of my profession by a primitive, opportunistic, and deadly intruder. My exemplary nursing career was abruptly and prematurely concluded by a tragic, yet preventable, act of extreme violence in a hospital ER, the last day that I ever provided patient care for another human being requiring my help in a hospital.

I have been rewarded in life, and my soul can rest without burden, for I have loved and been loved, helped perpetuate my species, and performed the ultimate sacrifice: I have given of my life so others could live. It was not the *brave* thing to do—it was just the *right* thing to do. This will be the footprint I leave on this earth, for I will surely be forgotten, as are the fallen leaves on a tree in winter. If this book is in print before my death, I will be complete and fulfilled, for this will be my legacy to the world, something to remember me by long after my bones have turned to dust...

CHAPTER 1

Shooters

"There are no rules. Thou shalt win at all cost"—
the tenth commandment of Specwar.

—Cmdr. Dick Marcinko, USN (Ret.), Rogue Warrior,
US Navy SEAL and founder of SEAL Team Six

Summer of 1968, Republic of South Viet Nam

The skids touched down hard and uneven on the hastily built steel-mesh heliport. It was well over 110 degrees, so hot that if you were to walk barefooted on the metal planks, it would blister the bottoms of your feet. Relative humidity was teetering near triple digits as well, so you never really dried out and the camouflage cotton BDUs (battle dress uniform) stuck to you like a second skin. The Huey, a UH-1 Iroquois Bell helicopter, shut down a few minutes later, after allowing the single 1,400 HP Avco Lycoming T-53-L-1 turbo shaft turbine engine to cool. The crew chief jumped out and did a walk-around to check for leaks and any new bullet holes. Its dirty olive-green skin was pockmarked with little green squares, "Band-Aids" covering recent bullet holes in the fuselage courtesy of Victor Charlie. The pilot, a warrant officer—my god, he was as young looking as me—removed his flight helmet and shook his sweat-soaked head from the heat, fatigue, and stress of war, much like a dog after an unwelcome bath, to remove the excess sweat from his short locks. Who knows where they came from last, but they must have received incoming fire because the door gunner, a kid with peach fuzz on his face and not much more on his head, went to resupply his ammo and police the brass scattered on the deck while the aircraft took on more fuel.

"I'm lookin' for a hop to Hué. Any chance you guys are headed up north?" I was actually on unofficial business, just going to visit a friend who was stationed near Hué, my first ever helicopter flight. No passport or official ID needed, just round eyes, a smile, and an offer of a free smoke. Smoking cigarettes was never popular with me, but I found out early on in the corps that when the call went out for "smoke 'em if you got 'em," those who smoked got to take a break; those who didn't kept on working, filling sandbags to build fortified bunkers against the frequent nightly incoming rocket attacks. Not that the bunkers would protect us from a direct hit from a 122 mm NVA rocket, but they afforded protection from unwanted shrapnel if one landed nearby. I learned to inhale with much effort and never really enjoyed it. Fortunately for me, just after my discharge two years later in '70, I had the willpower to stop cold turkey on July 4 and have never picked up another cigarette.

"It's your lucky day. Just so happens we're headed up that way if you can wait an hour or so. My crew needs to grab us some chow, resupply, fuel up, and hit the head. After we're refueled and my chief gives the thumbs-up, we'll be stopping at Phu Bai and Hué."

Thumbs-up, I thought. I felt like the *Sissy Hankshaw* of the Marine Corps, the first international helicopter hitchhiker, only my thumbs weren't any match for Ms. Hankshaw. This was way cool, just hang around the heliport and thumb a ride to anywhere in the countryside. I later became enamored with Sissy Hankshaw, a fictional feminist heroine born with mutant thumbs the size of Italian sausages, and savior of the endangered whooping cranes in *Even Cowgirls Get the Blues* by Thomas Robbins.

No lines, no boarding pass, and no E-Ticket required for the thrill ride of your life. For those too young to remember, E-Tickets were required for the best rides in Disneyland back in the '50s. An A or B-Ticket got you on to the Alice in Wonderland Storybook Boat or Mr. Toad's Wild Ride; an E-Ticket got you on the Matterhorn Bobsleds.

Since I was only nineteen, nearly the average age of the American combat GI in the Republic of Viet Nam, fighting to preserve democracy and Western civilization and to save these ignorant savages from the Communist insurgents from the North, I felt indestructible, immortal, the meanest motherfucker in the valley, fearing no evil, laughing and spitting in the eye of death.

I was still an *FNG*, a fucking new guy, in-country just long enough to find my way around my new home, Da Nang, host of one of the busiest air bases in the world, only most of the cargo transported was napalm, bombs, weary grunts, and no longer weary grunts in black body bags.

Da Nang, 85 miles (137 km) south of the DMZ, the 17th parallel dividing North and South Viet Nam, was a major port city situated on the South China Sea at the mouth of the Hán River in Quang Nam province, the middle of five provinces comprising I CTZ (I Corps), which was the Tactical Area of Responsibility (TAOR) of the Third Marine Amphibious Force (III MAF). Most of the fighting that took place in Viet Nam at the time was concentrated in this TAOR. The area surrounding Da Nang was the home of the First Viet Cong Regiment and the Second North Vietnamese Division. It was even more dangerous and confusing, because Marine Intelligence gave enemy estimates that were as inaccurate as the VC and NVA body counts. To further muddy the water, the VC and NVA (aka Vietnam People's Army) received large local support from the rural population. Areas that seemed safe during the daylight hours became deadly at night as the local, friendly farmers clad in black PJs, smiling and waving at you during the daytime, changed into their "VC black" PJs at night and sniped at Marines or launched 122 mm rocket and mortar attacks while some of us slept.

I was one of over 549,500 US troops stationed in the Republic of South Viet Nam in 1968 at the height of the military escalation under President Lyndon B. Johnson's watch. The Military Assistance Command Vietnam (MACV) commanding general, William Westmoreland, had recently requested from the chairman of the Joint Chiefs of Staff in Washington, DC, an additional 200,000 troops to combat the inaccurately reported figures of enemy strength, which the Central Intelligence Agency had underestimated previously by 50 percent. As one can guess, this was not a popular move by the president and secretary of defense, Robert McNamara, considering the growing antiwar sentiment pervading our country back home.

The First Marine Air Wing (1ˢᵗ MAW) was a large presence in Da Nang, and we were surrounded by the First Marine Division, the Seventh and Twenty-Seventh Marine Regiments, *and* we were Americans after all, who had never lost a war on foreign soil, so I felt confident walking around with the Marine strut, chest out, chin back, and robotic arm movements. I also was reminded early on that FNGs did all the shit work because we were not worthy yet; the "short-timers" were not going to risk their lives because they were rotating back to the "world," the US of A, soon. I wasn't out of boot camp that long, only slightly less than a year, only to realize that I was at the bottom of the pecking order, again. The credo in the Nam was "If you're going to die here, it's best to die early on so you do not suffer as long."

When my one-way ticket ride, a commercial Continental Airlines Boeing 707, landed in the middle of a rocket attack in August 1968 at Da Nang air base a month earlier, dropping off a horde of fresh cannon fodder, new troop replacements, I remember with vivid clarity the looks on the faces of some of the first American GIs I saw who had survived their thirteen-month tour and were waiting for their ride stateside. One of them offered me his *piasters*, the government-issue play money we GIs used instead of American greenbacks. He handed me a crinkled handful of this foreign-looking paper, free money, and I thanked him and stuck it in my pocket, somewhat unsure what he had just given me. His fatigues hung loosely on him; his tanned face was gaunt, the skin seemingly stretched around his facial bones, with hollow distant, fearful, distrustful eyes. He seemed to have a hypervigilance about him that allowed nothing to pass unnoticed. There was no longer the erect posture of a Marine, but the slumped-over shell of a man-teenager who must have seen death and destruction on a regular basis and taken the lives of other human beings as well.

Would I look like that in thirteen months? I thought. Hell no, I was a two-hundred-pound killing machine, here to kill Commies for

Christ and come home to ticker tape parades wearing a chestful of medals on my dress blue uniform, greeted by an anxious wife ready to suck the wind out of me and bear my children so they can grow up and do the same thing in another twenty years. I was a US Marine, the baddest, most feared fighting force in the world (no offense to my son and the US Navy SEALS!). Shit, was I in for the biggest surprise of my life!

"If you are coming along, get your shit in gear and hop aboard!" yelled the crew chief over the sound of the turbine engine spooling up. The door gunner was double-checking his M-60 machine gun, making sure it would be ready when needed, and it would be needed. The pilot and door gunner were talking to each other, probably talking pilot-speak, going over instruments and checklists; it was muted by the sounds of the now fully cranking Huey's single turbine engine.

The chief reminded me to "lock and load" but to keep my safety on my M16. "We don't want no friendly fire in the cabin. If I'm goin' to get greased, it's gonna to be by some cheesedick slope VC, and I'm gonna take a lot of them motherfuckers with me before I go!" I could live with that.

Although such speech is racially xenophobic and unacceptable, then and even more so now, warrior training in the Marines, especially during an active war, was singularly focused on dehumanizing the enemy using a myriad of not-so-pleasant names. We're all probably guilty as charged.

The Huey lifted off, nosed forward, and lifted effortlessly into the hot, humid air. The door gunner on the starboard side was already on the alert, ready for any suspicious activity; after all, he was a silhouette in the open doorway of a lumbering green target in a blue sky for every farmer with an AK-47 tucked under his black PJs.

About ten minutes into the flight, the serenity of the countryside below was abruptly interrupted as the door gunner opened fire on some rice farmers who were very exposed in the middle of several rice paddies. Apparently, they must have thought every American had read and adhered to the rules of the Geneva Convention. There were small children, mini-VC, around the older farmer-VC when the farmer decided to take a little target practice at one of LBJ's Texas instruments that I was a passenger in. Bad move. As the sizzling hot brass casings scattered over the deck and red tracer fire sliced across the azure blue sky, the one-ton organic garden tractor, a huge water buffalo, buckled and lurched forward as spots of red appeared on its left side, spilling two small children who were riding on its back; one was crushed as the beast fell onto its right side. The other one ran over and clung to the leg of one of the adults. Bad move. Both bodies jerked spastically as they were riddled with NATO 7.62 mm full metal jacket rounds from the M-60 machine gun. Two other VC returned fire but were easy prey for the door gunner and his Mike-60. I just sat there, speechless, not knowing what to do or say. I had just seen my first KIAs (killed in action). *Better them than me* was all I could think of. This Huey wouldn't need any more bullet-hole patches after this sortie; Charlie should have kept his head down and tended his rice or spent more time practicing his aim.

The serene beauty of the lush green countryside, momentarily interrupted by the roar of gunfire and five of its dead inhabitants, with its unending geometric patchwork of well-tended rice paddies, dense foliage, palm trees, and jungle, was breathtakingly overwhelming. The greens, reds, and blues were intense, almost surrealistic. The view from five hundred feet, flying above the farmland and villages, was so breathtaking; it was hard to realize the real reason why I was here. My country *needed* me to help stop the growing threat and the spread of Communism. If we didn't stop it here in Viet Nam, the old "domino theory" would unfold and countless other Southeast Asian countries would fall to the Commies. I was truly awestruck with this helicopter, amazed that something without wings could fly so swiftly, so gracefully, so deadly, and the perspective of the earth from this vantage point was out of this world. Definitely an E-Ticket ride!

The peach fuzz door gunner, still hyped from his recent kills, turned to me and said, "Ain't this fucking grand? Let's go get some more!" It had happened so quickly. I never fired a round, and it would have been difficult sharing the same door space. My time would likely come later. I urged him on and congratulated him, even offered him a Salem; after all, he had saved all our lives, but deep down inside, I realized that five living, breathing human beings and a beautiful water buffalo that minutes ago were peacefully tending their farmland had been senselessly killed. Many more lives would be lost on both sides, I was sure, before I got out of this country; that is, if I made it out alive. After all, I was the FNG.

I just couldn't get it out of my mind how utterly fascinated I was with flying in helicopters. This definitely was a turning point in my life! I made up my mind that very moment on that very day, if I ever made it back to the world, someday I would find work and fly in a helicopter. It didn't matter what I did; I just wanted to fly around and view the world from a bird's perspective, landing softly and effortlessly wherever there was space enough to park one of these amazing flying machines. I was *helplessly, hopelessly hooked on helicopters!*

CHAPTER 2

Short Final

It's not what you were, it's what you are today.

—David Marion

Summer of 1990, California, USA

"Medi-Flight 1, you have a scene flight to Olive and Shaffer in the Atwater area for an auto versus a school bus," the voice from dispatch over the Motorola radio clipped on my fanny pack resounded.

Adam and I sprinted toward the helipad from the emergency department (ED); our collective juices were flowing like the Yangtze River in monsoon season, pure adrenaline and testosterone, anticipating the worst from the initial dispatch. We had to run because our pilot, Geoff Frangos, was greased lightning getting out to the aircraft and firing up the twin turbine engines.

I was especially pumped, not because I hadn't handled major trauma a thousand times before in the ED and on ground ambulance, but rather because this was my first real scene flight since being hired as a flight nurse for Medi-Flight of Northern California. It was my special privilege to be the first person in the history of the training program, or so I was told, to be released with only my partner to assist me and orient me to the world of aeromedicine. In the past, after an extensive orientation and training program, the FNG would ride along as an extra person in the cramped helicopter and would have the luxury of learning and watching the regular flight crew handle the call while assisting as needed until he felt comfortable enough and the flight crew felt you were ready to be cut loose on your own. There was no fear, just slight apprehension and stress, which always make me function at a higher level.

I took the fire watch on the outside while Adam prepared the inside of the ship, while Geoff cranked engine numbers one and two. When Geoff gave the hand signal to disconnect the APU (auxiliary power unit), a huge, heavy wheeled battery cart that preserves the helicopter batteries and makes for quicker starts, I wheeled it to its designated spot and chocked the wheel. After a quick walk around the ship to ensure all hatches and latches were secured and no fluids were leaking from under the cowlings, I climbed into the portside seat, plugged in my headset, and secured my seat belt. Adam gave me a great big smile, his broad, pearly white teeth erupting beneath his ample blond cookie duster, as if to say, "You're going to do fine."

"Medi-Flight 1, your heading is 118 degrees for 23 nautical miles. Stand by for ground contact information." (A nautical mile is equal to 1.15 statute miles.)

"Flight Com, Medi-Flight 1 will be off in about one minute. We have one plus five-zero on fuel, three souls on board, standard flight plan," Geoff reported.

Before each and every takeoff, a standard preflight checklist must be thoroughly completed. In addition, the medical crew must preview the appropriate map to locate the scene. Fortunately, on most flights, the pilots know the general location by experience and repetition and could fly to most areas without all the sophisticated equipment on board. Still, it is reassuring to have pre-takeoff coordinates and a GPS (global positioning system), which, once entered into the onboard computer, can fly you to within fifty feet of your location.

"Roger that, Medi-Flight 1."

"Okay, you knuckleheads, you ready? Instruments and indicators are all in the green. Lights are on. Throttles are full forward in the gates. Bleed air is off. Just waiting for the goddamned autopilot light to go out and we'll be ready to blast out of here. Baggage doors, oxygen, and med bag?"

"Baggage doors checked and secured, oxygen is turned off, and med bag is on board and secured."

"Seat belts on?"

"We're both in tight. Chains are up, you're clear left and above."

"Okay, the damn autopilot light's out, we're out of here!" Geoff pulled pitch, and the miraculous flying machine was off to the races.

"Flight Com, Medi-Flight 1 is off the pad en route."

"Copy, Medi-Flight 1, at 1545."

"Modesto Tower, this is Lifeguard 84 Mike Hotel ["Lifeguard" status confers priority for medical transport aircraft in airport traffic areas (ATAs) and 84MH is the aircraft identifier located on the tail section]. We are requesting permission to transition the approach end of the field on a southeast heading at 1,000 feet, and we have Foxtrot."

"Lifeguard 84 Mike Hotel, permission granted. Winds are 310 degrees at 15 miles per hour. No reported traffic in the area. Report when you are one mile out." Just because there was no *reported* traffic in the ATA did not relieve the three crewmembers of their diligent duty to scan the area for unreported traffic, crop dusters, ultralights, or any other chopper-stopper "What are you guys going on this time?" asked the tower.

"Some bonehead decided to play chicken with a school bus," Geoff retorted while vertically hovering backward to about 300 feet above the helipad. This was another safety measure, which allowed a visual and forward approach back to the transitional parking area in the event of an engine failure requiring a quick autorotation to land. He nosed forward and headed north, quickly gaining altitude to 1,000 feet before turning right over the noise-sensitive residential areas around the hospital.

"Any Modesto-area traffic, this is Lifeguard 84 Mike Hotel. We are southeast-bound at 1,000 feet, three and one-half miles northeast of the airfield, crossing the approach end in about two minutes." Another redundant safety check and balance, just in case someone forgot to call the tower. Never can be too safe!

The critical times in flying are during takeoff and landing *and* when at low altitude (less time to pick a spot to land when shit happens) *and* when in the ATA, now called class D airspace (more chance of midair collisions). Our safety training reinforced this concept of situational awareness over and over. Radio discipline, that is, no inconsequential bullshit talk in the cockpit, should take place unless it is to report essential information like an ultralight closing on our heading at ten o'clock, eye level. The sterile cockpit in reality depends upon who is PIC (pilot-in-command) of the aircraft. Nevertheless, most of us respected this concept and practice it for obvious safety reasons.

After Geoff cleared south of the ATA with Modesto Tower, it was time for Adam and me to gather necessary information to mentally prepare for what will likely be a critical patient. Since I was the FNG *again*, I got to handle the outside fire watch pre-takeoff, handle all radio communications with dispatch and our ground contact at the scene, and assume primary patient care responsibility, normally all shared cockpit tasks. Each different EMS entity is on a different frequency, which requires total focus and concentration to ensure you are on the right channel and talking to the right person. "Flight Com, Medi-Flight 1 is ready for ground contact information."

"Medi-Flight 1, ground contact is Engine 92 on 154.400. I have further information for the medical crew when ready to copy." That was a heads-up for the pilot to switch off our "guard" frequency with dispatch. It has been determined from past EMS helicopter crashes the pilot should have limited information about the exact nature of the incident so as to prevent overly zealous risk-taking. When a call comes in for a three-year-old near-drowning victim and the weather conditions are marginal, pilots have taken greater risk in an attempt to complete the mission that would otherwise have been aborted. After all, most of us have children too. Anyway, every effort is made to sanitize the information given to the pilot; their job is to fly us to the scene and back safely—*period!* No need to let emotions interfere with the mission. Geoff already knew it could involve kids just by the initial dispatch information.

The flight to the scene took just a little over ten minutes flying at just over 120 knots. This is the time to try and mentally prepare oneself for the chaos and horror that is unfolding just minutes away.

It generally gets real quiet as each medical crew member goes over the important things like the ABCs (airway, breathing, and circulation), still the most overlooked of all essential, basic lifesaving maneuvers. I have always learned that if you do nothing more than the ABCs, you will never get into trouble; everything seems to take care of itself if you address the basics each and every time.

Adam looked over at me and our eyes met. There was this momentary flash of mutual respect that we were the best, and if anyone had a chance of surviving serious injury, they were going to get it today. Adam had been a paramedic for about five years. When he decided he wanted to work on Medi-Flight, he weighed around 270 pounds. One prerequisite to employment is the ability to weigh 200 pounds or less in full flight gear. Adam lost over 70 pounds to just to make weight; I had to lose only about 20 pounds before my job interview. Several crewmembers still belonged to the "*One Niner-Niner Club*" (199 lb.), but we somehow managed to make quarterly weigh-in.

Geoff was up front making strange sounds and Three Stooges imitations in the microphone over ICS (cockpit intercom system). The in-line communication control in our headsets had one hand-held switch; if you pushed it one direction, you talked to whatever frequency you had dialed in on the Wolfsburg radio. If you pushed it in the opposite direction, it transmitted only ICS in the cockpit. Woe to those who forgot which direction they pushed before talking. There is also another toggle switch on the Wolfsburg, which must be manually switched; up for Main, and down for Guard (Mom, our umbilical cord, Flight Com, the dispatch center from which all-important information emanates). So, when someone, like Stinky, the ever-flatulent paramedic Don Campell, leaned over a verbose, impolite, inebriate, recalcitrant patient several years later and said, "Shut your mouth, you little shit," everyone in dispatch as well as everyone in scanner land knew what was said when he inadvertently pushed the transmit button in the wrong direction.

The Mad Greek, Mr. Frangos, besides being quick to get up in the air, and doing it safely each and every time I might add, was one of our favorite pilots to fly with. He was basically a butt and leg man with a strong propensity for Guinness extra stout, stinky cheeses, and hot spicy food for which he pops Zantacs like Tic-Tacs and was the ultimate Stooge lover/imitator. He could break almost any computer code, program DOS better than I can recite ACLS protocols, and he was the computer wizard equivalent to the blind-deaf-and-dumb boy Tommy of Pinball Wizard fame. The Three Stooges shtick comedy was a shared phenomenon and fascination for Geoff and me when we were growing up back in the '50s. I have yet to run into Geoff anywhere, anytime, when he doesn't go off on a Stooge routine complete with hand and body gestures; his voice imitations are well-rehearsed and close to the real thing. Once during a shift briefing with another FNG years later, he gave a "brief" briefing by stating in Stooge voice, "Well, if we get a call, we'll go…and no Shemp in the cockpit." Curly Howard (real name Jerome Lester Horwitz), one-third of the Stooge trio, was by far the central catalyst for the shenanigans and the favorite of Geoff. After Curly died and others, like his brother Shemp, tried to take his place, it was like substituting Rush Limbaugh for Bill Clinton; the Stooges would never be the same again.

We scanned Mariposa frequency 154.400 as we got closer to the scene. "Mom" (our benevolent name for dispatch), in this case and by coincidence my wife of over nine months who was attending registered nursing school *and* working full-time in the ER, had previously relayed further information on the scene. There were two "immediates," or critical patients, and one "delayed," or moderate patient. Fortunately, there were only a few children left on the bus that afternoon, and once again, gross tonnage had won the battle: Bus 1, Car 0.

Geoff was again busy talking to Castle Air Force tower in Merced, our flight following once we left Modesto radar. At this particular time, air traffic in and around Castle was unusually busy, what with a Republican president with a thousand-points-of-light-machine-gun-hand, and a malodorous-maniacal-malevolent-murderous-madman of the Middle East threatening to take control of its southern neighbor's black gold. There seemed to be more than a subtle escalation in B-52 flights, this being the only B-52 pilot training center in the US. There's good news and bad news about B-52s: good news is they are s-o-o-o-o big you can't miss seeing them; bad news is if they did hit us, it would be like hitting a butterfly on your windshield. Besides that, our LZ, or landing zone at the scene, was just about a mile off the departure path north of Castle AFB, and there were numerous other military aircraft besides the r-e-a-l-l-y b-i-g o-n-e-s to look out for in addition to light air traffic from Merced airport a few miles to the east.

Time to contact our ground personnel. "Engine 92, Medi-Flight 1."

"Medi-Flight 1, this is Engine 92, copy you loud and clear. Go ahead."

"Engine 92, Medi-Flight 1 is two minutes out from your location. We have you in visual contact. Ready to copy LZ information."

"You will be landing just east of the accident scene in a field with short grass. It is flat, and we have watered it down for you. There are no HAZMATS [hazardous materials]. There are power lines running east and west on the south side of Olive, and power lines running north and south on the west side of Shaffer Road."

"Copy that, Engine 92. Could you give us wind speed and direction, please?"

"Sorry about that, Medi-Flight 1. Winds are out of the north-west at 5 to 10. The LZ is secure and ready for landing at your discretion."

As part of our Safety Program and Community Outreach, our company flies to every fire, rescue, law enforcement, search and rescue, and ski patrol base in our service area, which covers several thousand square miles, to teach helicopter safety classes. We try to return every other year to give updates, reeducate, and train new employees. They are our eyes and ears on the ground, and we do not land, except under special circumstances, without a landing zone officer to prepare and secure an LZ for us to land safely. Our flight crews present a fifteen-minute video that briefly covers everything that is covered in the class, which is theirs to keep. Then a didactic portion is given and is supplemented with a slide and video presentation. It is after that that the fun really begins. They are given the opportunity to practice what they just learned for real. A preselected LZ, surveyed by a few select LZ training personnel weeks before, is set up just like a real scene LZ. One of our crew assigns three "patients" and three "passengers" to fly with us. The helicopter is dispatched to the training site, and three LZ officers are given the opportunity to assist in landing the helicopter. When we land, we stay "hot," with the rotors turning, while several of their personnel load the patient and passenger in the helicopter. We take off, fly around for five minutes, and repeat the procedure for three go-arounds. After this, the helicopter lands, shuts down, and the class gets to meet the on-duty crew (yes, we are still available for real missions and are sometimes called out during the training exercise) to ask further questions, view the aircraft, and go over the emergency controls in the cockpit which were covered in class. In addition to the usual handouts, each person is given a laminated card with information on how to select a proper LZ or helispot, proper radio report information required before landing, and dangers to avoid around helicopters with rotors turning. Everyone has fun, everyone learns, and our job becomes easier and safer.

"Engine 92, Medi-Flight 1 copies. We are going to circle overhead a few times to familiarize ourselves with the obstacles. When the pilot has re-conned and feels comfortable, we will recontact you." *Flip the switch on the Wolfsburg from main back to guard,* my mind tells me subconsciously. "Flight Com, Medi-Flight 1 is overhead with ground contact established. We will be landing shortly."

"Medi-Flight 1, Flight Com copies." replied my beautiful wife Karen.

Geoff circled, banking to the right so he could see the reported obstacles. Time for the prelanding checklist. "Okay, instruments are all okay, bleed air is off. I have all the obstacles in sight. Approach path will be from the southeast to northwest. When I clear those power lines to the south, I'm going to swing my tail to the right so I can keep my eyes on the gawkers lined up along the highway and give you guys a safer approach back with the patient. Got the strap on my lap, how 'bout you two?"

"We're both in tight. If you're ready, I'll call Engine 92 for final."

"I'm ready. Let's go kick some ass!"

"Engine 92, Medi-Flight 1 is ready for landing. We will approach from the southeast to the northwest. If the LZ is still secure, we will be landing on this turn."

"Medi-Flight 1, this is Flight Com. Be aware, you are still on Guard frequency," reported my new bride.

Doom on you, dumbshit, I thought to myself. I forgot to switch back to main before talking to my LZ officer. I flipped the switch back up to main and repeated my previous transmission. Engine 92 acknowledged. Now, I had to flip the switch back down to guard *again*, to let Mom know that we were ready for landing. Jesus, I hadn't even seen or touched my patient yet and I was stressing big-time. So much aviation crap to remember; the patient care portion would come naturally, I was sure. Doom on you again, shithead. I remembered to flip the toggle switch back up to main this time. Before talking to Engine 92, I flashed back (not the LSD type) to my pre-nursing mandatory reading primer, *The House of God*, by Samuel Shem. Laws of the House of God, Commandment III states, "At a cardiac arrest, the first procedure is to take your own pulse." I took my pulse. The storm looming on the horizon was about to unleash all of its pent-up fury on me. I felt queasy. Suddenly, I realized that even patient care was going to be a stressful event today. Adam glanced over and saw me taking my pulse. Smiling, he keyed his ICS and said, "Don't worry, Ron, I won't let anything bad happen." I was ready.

"Yaaaahhhh-aaahhhh-aaahhhh! Why, you numbskulls! Moe, Larry, cheese! Calling Dr. Howard, Dr. Fine, Dr. Howard!" Geoff, our Stooge-loving pilot, was ready.

"Engine 92, Medi-Flight 1 is on short final for landing!"

CHAPTER 3

To Every Season

Those who do not feel pain, seldom think it is felt.

—Samuel Johnson

"Copy, Medi-Flight 1, short final for landing."

"Below 40 door?" I asked Geoff over ICS.

"Go ahead."

Geoff approached from the southeast, passing over the east-west power lines on Olive. I had opened the port (left) side sliding door to gain a better viewing advantage of the scene and the approaching power lines. Company policy allows the medical crews to open the sliding door below 40 knots, even though the aircraft is designed to withstand speeds of nearly 110 knots before the door theoretically will be swept away from wind shear. In Viet Nam, the side doors were always open. We crewmembers don't do anything without checking with the pilot first when it comes to affecting or potentially affecting aircraft performance. Even if we need to lean forward to perform patient care, or if the starboard (right) side crewmember needs to lean over the patient, who is transported on the port side, we advise the pilot first so he will be aware of subtle changes in the weight and balance of the helicopter. This probably is not a problem with larger aircraft; however, with our medium-sized Aeorspatiale TwinStar, performing the above maneuvers without advising the pilot's knowledge will certainly get his attention quickly.

"Tail's clear of the power lines. There's no FOD blowing from the rotor wash." FOD, an acronym for foreign object damage, relates to objects in the immediate landing area that can be lifted from the generated rotor wash, twirled around, and enter through the protective screen on the intake side of the turbine engines, causing very expensive damage. It also includes trash, paper, plywood, and other objects, which can become dangerous flying projectiles that could injure the ground rescuers, curious onlookers, or the rotor system. This is one of the items covered under our Helispot Training classes, and the fire departments are very diligent in clearing the area prior to landing.

The one problem we do encounter often, however, is dusty landing zones, even though they may appear to be wet down adequately. The turbulence generated by the main rotors can create winds up to 50 mph. If we try to land and churn up a lot of dust, it can create a dangerous "brownout" situation by blinding the pilot or creating temporary loss of equilibrium and inability to see objects outside the aircraft for visual reference necessary for control so near to the ground, not knowing which way is up. Unfortunately, being very close to the ground, the margin for error is minimal, and a hard landing or a crash is not worth the risk. So, when we find ourselves in a situation where too much dust is blowing, the pilot will abort the landing, circle the scene until more water can be applied, or look for another alternate landing site. The other hazard with dusty LZs is the FOD problem, which does not make for happy mechanics, who are tasked with taking the aircraft out of service for several days. They get crabby. Then, the flight crew doesn't have a helicopter to play in for several days, and they get crabby. The program director has to explain to his boss (hospital administration) why we had to spend $50,000 for turbine parts; he yells at him, and he gets crabby. That helicopter can't bring patients back to the hospital (fortunately, we do have three helicopters), revenue cannot be generated, and the board of directors get crabby. All these crabby people go home and get crabbier and yell at their dogs. Except the dogs; dogs don't get crabby. I learn something from my dogs every day. They don't talk back, have undying loyalty, seek constant affection, and don't nudge your significant other awake when you sneak in the house at 3:00 a.m. after being out with the guys, drinking tequila and smoking cheap cigars!

Geoff hovered, kicked the tail to starboard, and set us down parallel to Olive, facing west with a full view of the chaos a few hundred feet away. I double-checked the switch on the Wolfsburg radio to make sure it was down to Guard, unbelted, grabbed the ample med bags, took a deep breath, and stepped out. First duty is to greet the LZ officer, find out where I needed to go, and ensure that he is clear about his responsibility for guaranteeing helicopter security while we were on the ground. He said he thought my patient was down by the school bus, about 150 yards north, so I fast-walked down Olive, stepping over 1½-inch charged fire hoses, car parts, and broken glass, until I found someone in a Riggs Ambulance uniform who was attending to a patient on a backboard next to the demolished car, introduced myself, and asked if this was the patient they wanted us to take.

"No, we're transporting this one. Your patient is back there," he said, pointing back southeast toward the helicopter. Sure enough, while I was walking to the accident scene, another medical crew with our patient had sneaked around one of the fire engines, so we passed without seeing each other. From one hundred feet away, I could see someone at the head of the gurney "bagging" the patient with a BVM device (bag-valve-mask), not a good sign.

Now I had to sprint to catch up with them before they got too close to the helicopter because I still needed to get a verbal report on the mechanism, injuries, vital signs, and treatment they had initiated; then, I had to perform a rapid primary survey, the ABCs, and an even briefer secondary exam.

Since I had to run, and since I was already amped to the max even before we landed, handling all the aviation portion of the flight, I was as clammy as my patient, and out of breath, which the patient would have been, literally, had the paramedic not been breathing for him. When I caught up with them, I could tell they were stressed also. They didn't want to stop, and the gurney kept moving quickly toward the helicopter, which was only about fifty feet away now.

Suddenly out of nowhere, Adam, a huge imposing and intimidating teddy bear, appeared next to the patient and grabbed the gurney. They got the message.

"Wait here for a minute," I gasped to the Riggs medic. "Tell me what you've got while I check the patient out."

"We have a twentyish-year-old male who was the nonrestrained driver of the car you saw. He was driving real fast down Olive and, for reasons unknown, hit the school bus. He was pinned in and unconscious with agonal respirations when we found him. There's alcohol on his breath. Vitals are BP 66 over 40, pulse 150, and we're assisting his respirations. We tubed him as soon as we got him out of the car. The windshield was spidered outward and the steering wheel was destroyed—probably took it right on the chest."

Intubation is the airway of choice for someone unable to support or maintain his or her own respiratory drive; thus, they "tubed" him. This is without question the most important lifesaving prehospital procedure we provide for our patients. It is the *A* of the ABCs, and without A, one cannot proceed to B or C. Remember this point, because it is the most basic of concepts taught in basic CPR (cardiopulmonary resuscitation) training, first aid, EMT (emergency medical technician), paramedic training, nursing school, and, I presume, medical school. You will see this later many times and realize how often it is overlooked and realize its lethal significance.

"What are his injuries?"

"Didn't have time to look real close. We really had our hands full, the scene was a zoo! We just tubed him, started an IV, and C-spined him. Then we saw you guys landing, so we loaded him on the gurney and started heading this way."

"Where do you want him to go, and how much does he weigh?"

"He can go back to Memorial, and I guess he weighs about 175."

"Geoff, Ron. Patient weight 175, and we're going back home." These two pieces of information are imperative for the pilot; it enables him to compute weight and balance and file his flight plan and manifest with dispatch. The sooner the pilot gets this information, the sooner we can get off the scene.

"Roger-dodger, going home with one," Geoff replied.

"Okay, give me about a minute to do a quick PE [physical exam], and then we can load him." First priority (once again ABCs) is to check the "tube," or endotracheal (ET) tube, for proper placement to ensure it is in the trachea and not the esophagus. I placed my stethoscope over both sides of his chest and auscultated breath sounds, then over the stomach to listen for air sounds. No stomach sounds—good news. Breath sounds heard over the chest but more diminished on the left side. Now, does he have a pneumo or hemothorax on the left, or is this a right mainstem intubation? The 8.0 mm ET tube was taped securely in the mouth with the small number "26," indicating 26 cm, on the side of the ET tube at the location of his lips. *Right mainstem,* I thought to myself. "We need to pull the tube back slightly," I said to no one in particular. Adam heard me though, and the 10 cc distal cuffed balloon was deflated, the tube was slowly pulled back to 24 cm, and then reinflated. This time, lung sounds were equal bilaterally, but they still sounded like shit. Lots of rhonchi (coarse wet breath sounds). Next, I pulled out an End-Tidal CO2 monitor out of my fanny pack and disconnected the BVM from the ET tube just long enough to insert it between the two and reconnected the system. The purple center turned yellow after two breaths, indicating expired carbon dioxide. This simple, compact, inexpensive device utilizes a nontoxic chemical indicator strip that changes from purple to yellow with inspiration and expiration, indicating expired carbon dioxide from the trachea. When it turns yellow, it indicates expired CO2 from 2% to 5% (15–38 mmHg), indicative of proper endotracheal intubation. If the tube were in the esophagus, which leads to the stomach, the indicator strip would have remained purple with no color change. Great, we were definitely in the right hole.

ABCs now out of the way, I needed to perform a rapid secondary assessment. This consists of a head-to-toe, visual, and hands-on examination to determine extent of injuries. A secondary survey under controlled conditions can take several minutes, much like an exam your physician performs during an annual physical. A field exam by an experienced paramedic or nurse takes about sixty seconds. During that time, we need to assess life-threatening injuries, prioritize a plan of care, and implement that plan, most of it en route to the hospital. Sometimes treatment of injuries that are not life-threatening are noted but not initially addressed if there are other high-priority issues such as a bloody, unprotected airway. The ABCs are a scene priority; all else can be performed in flight.

His head revealed a large laceration in the scalp that exposed his skull and was deep and gaping but was not bleeding profusely. Pupils were dilated at 5–6 mm and sluggish to light. His face was covered with blood, so it was difficult to determine if blood was coming from the scalp wound or his nose or ears. No big deal now anyway. Facial bones felt intact. Some front teeth missing, mandible stable. His neck was in a rigid cervical collar for stabilization of the cervical spine, along with the backboard, straps, tape, and neck wedges, which is routine on most major trauma patients. His trachea was midline; that's about all I could see with the C-collar on. His chest I had already checked when verifying ET tube placement. It felt stable, but he probably had some chest wall damage from the sounds of his lungs. His abdomen was another matter. It felt firm to palpation, and there was already bruising across his right upper quadrant over the liver. Since he was unconscious, there was no way to ask if it hurt—I knew it did; he just couldn't tell me from wherever he was in his traumatic dream state. There was crepitus, a nasty crunchy feeling one feels when broken bone ends grind together, when I checked his pelvis. Right leg okay. Oops, open fracture of his left tibia, midshaft, ankle seriously angulated and broken too. There was very little bleeding from the hole in the leg where his tibia (shin bone) stuck out, along with adipose and muscle tissue; ditto for his ankle, which was facing west when it should have been facing north. Distal pulses were weak, but at least they were present. This guy was dying! No time to waste placing a splint on his lower leg when we were ready to load; we just placed a dressing over the wound. That's not what was going to kill him. First and foremost was addressing "A," which would kill him first, but the "A and B" were already addressed; "C" needed my immediate attention now. My biggest fear was that he would exsanguinate, a fancy term that means bleed to death, if we couldn't get him to surgery quickly.

"Okay, I'm satisfied, let's get the hell out of Dodge!" I screamed over the sound of the turbines and rotors. The whole primary and secondary exam took less than two minutes, including repositioning the ET tube, and now I knew what I was faced with. This time was very well spent. Had I not taken the time, I would have been working with too many variables and unknowns. God help us all if the ET tube would have been in the esophagus and I didn't catch it. He would have died before we lifted off from the scene. Guilt, remorse, blame, and lawsuits would come later.

"We will load him feet first. Make sure your chinstraps on your helmets are secured. I need four persons to assist with loading. The guy bagging the patient will call the shots; hold on with both hands and don't let that tube move or come out! Let's go." I was starting to feel better. Automatic mode had kicked in when I finally reached my patient, and my years of training and my assertive personality just became second nature.

We loaded him "hot," with the rotors turning, secured him to our gurney with seat belts, hung his IV up, and Adam bagged him while I went back into aviation mode for a few seconds. After a quick walk around to check all doors and latches, I climbed in and secured my seat belt. I took over ventilations while Adam belted himself in and reconfirmed ET tube placement. Geoff had called Mom to give the manifest and ETA while we were out of the helicopter doing our thing.

He went through the takeoff checklist by rote memory. Baggage doors all secured, lights on, oxygen on, med bag on board, bleed air off, seat belts on. "Engine 92, if the LZ is secure, we will be taking off in one minute."

"All secure, Medi-Flight 1. Have a safe flight."

Next, Geoff called Castle AFB to advise their tower of our intentions. No need to get sucked into the engine intake of a B-52 since we had gotten this far, and we were going to take off right near the departure end of the main runway of a busy air force base. Castle acknowledged and gave us "Lifeguard" priority status. We could only hope all the pilots got a good night's rest, were not hung over from the night before, and were paying attention to business and not playing grabass with the female staff on board. We lifted off; Geoff turned his tail left and took off to the north over the open field. After we had reached cruising altitude, he cleared the radio with Engine 92. "Engine 92, this is Medi-Flight 1. We are clear of your LZ. Thanks a lot for all the help and the great LZ. See you on the next one." He changed frequencies and notified Mom that we were off the scene and en route to Memorial.

Adam and I were busy in back. We had twelve minutes to get a lot of work done and try to keep this young man alive long enough for the surgeons to play their part. The IV the medics had started on scene we placed in a pressure infusion bag, much like a long BP cuff, and inflated it until the indicator gauge went from green to red, then opened the roller clamp wide open on the IV tubing. Great IV, a 14-gauge; the normal saline flowed through the drip chamber in a steady stream. He needed another one, and Adam was already setting it up. He swiped his arm with an alcohol prep after applying a tourniquet around his right upper arm. Fortunately for us and the patient, and despite his impaired hemodynamic state, a vein miraculously appeared. Adam nailed it on the first attempt with a 16-gauge, popped the tourniquet, removed the needle, carefully placed it in the red sharps container (no need risking our lives getting stuck with a contaminated needle!), and hooked up the IV on blood Y-tubing. When he had it secured with tape, this one was opened wide also and placed on a pressure bag. What he really needed was blood, but until then, isotonic normal saline would have to suffice. It's about a 4:1 replacement ratio with crystalloid solutions; it requires four liters of normal saline or lactated Ringer's to be equivalent to one liter of blood in terms of volume expansion. Also, crystalloids do not carry oxygen molecules like the heme molecule on our red blood cells. Too much IV fluid given before blood is administered and one risks other complications like ARDS (adult respiratory distress syndrome), DIC (disseminated intravascular coagulation), fluid overload, electrolyte imbalance, and hypothermia. These sequelae are what the ICU nurses have to deal with for the next several days, weeks, or sometimes even months, for those patients who survive beyond the ED and the OR.

"So, Ron, what do you think?" Adam asked me.

"This guy is really FUBAR [fucked up beyond all recognition], Adam! He has a giant head lac, a closed head injury, probably bilateral pulmonary contusions or hemos, high probability of a liver laceration, a fractured pelvis, and of course, the obvious open tib-fib and ankle fractures. I wish we could fly faster."

"Why, you numbskull, I'm flying as fast as I can. Maybe if Adam jumps out, it'll lighten our load a little."

God, I love flying with this crazy man. He can cut through the stressful bullshit and make you laugh when you're looking death in the face. This was nothing new for him. Geoff had seen the face of death many times as well, long ago in the jungles of Viet Nam too, as an army combat Huey helicopter pilot. He still possessed the damaged dash instrument on the Huey that saved his life when an enemy round lodged in it just inches from his chest during a firefight twenty-five years prior.

While I continued to ventilate our patient, watch the IVs, and monitor his vital signs on the monitor screen, I realized it was time to call our base hospital on the radio and give them a heads-up so they could prepare for the task of trauma resuscitation and notify the surgeon, neurosurgeon, surgical team, respiratory, lab, social services, x-ray and CT scan, blood bank, and anesthesia. I switched the frequency preselect dial to 155.385 on A-11 of the Wolfsburg, flipped the toggle switch up to main, and keyed the mike. I did it right this time.

"Memorial Medical Center, Medi-Flight 1 on VHF with code 3 trauma!"

"This is Memorial Medical Center, MICN [mobile intensive care nurse] Ekstrum. Go ahead, Medi-Flight 1."

"Memorial, this is Medi-Flight 1, MICN Martin with Paramedic Christianson. We are en route with a six-minute ETA for a hot offload. On board we have a multisystems trauma patient, from an MCI [multi-casualty incident] in Merced County with an approximate twenty-year-old male patient weighing eighty kilos. He is unconscious with a Glasgow coma score of six. There is no eye opening, no verbal, and he withdraws to pain. Mechanism is a high-speed MVC into a school bus. He was the unrestrained driver and was not ejected

35

from the car. There was major passenger space intrusion, windshield and steering wheel damage. His injuries include closed head, chest, abdominal, and pelvic trauma, and open extremity fractures. Current vital signs are BP 95 over 62, pulse rate 132 with sinus tachycardia on the monitor, respirations assisted at 20, pulse oximetry 92% on 100% oxygen. He is in full C-spine precautions, two IVs of normal saline running wide-open on pressure bags with 2,500 cc infused thus far. He is intubated with an 8.0 ET tube. His vital signs have improved significantly since we left the scene. Do you have any questions or further orders for us?"

"Medi-Flight 1, Memorial copies twenty-year-old major trauma patient intubated and in traumatic shock. Sounds like you have your hands full in back. No further orders. We have called a trauma alert and will be waiting for you on the pad for a hot off-load in about five minutes. Memorial North clear."

The last major nonmedical task now completed, I could turn my full attention back to the patient. Well, not just quite yet.

"Geoff, I've got traffic at our eight o'clock, low but gaining altitude, converging on our heading!"

Shit, just when you think everything's just about back to normal, something else demands immediate attention. That's life in aeromedicine, continuous challenges from all sources, always demanding keen situational awareness, always titillating and exciting all five senses, and always testing your sixth sense, your "intuitive gut" feeling. The environment is exciting, challenging, and yes, fun; however, it is a very precise and unforgiving environment with little margin for error. There are no replays or retakes, Hollywood. If you screw up, you can kill yourself, your team members, and possibly those on the ground below.

"I see that little dipshit cocksucker crop duster. No fucking radio, no contact with the tower. Sure would be nice if that shithead would give us good guys a heads-up when he's out here spraying!" Geoff took evasive maneuvers and banked right while almost imperceptibly pulling up on the collective, which increased our altitude, giving us some breathing room between this totally obtuse, unobservant renegade.

When we were clear of the crop duster, I performed another visual scan outside the aircraft to look for other potential targets, all the while bagging the patient rhythmically, *squeeze* one-thousand, two one-thousand, three one-thousand. *Squeeze* one-thousand, two one-thousand, three one-thousand. My mind drifted, thinking about all that had transpired in the last twenty or thirty minutes, trying to dissect each moment, freeze-framing each event, trying to find pitfalls and errors made, trying to determine what I would do next time to make it better, quicker, faster, more efficient. I searched my soul trying to understand why this particular incident happened at exactly the precise time it did, in that exact location, to these individual persons. Was alcohol an underlying factor, or would it have happened anyway? Was fate extending its dark hand over these individuals, regardless of whether the alcohol that had numbed this poor guy's senses and impaired his psychomotor skills such that he could not safely operate a motor vehicle? Or was it a prearranged, premeditated suicide attempt on his behalf with no thought of the full consequences of his actions, and how they would play in the big picture, which involved several other injured persons, their families, their friends, their schoolmates, the fire department, paramedics, nurses, doctors, social workers, law enforcement, coroners, funeral home directors?

As my mind unconsciously struggled to sort out these unanswered questions, another channel in my brain was simultaneously tuned in to the oldies-but-goodies station, KWTF (K-What-The-Fuck), and they kept playing the same tune, over and over, an old Byrds number 1 folk-rock legend, adapted by Pete Seeger from the book of Ecclesiastes in the Old Testament and recorded on September 9, 1965. The vocal trinity consisted of Jim McGuinn, an Old Christy Minstrels member; Gene Clark, who abruptly and unfortunately left the Byrds in the following year; David (I-Don't-Have-A-Drug-Problem) Crosby, who now sported an abdominal scar and some dead donor's liver in his right upper quadrant; and accompanied by Chris Hillman on bass and Michael Clark on drums.

The song, an instant number 1 hit on the charts, was recorded just as my brother had enlisted in the Marines Corps and I was a soph-

omore at Rosedale High School in Kansas City, Kansas, not far from
Em and Henry Gale and niece Dorothy, and a devout Christian in
regular attendance at YOU BAD DOG Church (Ye Olde Unitarian
Baptist Anglican *Dyslexic* Diocese of *Dog*), just learning about Viet
Nam, the cultural revolution, the sexual revolution, the escalating
racial and generation tensions, and the rising antiwar sentiment
growing in America. The Byrds would later introduce '60s-style acid
rock to the masses long before other rock groups; it would not be
until the summer of 1969, after I had returned from Viet Nam (the
first day after coming home to the "world," actually!) that I would
experience the meaning of this. Oh well, Kansas was several years
behind California in grasping the undercurrent of social change back
then.

The volume cranked up on channel KWTF until it occupied
the center of thoughts and feelings, and the words rang stentoriously
in my conscious mind.

> *To everything, turn, turn, turn.*
> *There is a season, turn, turn, turn.*
> *And a time to every purpose, under heaven.*
> *A time to be born, a time to die.*

The young man who lay in front of me, clinging to life by a
thread of hope, and in whose hands I held a great responsibility for,
opened his eyes and looked up into mine for a brief second. It was
the bottom of the ninth inning, down by three with the bases loaded,
two outs and two strikes. His eyes in that glimmering second pleaded
with mine to pitch him one belt high down the middle of the plate.
Sorry, I thought, *I would if I could, but this is not a call I can make. It
comes from much higher up the administrative ladder.* Would he die in
the spring of his season?

> *A time to die, turn, turn, turn.*

Of the many times I prayed, this was one of them. I prayed to
God for this man's life to be spared, for his family to be spared the

grief of a sudden, unexpected, unnecessary, traumatic death, another alcohol-related highway fatality statistic. There would be suffering enough even if he survived.

The lyrics continued over and over until suddenly I was jolted back to present time. Geoff's voice cracked over the ICS as he spewed out the prelanding checklist as we prepared to land at the hospital. "Instruments are still working, landing and approach path I'm familiar with. We won't need the loudspeaker, bleed air's off. You knuckleheads still strapped in?"

"We're both in tight, patient's still strapped."

Geoff cleared with the airport on the tower frequency.

"Flight Com, Medi-Flight 1 is on short final for landing at the hospital." I crowed, relieved that this acid test was nearly drawing to a close.

"Medi-Flight 1, Flight Com, be advised you are still on the Med Net frequency."

"Damnit to hell!" I yelled, fortunately over ICS and not for all the San Joaquin Valley scanner freaks. No bother calling Mom again; they knew already where we were since they were scanning the Med Net frequency also.

Adam just leaned back and smiled. He was right. Nothing bad happened. The FNG had passed the acid test. It was true, I had made several minor errors, but they were easily correctable and did not violate flight protocol or patient safety.

We touched down, and Geoff adjusted blade pitch while the turbines cooled down. He punched the timer clock on the console, timing the required two-minute cool-down period before he could safely shut down.

"Flight Com, Medi-Flight 1 has landed at Memorial." On the correct frequency, I might add.

"Copy, Medi-Flight 1, at 1618. Your flight number is 6901."

The pitcher looked into the catcher for the signal. He checked the runners. He nodded to the catcher that the signal was okay. He looked at the batter. The batter, whose life depended on this next pitch, grasped the bat tightly and stared back with equally fierce intensity. The pitcher slowly went into his windup.

A time to kill, a time to heal.
A time to laugh, a time to weep.
A time for peace, I swear
It's not too late.

I unbelted, jumped out, rotated the gurney outward, took the seat belts off the patient while Adam bagged him, took the two IVs down from their IV hooks, and motioned for the trauma team to come over from their protective area behind the wind blast shield. We off-loaded him "hot" and quickly rolled the gurney toward the vast assemblage of professionals waiting in the ED to take over with the trauma resuscitation. The RT took over ventilating Mr. Doe while another nurse hung up the IVs on the gurney's IV pole once outside the rotor system. I gave a brief report to them while we rushed down the hallway, making sure no lines or tubes got pulled out and that nobody dropped the monitor on the floor. We swung around the last turn, down the long corridor and into the trauma room. There stood two ED docs, the trauma surgeon, a neurosurgeon, an anesthesiologist, two ED nurses, four RTs (no one knows why so many show up, they just do), an OR nurse, a lab tech, two x-ray techs with their portable x-ray machine, a social worker, an ED admissions clerk, and Trish, our trauma services director, the quiet watcher in the corner of the room, preparing to evaluate the trauma alert and the organized chaos about to begin.

There is a season, turn, turn, turn.
I swear it's not too late.

I would find time to weep later. And here comes the pitch!

40

CHAPTER 4

Play Ball

It ain't over till it's over.

—Yogi Berra

Summer 1967, Kansas

I swung at the hanging curve ball, shoulders and arms fully extended, wrists rotating just as the ball went over the middle of the plate belt high and the thirty-three-ounce bat connected smartly with a solid *thwack!* The pitcher nearly fell over backward, trying to look back over his right shoulder toward left-center as the pitch he had just thrown proceeded about fifty feet beyond the fence in a line drive, a distance of nearly four hundred feet. Not bad for an eighteen-year-old country boy from Kansas. Pee Wee Reese's radio sports announcer partner Dizzy Dean would have described it as a "frozen rope, pawdners."

It was the bottom of the ninth inning of the last game of regulation baseball I would ever play, and it was a memorable way indeed to leave a sport that I lived, drank, ate, and dreamed about for the last eighteen years. I was a walk-on player and short-timer, so I had not told the manager of my team that I had already enlisted in the Marines while still in high school three months prior. My final hit was not only a towering home run but a grand slam home run, the first and only one I had ever hit, and my walk-off homer won the game. Oh, I had hit several home runs, but never the *coup de grace,* the ultimate hit. Most of the ball fields we played on were open fields in the park with no fences. To hit a home run, you had to race around four bases at full gallop before the outfielder caught up with the ball and tried to throw you out at home. No home run trot and hat nod to the sparse crowd. I think, rather, I *know* I could have gone on to the Major Leagues to play professional baseball, had my fate not taken another path. Since I was old enough to grasp and toss a ball, baseball was my life. Good genes and good fortune equated to pure, raw, natural talent. From sunup to well after sundown, I played baseball, most of the time with my childhood neighbor and best buddy, David Peterson, an outstanding all-sports athlete who went on to excel and set track and field records in college, became a professional photographer, and won a Pulitzer Prize in photography. I played baseball, football, basketball, and track, the "all-season" athlete, but baseball was my one and only love. Our team was always good, we won several championships, and I made All-Star several times. My batting average the last two years was well over .400, and I led our team in homers and extra base hits. On defense, I generally played center field, same as my boyhood idol, the Mick, but liked to play third base equally as well. My power lay in the fact that I had a throwing arm similar to another legend, Roberto Clemente, who could throw a baseball from deep right field all the way to home plate on a perfect one-hop, and the ball would never get more than ten feet off the ground. Players simply did not try to take that extra chance if the ball was hit to me, because their chances of success were severely decreased, and more often than not, I won the mental and physical battle. You're out of there, sucker!

Growing up in Kansas City afforded me ample opportunity to watch professional baseball at Municipal Stadium, home of the Kansas City Athletics. My favorite team, and most of America's favorite, the New York Yankees, came to town several times each summer, and my parents would drive me to the stadium; give me three dollars for a general admission ticket, hot dogs, Coke, Tootsie Roll, and a few cherry-flavored snow cones (God, you could sure get a lot for a few bucks back then!); drop me and my baseball glove off; then probably go back home and screw their brains out while I was in heaven watching my childhood idol, Mickey Mantle, son of Mutt Mantle, single-handedly decimate the As from both sides of the plate. I loved the pinstripe blue suits they wore (they wore gray uniforms with blue lettering when playing on the road) and vowed that someday I would wear Yankee pinstripes. That was before George Steinbrenner bought the Yanks!

After my rare home run trot around the bases, I sadly informed my manager I was leaving in three days for Marine boot camp and quietly said goodbye to my fellow players and left the ballpark. As much as my dream awaited me, I had another more important job to do first; baseball would just have to wait a few years, much to the detriment of the Yankees and millions of adoring fans. I answered my calling, my duty, to preserve and protect the Constitution of the United States of America; to defend it against all enemies, foreign and domestic (more about domestic "enemies" in a later chapter), so help me God. I passed up college academic and sport scholarships to defend my country from foreign aggression. Doom on Mr. Shithead!

World history was one of my favorite classes in my senior year of high school. Not so much so because I loved world history, but because Charlie Case taught the class. He was also a basketball, football, and track coach, but that wasn't even the reason. He led his class and gained our respect by honesty, integrity, and leadership and by being a friend. He was an inspiring teacher who made learning fun. Since we were learning about world history, and since Viet Nam was part of the world, and since we spent a lot of class time discussing current world history as well as the past, I made it my personal project to learn everything there was to know about Viet Nam. It made sense. I had already joined the Marine Corps on April 15 of 1967, on the deferred plan, two months before graduation, and had wanted to join since my brother joined two years earlier. He kept telling me, "Don't join the Marines!" Well, I knew he must have been trying to keep all that good stuff for himself; otherwise, he wouldn't want me to join up with him. It seemed okay to postpone my baseball career for a short time. My job was first to go over to Viet Nam and kill all the communists I could who were trying to take over the world, then come home, buy a house, get married, have 2.5 children, and get my ass deep in debt, just like our government.

When not playing or watching baseball, like at night, when it was snowing outside, or when I was not in school, I was hooked on watching classic war movies starring John Wayne, Spencer Tracy, William Bendix, Broderick Crawford, and Audie Murphy. Movies about our great battles and triumphs during World War II. The movies were in black-and-white (I put this in for you young readers who never knew anything except color TV, HDTV, remote control, and 3D), and we only had three (yes, 3!) channels, and no remote control. Believe it or not, kids, you had to get off your lazy butt and physically turn a dial to change TV channels! The American GI was my idol second only to Mickey Mantle. The good guy, a benevolent hunk who always had a cigarette smoldering out the side of his mouth and a cup of joe in hand, somehow managed to find the only woman west of Hawaii and fall in love, get shot up, but not too bad, and come home to marry his sweetheart amidst a flourish of marching music and welcome-back-GI-Joe parades. This didn't sound like too bad of an avocation to baseball. The Marines were always first to fight, the meanest and leanest, the most awesome fighting force in the world (once again with apologies to my son Forrest and the SEALS!). I wanted a piece of that action.

I left for basic training in mid-August 1967, just a few weeks after the famous Grand Slam, leaving Kansas City by train en route to MCRD (Marine Corps Recruit Depot), San Diego, with several stops along the way. At each stop, a few recruits would jump train, run to a liquor store, and buy all the cheap booze with money we managed to scrounge up at the time. I learned to dislike gin at the early age of eighteen in Albuquerque, New Mexico, where we stopped to pick up three Pullman cars full of young Navajo Indians, also on their way to MCRD, San Diego, and several bottles of cheap gin. We drank gin and 7-Up all the way through the southwest and awoke that next fateful morning all terribly hung over and smelling like a juniper forest. We were promptly shuttled from the train onto awaiting olive-green buses with black lettering and driven a short distance to MCRD, San Diego.

The doors of the bus shuddered when they opened. In stepped the biggest, meanest, angriest-looking staff sergeant with a Smokey the Bear hat wearing green fatigues with starched creases in the pants and shirt sleeves that could cut through the toughest buffalo steak. He looked around for a few seconds, and then he yelled out a command so loud that I believed my head would split and shatter much like the crystal glass on the Memorex cassette tape commercial. Doom on (cheap) gin! It would never again pass my lips for another three decades since that pretentious night in Albuquerque. That was when my wife, with the endorsement of Dick Marcinko (refer to chapter 1), introduced me to Bombay Sapphire gin in my later life. Dr. Bombay and I have since become close friends and drinking buddies.

"What are you wormy pukes looking at!? Don't look at me! You aren't even worthy enough to see me! Get your worthless fucking asses off this bus now, and line up on the yellow footprints outside! Move—now, you pussies! Go!"

Caught up in a state of mass confusion and disbelief, we all jumped up at once and fell over each other trying to get out of the bus at the same time. Imagine yourself on a bus that suddenly bursts into flames, and everyone panics, as expected, and tries to get off the bus at once, clawing and pushing to get off before being burned to death. That is what this Charlie Foxtrot, aka Cluster Fuck, looked like with forty-five of us simultaneously running for a single exit door twenty-eight inches wide.

Marine boot camp had suddenly and recently experienced an increased need for more bodies to replace those returning with toe tags as the American body count continued to increase with the escalating war. It previously encompassed twelve weeks of basic training. Training, it now turned out, was reduced to eight weeks, but we were supposed to learn the same amount in one-third the time allotted. It seemed like the drill sergeants were making up for that lost time by rousting us out of bed before the rooster had made his rounds to the chicken coop and decided to crow, boasting his amorous deeds. We were up way before dawn, doing what recruits do. I won't bother chronicling the events of boot camp. If you want to know what it was like, watch *Full Metal Jacket* some time; Stanley Kubrick nailed it! The first half of the movie very realistically details the physical and mental challenges experienced by recruits. This is not to say that harsh discipline does not have its place. The drill instructors, or DIs, had only eight weeks to mold weak, shapeless, individualistic lumps of protoplasm from every conceivable walk of life into an integrated team of trained killers who feared nothing and would obey orders without question (well, most of us anyway). However, there were extremes to both the physical and mental abuse imposed by the drill instructors, one who was, in my mind, a crazy absolutely sociopathic demon who enjoyed inflicting pain and suffering at every opportunity to any recruit who screwed up. Suffice it to say that not everyone who started out in my platoon made it to graduation day fifty-six days later.

Fortunately for me, my brains and common sense kept me out of too much trouble, and I had little problem learning and adjusting to military life. I was selected as one of four squad leaders in my platoon, giving me charge of fourteen men in my squad and allowed me to be first in line in our platoon marches. Some of the men in our platoon #1042, and surely our platoon was no exception, could not even read or write their name. The draft was very nonselective back then, and if you had two good feet, one good eye, and a trigger finger, your ass belonged to Uncle Sam.

Graduation day was a proud day. We could finally be called "Marines," no longer pukes, scum, cocksuckers, peter puffers, recruits, and various other unmentionable names our DIs called us. My record was clean; I scored well on my tests and was promoted to PFC, private first class. The day or so before graduation, we got our MOS (military occupational specialty) and our duty assignments. I was assigned to 4011, computer programmer; I signed up requesting to be assigned 0311, a grunt, the infantry. This is what I had joined the Marines for, for dog's sake! If I had wanted to play with computers, I would have joined the Air Force or stayed home as a civilian and made more than eighty-six dollars per month, my monthly USMC salary. Needless to say, I was very disappointed and would not take this lying down. How dare they do this to me? I would come to know how Lieutenant Dan felt when Forrest Gump carried him out of the jungle during the air strike he had called in on his own position. Forrest had robbed Lieutenant Dan of his destiny, to die like every one of his military ancestors, on the field of battle. The Marines had just robbed me of my destiny to become a real American hero. How dare they!

From MCRD-SD after graduation, we moved up the coast about thirty-five miles to Camp Pendleton. This base extends from Oceanside on the south to San Clemente on the north, location of the western white house for my soon-to-be commander in chief, Trickie Dick Nixon, the one who finally brought "Peace with Honor" to the "police action" in Viet Nam. It was here that we would receive four more weeks of intensive advanced infantry training, where we got to fire most of the weapons in the Marine arsenal, learn patrol tactics, and fight simulated battles in VC villages. For a while, it seemed I could do what I had prepared for, to kill VC, the enemy of my country. Despite the twenty-mile forced marches every day up and down the brown chaparral-covered hills, crawling around in hot, dusty ant-infested earth, and eating C-rations left over from the last police action in Korea fifteen years previous, I had a great time. This was fun shit!

A friend of mine, Terry S., who ended up serving later with me in Viet Nam, shared neither my enthusiasm nor my philosophic beliefs about the war *at the time*. He "accidentally" shot himself in the foot with his M-14 rifle, thinking that would get him out of the long marches and going to Viet Nam. Wrong and wrong. He was forced to march along, albeit somewhat more slowly and at the end of the platoon, and he ended up in the land of early promotions less than a year later. Promotions generally came at preestablished time intervals after certain criteria were met, along with good evaluations. In Viet Nam, the climb up the ol' career ladder could be hastened along quite quickly, thanks to Victor Charlie or the NVA. If you were a corporal and Jack, your platoon sergeant, got waxed, you suddenly found yourself supplanting Sergeant Jack-in-the-Box and given a field promotion to sergeant.

My time was not yet to come. After Camp Pendleton, I was assigned to computer programmer school in Quantico, Virginia, home of Marine Officers Candidate School (OCS) and the nearby FBI training academy. What a dipshit I was, in retrospect, of course, hindsight always being 20/20. I braved the chain of command on several occasions attempting to convince my superiors to let me be a grunt in the infantry, to no avail. One sergeant major told me his decision to deny my request would likely save my life and that I would one day thank him for it. Thanks, Sergeant Major!

I finished the class near the bottom of fifty students, even though I possessed the intelligence and understood the course material but lacked motivation, merely because I did not want to work with or around computers and talk in binary code like C3PO; I wanted to carry an M-14 and kill commies. From Quantico, I was transferred to MCRD, Parris Island, South Carolina, the East Coast equivalent of MCRD, San Diego, just outside Beaumont, South Carolina. That was my punishment for being a self-appointed smart-ass, I presumed. If God were required to give the planet Earth an enema, I think he would have placed the probe in Parris Island. My wish came true not long after my assignment at this swampy, temporary duty station. I got my orders, *the* orders, to go to Viet Nam.

A brief stopover in Kansas City to visit my parents and tell them not to worry, everything will be okay, and then it was off to Camp Pendleton for two weeks of jungle warfare training. This was really great fun. We got to play soldier twenty-four hours a day, set up listening and observation posts, establish a base and set up perimeter defenses, practice tactics and warfare, learn navigation and map and compass reading, and do lots of mock ambushes and village clearing exercises. We shot at pop-up targets in black pajamas that didn't shoot back. That would surely change in a few weeks!

It was on one of the last days of training that will remain in my memory for decades to come. The first day I ever hallucinated was the day after our simulated internment in a life-sized VC prisoner-of-war camp, long before I even knew what LSD was or could spell *psychedelic*. A barren level patch of dirt one hundred meters square was surrounded by a ten-foot-high barbed-wire fence with concertina wire topping, and four turrets with armed sentries at each of the four corners. Everything was removed from us except for our boots, pants, and dog tags. We were marched into the compound and forced to stay there all night, not allowed to talk to each other, and were given one small serving of rice at night. Thank goodness it was August; at least it was warm at night. Pretty fair treatment compared to what our POWs really had to persevere, some of them for years; however, for fat, spoiled American GIs accustomed to three meals a day, weekend liberty, and all the booze and pussy we could afford, this was torture! The next day, we were taken on a forced march for several miles, once again without food or drink. Dehydration and hypoglycemia, both terms and concepts unknown to me at the time, crept up on me during the march under the hot sun about midday. I was walking down a narrow path along a hillside, and suddenly, a cliff appeared directly ahead, so I hit the deck to avoid falling into the abyss to my apparent death. I was told later that I saw many other imaginary objects before the medics tended to me and brought me back to reality.

Marine Corps Air Station, El Toro, just south of the Magic Kingdom of Disneyland, was the last sight of America I saw before my thirteen-month tour of duty began in the Republic of Viet Nam. I ceremoniously kissed the ground just before boarding, not knowing if I would ever see America again. We made a stopover in Hawaii and were allowed to exit the aircraft while it refueled and walk into the terminal to stretch our legs, which was cordoned off with rope in our specified area and had several armed MPs standing watch, I presume, to ensure no one went AWOL in Pineapple Land. Our second and final stopover was in Okinawa, which was where my brother was stationed at the time. For reasons unknown, we spent the night there before continuing on to RVN. I was allowed to visit my brother Rich, now a sergeant, who absconded with a jeep and drove us into town to visit the local nightspots and get some trim. I remember drinking several layered mixed rum drinks for the indecent price of thirty-five cents each and having several very friendly ladies sit on my lap and grind all over my groin, but I got so shit-faced drunk it was all I could muster to crawl back to the jeep. Rich got me back to base alive and breathing, but not much else. My traveling companions who were forced to remain in quarters all night were all green with envy; I was greener than Kermit the Frog.

The next morning, I boarded a commercial airplane, a Continental Airlines 707, and took the short hop to Da Nang, RVN—hungover but alive. F-4 Phantoms lined up on the tarmac, waiting to launch an airstrike somewhere in support of our troops; helicopters of all shapes and sizes flew in all directions. In the distance could be heard explosions and puffs of black smoke in the hills surrounding the bustling air base, some landing dangerously close to the air base (the bad guy's rockets!). Their bombs or ours, it didn't really matter. Reality had set in for the first time. No more simulations. What did matter is that real bullets were being fired, and the bad guys shot back now, with real bullets. Anyone who didn't have round eyes was a potential VC, and they all wanted to kill me and every other Marine who got off the plane. For this adventure, I gave up a scholarship to play baseball?

CHAPTER 5

In Country

I love the smell of napalm in the morning. It smells of...victory!

—Robert Duvall, in *Apocalypse Now*

The average age of the combat soldier in Viet Nam was nineteen. I also was nineteen when I spent my thirteen months in RVN. Just a sheltered, Baptist country bumpkin from the Midwestern United States, one day in the most industrialized, powerful country in the world, suddenly awakening the next in an underdeveloped, third world country engaged in a civil war. The diversity between cultures, language, weather, economy, government, and social structure presented a cultural shock, which was not properly addressed in any of our training and for which very few of us, if any, were prepared to deal with adequately. We were forced to assimilate these differences by trial and error.

As I iterated earlier, as the FNG, I expected to get a lot of the "shit jobs" when I first arrived. Kitchen patrol, or KP duty, was quite an adventure. We either bought a lot of local produce, or it was purchased at bargain basement prices in the US, because the lettuce, potatoes, and other vegetables that I had to clean and prepare each day were nothing like I had ever seen growing up as a child. Worms, larvae, slugs, and other creepy-crawly creatures I had never seen were discovered cutting into the lettuce heads. Everything had to be washed thoroughly before it was fit to serve to the troops. The mess hall was about a mile away from my stalag, or "hooch," where I would call home for most of the next year. I was content to walk there each morning before everyone awoke; it was late at night when it was a little scary, walking back to the hooch all alone, cutting through narrow paths in the dense foliage. One thing I remembered in my training was to never establish a routine. I decided to heed this advice, even within the "safe" confines of our base compound. One should never take the same route twice, so I began the first exploration around my new neighborhood.

One night around 2200 (that's ten o'clock p.m. in civilian time), after cleaning up the kitchen, I decided to take a new route back. I had walked about a quarter mile when I heard what sounded like a movie playing, so I followed the sound until I saw a tiny makeshift screen outdoors with several seats in front of the screen. Sure enough, *The Good, The Bad, and the Ugly*, with Clint Eastwood (Good), Lee Van Cleef (Bad), and Eli Wallach (Ugly) was playing on the screen, so I sat myself down and began watching Clint. It was a moonless dark night, so I didn't realize what I had stumbled onto until "half time" when reel number one ran out and the projectionist had to load reel number two. The lights came up, although none too brightly, and I noticed that I was the *only* one without silver or brass on my collar. It didn't take most of the officers, major and above, to notice me either. When they asked me what I was doing there, I explained in my best FNG voice that I just saw the movie and decided to watch it before turning in for the night. They all had a good laugh, told me to stop saluting, sit down, have some popcorn and a beer, and watch the second half of the movie. Right friendly officers, they were!

Sanitation was not what I had experienced the first nineteen years of my life. I guess my company was lucky in that we did have showers, sometimes. I don't know whether they purposely made us take cold showers to try and reduce our sexual drive, or if there wasn't really any heat for the water. Our bathroom facilities consisted of a fifty-five-gallon drum cut in half and buried in the ground with a wire mesh screen covering it for urinating. The wire mesh was large enough for the flies to enter and leave at their leisure, and small enough that when you took a leak, it splattered in a fine mist all over your legs. The problem with these portable urinals was, when the monsoon season began in earnest around December and rained virtually nonstop for several months, the water table rose anywhere from eighteen to twenty-four inches and you couldn't even find the submerged urine barrels. Our hooches were elevated about sixteen inches off the ground to accommodate the monsoon flooding, but there were days on end when the water level was higher than sixteen inches and water simply ran through each hooch, so it didn't matter where you drained your lizard. Usually we would just open the door and let it fly outside, only to run right back in the hooch. Since our hooches were like floating islands, those rats that earned their Rat Scout Swimming Merit Badges swam to the nearest island and set up housekeeping with us. Never have liked rats!

Cat is a more sizable likeness when comparing the Viet Nam swamp rat to our domestic house cat. Some rats, those fortunate enough to take up residence in the mess halls, or the real lucky ones who resided at the USG Da Nang dump where we disposed of food too unsuitable for human consumption, grew to several pounds. Some I saw in the mess hall were so fat they actually *waddled*. When I got to go to the dump, another FNG task, I was told to take my M16 along. At first I thought it was just in case we might encounter VC. *Au contraire, monsieur.* We found the M16 a most entertaining pastime for taking target practice at the slothful, lethargic, overfed, cat-sized rats. Fortunately for us GIs, and for me in particular, the rats were not the Hollywood version rats, the bold, aggressive, type-A vermin who attacked humans and tore flesh off bones.

The mosquitoes took the Academy Award for that behavior. Mosquitoes were big and bad enough to land on a mosquito net, a pseudosecurity barrier that covered our rack (bed), pry the stitching open with as little effort as Superman bending steel in his bare hands, strut inside, park her pointed proboscis in a capillary bed, draw off a few cc's of blood, and fly away to tell her sisters what an easy score she'd just made. We were lucky indeed if Ms. Anopheles didn't leave behind a few protozoan friends of the *Plasmodium* variety, the bug responsible for transmitting malaria, especially those, like me, who got very ill from taking the weekly quinine tablets with the evening meal. I had to stop taking Quinine because of the horrible side effects.

One night a few months later, just before I was supposed to go to on duty at 2300, I developed an acute onset of chills followed shortly thereafter by a fever of 105 degrees Fahrenheit (40.5 degrees Celsius). My body ached, and my head felt like it was going to explode. Then the bloody explosion began; only it was via the back door. I could not even hold the forward progress. It was like Emmett Thomas running through the defensive line of the Miami Dolphins cheerleader squad. My "boss," a staff sergeant E-6, thought I was malingering, since by this time I was labeled a recalcitrant-shit-bird-troublemaker, one in a group of six other enlightened free thinkers in my company who began questioning the incongruity of war, and proceeded to literally kick me out of my soaking-wet bed, grabbed me by the scruff of the neck, and tried to force me into one of the ubiquitous idling M35 deuce-and-a-half six-by-six trucks waiting nearby. It was the monsoon season, and it was pouring rain so hard that it was hard to see far ahead. The water level was above our knees, and it flowed freely through our elevated hooches, forcing all of God's slithering and creepy vermin to share our living space. When he felt my hot skin and soaking wet fatigues (doh!) and saw my pale chalky-white skin in the headlights of the truck as I DFO'd (done fell out) or passed out cold on him, he took the quickest route to the local *bác si*, or doctor of medicine. I learned that night what a trainee and a preceptor was when the bac-si, a Navy lieutenant, gave step-by-step instructions, at *least* three times, to the young medic on the proper technique for starting an IV.

The bac-si, a young doctor in his late twenties and probably not long out of medical school and likely a draftee, asked me all the usual questions, including, "Do you take your quinine tablets regularly?"

"No," I answered weakly, "they make me sick to my stomach."

"Well, son, we need to get you to a hospital, you're pretty sick. You have many of the symptoms of malaria."

"My sergeant thinks I'm fakin' it. Could you tell him I won't be able to make it in to work tonight?"

"No problem, son. What was your name?"

"Lance Corporal Ron Martin, sir. Thanks. And thanks for making me feel a little better." I don't know what he gave me, or the greenhorn Navy medic gave me, but I was floating above the bed either from drug-induced euphoria or just more delirious from the fever. That night turned out to be the beginning of a long relationship with Dr. Young. Not only was he available most any time, day or night, for my physical ailments of which there were many (sprains, immersion foot, fungal infections, lacerations, etc.), but he also tended to the spiritual and psychological needs and sickness that afflicted not only myself but most young Americans in that war. An attentive ear sometimes was all that was needed.

I was taken by an old ambulance dating back to the Korean War to Da Nang Hospital and placed in a long, dreary-looking Quonset hut with about twenty-five or thirty other young GIs. The good news was that because I had uncontrollable bloody diarrhea, I was given the bed closest to the head. The bad news was that I was so profoundly dehydrated when I first arrived I could not even get out of bed or stand up without DFO'ing, so guess where yours truly went? The intake from the IVs could not keep up with the output, so I was given Paregoric, a clear, amber, acrid liquid containing 15 mg of opium, every few hours, for several days until the diarrhea slowed from a sprint to a slow trot. That and unknown IV antibiotics I received every four hours finally got the upper hand on the salmonella poisoning and its odious symptoms. Once I was physically strong enough to get out of bed and run to the head, *they* discovered I was also physically strong enough to make my own bed and mop the floors each morning, with IV pole and roll of toilet paper in tow. And I thought the Navy swabbed decks, not Marines! Well, it turned out I didn't catch malaria despite my noncompliance with quinine. I had contracted a severe case of salmonella poisoning from eating in our own mess hall. I decided then and there I was going native.

During my two-week stay at the Da Nang Hilton, I saw some pretty gruesome injuries come and go; many of those who left went out "ala toe tag and black body bag." The final days were nicer, because I got to see my first "round-eyed" women in some months. Some American and Australian nurses and volunteers would make the rounds and talk with us, play games, sing, and play guitar, whatever they could do to cheer us up and aid in the healing process. I had a constant boner gawking at these beautiful nurses! It was great to get out of there despite the easier routine.

When I got back to my unit, I explained to my mama-san that I wanted to eat with her and learn the Vietnamese cuisine. On my "days off" or downtime, I began visiting the villages around Da Nang with some of my friends. We met and became friends with some of the locals, and thus began my Vietnamization. Armed with pockets full of gum and hard candy, my Minolta SRT-101 camera, and M16 in tow, we moved around the local villes or hamlets in small groups, not posing a visual threat to the locals. I'm sure some of the local black-clad boys and girls smiling at us during the day assumed the persona of VC by night, but that was the way of Viet Nam. I fell in love with all the children, taking lots of pictures of them and bringing back pictures to give to them as mementos. It meant a lot to the elders and made me feel like I was in some small way giving back for all the evil horrors of war brought on by our presence here. Actually, this philosophy was encouraged from the beginning of my tour and was supported by Marine Corps generals Lewis Walt, Victor "Brute" Krulak, and Wallace Green Jr. They felt that if the Marines could win over the hearts of the locals by providing security to the villages, we could cut off the VC/NVA main source of strength, the population centers in the lowlands. On our days off, we were *strongly encouraged* (military speak for *you-have-no-fucking-choice*) to enter the local hamlets and volunteer time at relocation (refugee) centers, schools, orphanages, and hospitals, just as we were *strongly encouraged* to buy US savings bonds and give blood on a regular basis.

I spent most of my free time in Nam-O, about ten clicks south of Da Nang, and Hai Van Pass between Da Nang and Chu Lai. We were welcomed just like family and hung out in the village, swimming, playing with the children, drinking hot Tiger Beer, and eating the local cuisine. Our diet consisted of lots of rice, some noodles, and assorted local vegetables mixed and cooked in with the rest. Often times, there would be ocean fish caught locally or traded at the market, and on several occasions there would even be meat, cut up in tiny cubed pieces, cooked in with the rice or noodles. We just ate and never questioned what we were eating because we were content, and it was a sign of disrespect to turn down food from people who barely made the equivalent of thirty dollars in annual income. One day, however, I did ask Lindas, our contact and best friend in Nam-O, what the meat was we had eaten. Foolish me, I would have easily guessed if I had worked animal control in town. The dog *pup-ula-tion* varied from month to month. There were also the ubiquitous, omnipresent aforementioned cat-sized rats, which cooked up quite nicely with curry and ginger root. Even after I discovered what I had been eating, I didn't really care. At least I never contracted salmonella poisoning again. Amazingly, when I arrived in Viet Nam, I weighed over 210 pounds. When I got home and stood on my parent's scales, I weighed in at 145 pounds. The weight loss went unnoticed by me because I never saw a scale nor had a mirror to stand in front of to look or compare, plus, it just didn't matter at the time. My mom nearly DFO'd when she looked upon her emaciated son for the first time in over a year. She said I looked like a POW! I couldn't understand what she was so worried about; I was alive after all! The last six or seven months in country, I don't believe I ever again crossed the threshold of an American mess hall.

Besides the preoccupation of dying at the hands of the enemy, I experienced another fear, or rather phobia, while I was visiting one of the local hamlets north of Da Nang. John "Fish" and I were visiting with some local Vietnamese who were loyal to GIs when one middle-aged mama-san came running in with a frightened look on her face, yelling, "VC, VC come! Hide now!"

John and I looked at each other. Our weapons were in another room some distance from where we sat. We decided discretion was the better part of valor, and we did not know how much time we had before the VC came in the hut or how many there were. Gilbert Chesterton once said that "courage is almost a contradiction in terms: it means a strong desire to live taking the form of readiness to die." I was ready to die for my country long before I arrived, but I also had a stronger will to live.

"Come quick! Go now!" the mama-san quietly whispered. She led us and two Vietnamese boys to a "hidden door," which contained a false wall space, although not very large. They were afraid the VC or NVA would take the two young boys and force them to join their army. There would surely be assassinations as reprisals to the village elders if they were found harboring Americans, so we all had something to lose.

The hidden space dimensions were about thirty-six inches high by thirty inches wide by six to eight feet deep, running the length of the wall. It felt like being stuffed into a dishwasher, and the dimensions of the concealed space were engineered for much smaller persons than American GIs. The four of us were crammed into the dark cave, forced to sit scrunched up with our knees in our chest and head flexed into the chest to fit in the tight space. Not a minute passed after mama-san had closed the hidden door when we heard several heavy footsteps in the hut and a male voice speaking boldly to the villagers. There was a heated exchange of unintelligible garble, and then the boot-steps entered the room directly outside where we were hidden. More words were exchanged between the villagers and the male interrogator. The voice of the VC/NVA regular became louder with a hint of suspicion, even though I didn't understand much Vietnamese at all, as he questioned the locals. I felt sure they would smell us and sense our presence, so even if our hiding place weren't given away, we were going to die anyway. My twisted logic at the time felt it better to die quick than to become a prisoner of war (POW).

I always found it very interesting that a Vietnamese child of six could ride atop and control a two-thousand-pound water buffalo working in the rice paddies. I learned to give them a wide berth early in my tour. Something about the odor of Americans seemed to alter their normally placid demeanor to one of tenacious defensive action. I was charged and chased a few times, narrowly escaping on those frightening occasions, thus gaining a healthy respect for them and giving them plenty of distance. My M16 might stop most bad guys, but it would probably take several rounds or a very well-placed shot between the eyes to stop a charging water buffalo. I sometimes wondered if I were trampled by a water buffalo, would I be "killed in action"? We were instructed to never wear aftershave, cologne, or anything scented, for obvious reasons. It wasn't like we got dressed up to go out cruising for chicks. Better to smell like the stench of rotting flesh to blend in with the environment! Yet there is a subtle difference in body odor of different ethnic groups, strongly influenced by diet, and just using soap to shower with gave us a distinctive odor, also likely influenced by our heavy Western diet. To the perceptive individual, who is always in a higher state of hyperarousal as a defense mechanism to survival, some Vietnamese could actually smell Americans without seeing them.

The experience in the hiding space was one that I will never forget as long as I live. Besides being very hot and humid, well over 110 degrees, it was nearly pitch black and extremely uncomfortable to maintain the slumped-over position we were in without being able to move. Time seemed to slow to a stop. My senses were pressed into a state of hyperawareness. Each bead of sweat on my body was counted, inventoried, and stored in memory as they trickled in unison over my body. My rapid heartbeat was palpable in every part of my body and throbbed in my forehead like a locomotive churning up a steep mountain grade. My sense of smell was heightened, so I could smell the cotton in my fatigues, the cowhide in my boondocker boots, the mold and mildew in the dirt floor, the rat 'n' rice stew brewing outside on the open stove, the gunpowder in the AK-47 about to wax our collective asses. I sensed that this must be the added sensory perception that blind people must experience, having lost the most precious of the senses. I could feel the tension in every muscle in my body as it strained under the unnatural position it was in, and the counter-tension it had to equally express in order not to move one millimeter, which would make a sound and give away our position. The bowels were turned completely off, a result of the sympathetic autonomic nervous system pumping out extraordinary amounts of endogenous catecholamines, not making a sound. My anal sphincter puckered so tight a lubricated paper clip wouldn't pass. My mouth was dry, and I felt like I had to urinate, even though my scrotum was so tight in this contorted position that the family jewels had to be somewhere north of my diaphragm. The only organ that was sensory-deprived was the sense of sight, which was probably a good omen, since I would have probably totally fucking freaked had I known what else had taken up residence in our dark hiding place. It was the sense of touch that gave away its location, while the bad guys were only a few feet away just outside the hidden door, still interrogating the locals.

The dinner-that-got-away, a huge black (everything looked black inside there!) rat climbed over my nearly numb, cramped legs and sat in my crotch area, which was only inches from my face, sniffing and doing what rats do. Besides my fear of being in small confined spaces, and like most civilized inhabitants of the planet with the exception of laboratory scientists and geeks, I share a similar dislike and disgust for wild rats. My primitive fear of rats, coupled with the dread of dying in a nameless hamlet in a foreign land halfway around the world, transcended into an intuitive understanding between the two of us. We both sat transfixed in this dark hellhole, looking at each other eye to eye in the darkness, his front feet now positioned on my chest, tail hanging down between my legs, sniffing each other, nose to nose, animal to animal, mano a mano.

There suddenly came an understanding between man and beast; I wouldn't scream, and he wouldn't bite me. We both wanted to live! I didn't know what John or the two young Vietnamese boys were thinking, but somehow I felt they were experiencing the same emotions. It is unknown how much time we actually spent in our hiding space. I know it seemed like hours, but it more likely was less than thirty minutes before the voices of the VC/NVA trailed off and they moved on to more important business out of the village.

Finally, the door opened and friendly faces, not an AK-47, greeted us. The rush of fresh hot, 110-degree humid air seemed like a cool ocean breeze after being locked in that tight space with no circulation. Our bodies were wet and stiff, and it took several minutes before I was able to stand upright, longer still to stop shaking. I brushed the rat feces off my wet fatigues, but it still left a stain. Fortunately, I had not done same, and my SPF (sphincter pucker factor) was still in triple digits.

"VC gone, you lucky luck GIs," mama-san said, her lips surrounding the betel nut-blackened teeth now in an upturned smile. "Here, we hide guns. VC no find. Lucky GI. Better go now. Beaucoup VC come, be back soon. We show you way out." The mama-san handed us our M16s, patted us on the back, and allowed us to leave out the door after her spy at the end of the village gave the all clear sign.

I looked at John, who was clearly as shaken and soaking wet with sweat as I must have been. "That was a close fucking call, man!"

"I'll say. I don't think I've ever been so scared."

"Let's get the fuck out of here, pronto!" We followed our guide through a narrow seldom-used path, trusting our lives to a teenager who had just helped spare our American asses. Nevertheless, our weapons were at the ready with the safeties off. We had no choice at the time. This was their backyard, and if they had gone to such trouble, risking their own lives in the process, to save our hides, there was no reason not to trust him. Up to this point, I had a rather cav-alier attitude about traveling around the small hamlets and villages surrounding Da Nang, feeling overly secure in an unsecure combat zone. That all changed after this close encounter. It was one ter-ror-filled hour we would live to remember.

Needless to say, John and I made it back to base safely and took extra precautions each time we ventured out into hostile territory, if even to visit the friendlies. To this day, I have not conquered claus-trophobia. When I was injured several years later and asked to enter the magnetic resonance imager, or MRI (a high-tech diagnostic non-invasive nuclear imaging device that takes well-defined radiographic images, creating a three-dimensional image of internal tissues that cannot be seen with other radiological techniques), I had refused to enter on the first attempt. The MRI requires one to lie in the bore of a cylindrical magnetic resonance machine, much like a bullet in the muzzle of a rifle and nearly as tight. Large persons like me actually have to squeeze our shoulders together to fit in the cylinder. The procedure requires one to lie completely still for upwards of ninety minutes, all the while accompanied by a very loud cyclic metallic clattering. It took several minutes to explain to the technician why I couldn't go in there without going into specifics, although I would have enlightened him had he insisted. If not for the wonder of ben-zodiazepines, more specifically, liberal amounts of Versed given IV,

I would not have gone in the MRI. The Versed induced a euphoric state of I-don't-give-a-shit, with the added IV side effect of amnesia, so I didn't recall the procedure. Nevertheless, that experience years ago still creeps in and haunts my psyche from time to time.

After that day in the false wall hiding space, I always asked beforehand what the carte du jour was in the rice or noodles when served by my Vietnamese friends. I didn't want to eat my comrade-in-arms-rat after the intimate experience we both had shared.

Suffice it to say that my experience in Viet Nam was not at all glorious or heroic, nor was it without experiencing death, tragedy, or killing up close and personal. I've lamented my actions and felt remorse, guilt, and regret for fifty years. My story will now finally reach others' ears, and hopefully my revelations will help provide closure, peace, and give others who know me a clearer understanding of how my experiences helped shape my future. I did not return with a chestful of medals and ribbons, and there were no crowds waiting to cheer for us or line up for welcome-home parades. Quite the contrary! I did have the ill-fated opportunity to see death of my fellow GIs firsthand, stop the beating hearts of other human beings, and witness travesties of human destruction beyond the realm of understanding and comprehension. No Purple Heart or Medal of Valor decorates a plaque in my home. The closest experience I encountered during my entire thirteen-month tour of duty was when I was blown backward off a twelve-foot rooftop and landed momentarily unconscious with a head injury and small piece of shrapnel imbedded in my left leg after a fire blew up an ammunition storage area nearby. The impaled metal barely left a blood spot on my camos. Over 351,000 US troops received the Purple Heart in Viet Nam, 58,220 of them awarded posthumously. Not exactly the kind of club I that wanted to become a member.

Twenty years later, during a surprisingly slow night shift in the ER at Fresno's Level I Trauma Center, Valley Medical Center (now Community Regional Medical Center), I asked one of my coworkers if they would like to cut out the metal in my thigh and practice easy noncosmetic suturing. The night shift began with a flurry of activity the evening of October 17, 1989. Two of our children were seated in the right-field bleacher section of Candlestick Park for the third game of the Bay-to-Bay World Series between the SF Giants and the Oakland As. Mother Earth released her unrivaled powers with a 6.9 magnitude earthquake that created large-scale death and devastation all around the Bay Area. The hours of not knowing whether our children were unharmed were stressful enough. It was compounded even more by the external disaster alert to anticipate impending mass casualties. My kids were not injured, and amazingly we received no immediate patients from the Loma Prieta Earthquake.

Around 0300, the ED slowed. Carolyn and Krazy Kathy gathered scalpel, hemostats, 2% lidocaine, and a suture set. After twenty years of hiding in my left thigh, the metal, I believe, had migrated close to the surface of my skin. Its movement may have been facilitated by the giant magnet in the MRI scanner. Each time I had an MRI, it could be felt tugging on the soft tissue and it was becoming bothersome. After several minutes of slicing, probing, and exploring, KK grabbed it with a pair of hemostats, and out it came!

One of the pearls of wisdom I vividly remember from our advanced infantry training just before deployment came from the lips of one of our gunnery sergeants that gave me the collywobbles.

The gunny said, "The gooks are so sneaky that they can crawl up behind you and slit your throat while you're asleep without making a noise."

That really creeped me out big-time. I had come to terms with getting shot and killed or being blown up by a bomb into a red mist. I wouldn't feel it or have time to contemplate the future. The thought of having my throat slit just gave me collywobbles. I always had my rifle next to me or in bed with me.

One night in late 1968, I had sneaked off base to visit Dog Patch, a village just outside the east gate, to visit a young lady named Mai Li to release some of my teenage angst and sexual tension. We became close, but both were accepting of the fact that nothing could come of the relationship other than a few hours of distraction and pleasure in a war-torn country.

After spending several hours with Mai Li, it was time to hoof it back to the base before daylight. We were not authorized to be off base at night, so it was imperative to be cautious and stealthy. Amazingly, no sirens or rocket attacks on the air base occurred that night. I was quietly walking down a different narrow trail when suddenly I heard a not too distant gunshot from my six o'clock and then felt the bullet zip through the dense foliage close enough to get my undivided attention.

"Probably shooting at me!" I shouted to myself, body now in hyperdrive, autonomic nervous system pumping out catecholamines causing my eyes to dilate even more in the dark, heart rate increased, more blood dispatched to the lungs. Not knowing the shooter's exact distance and location was unsettling, or if I was even the intended target, so I dove into the nearest dense undergrowth next to the trail to seek cover. And I sat quietly, focusing on controlling my breathing and trying not to hyperventilate. I decided to wait in my position and wait for my hunter to make a move, a sound, a shadow. The seconds turned to minutes, the minutes turned to hours, but in reality probably no more than ten minutes had elapsed when I heard the soft footsteps of someone walking stealthily down the trail.

"'Twas curiosity that killed the cat, but 'twas urinary urgency that killed the stalker." He stopped very near to my position in the dense foliage facing the opposite side of the trail and looked around, then leaned his foreign-looking carbine against a large palm tree and began relieving his full bladder. With both of his hands now occupied with more urgent micturation matters, I decided to make my move while he was preoccupied and unarmed, and do it without making any noise. Surprise, size, and an empty bladder were strong assets, giving me a decisive edge.

It was a quick three strides to reach my unsuspecting victim, and my left arm encircled the man's head and neck, pulling upward and backward, exposing the full neck anatomy. My right hand grasping the K-bar knife simultaneously slashed deeply from just below his left ear and continued its course to the other ear. He dropped like a rock, hands still holding his dick. Blood literally gushed everywhere and on the ground.

The experience caught me by surprise as I had never expected to kill someone with my own hands, and the feeling of slitting someone's throat is *the* creepiest sensation I've ever felt in my life and the experience still disturbs me. Maybe my wife now will understand why I've slept with Smaug under my pillow every night for decades. Nope! Not happening on my shift. I don't watch "slasher" movies, and I wore turtlenecks for years after coming home. As if a thin layer of cotton could protect my neck! One of the monikers assigned to the Marines was "Leatherneck," a term that originated from the wearing of a leather collar around the neck to improve posture, an early nineteenth-century military fashion trend. Legend has it that it was worn to protect Marines from swords and scimitars, and it was adopted three years before the Barbary Wars in North Africa when Marines stormed the "shores of Tripoli." I still have a few decades-old turtlenecks folded neatly in Fibber McGee's closet somewhere.

Paradoxically, decades later while working as a flight nurse, I was again cutting people's throats, only with guided precision and a number 11 scalpel blade over the cricothyroid membrane to provide emergent airway access via surgical cricothyrotomy! I performed several of them during my nursing career, and it's still always the scariest and creepiest procedure I've ever done on living patients. Every one of them triggered flashbacks from my earlier experience at age nineteen.

I dragged him into the dense overgrowth and tossed his rifle well away from his body in the jungle growth. My body was numb. I had just killed a human being I did not even know. I still lived, and that's what really mattered at the time. The duty of a soldier is not to give his life for his country, but to make the enemy give his life for his country!

When I got back to my hooch, I went to the head first and washed all the blood off my left arm and cleaned up. When I finally climbed into my rack and secured the mosquito netting around it, sleep evaded me while I replayed the events of the last few hours over and over in my head. Thoughts of my lustful encounter with Mai Li never entered my mind; rather, I was overwhelmed with feelings and emotions that I had no control over and was completely unable to process. My actions had saved my life, yet I took another's. Confusion, guilt, broken commandments, antithetical to my Christian upbringing; my life would never be the same. I was not proud of what I had done and never sought bragging rights. I just stashed that horrible experience in long-term data storage. The nightmare of that encounter still disturbs me! I never revealed this dark tale to anyone for years, riddled with shame, guilt, and remorse. This creepy experience and the gunny's ominous warning were influential catalysts to justify sleeping with Smaug, a loaded semiautomatic fire-breathing pistol under my pillow all these years.

The now infamous headline-grabbing incident at the hamlets of My Lai and My Khe, in the Quang Ngai Province south of Da Nang, which took place months earlier on March 16, 1968, resulted in the massacre, rape, and mutilation of several hundred (sources vary from 347 to 504 killed) *unarmed* Vietnamese women, children, infants, and elderly. Members of the US Army's Charlie Company, First Battalion, Twentieth Infantry Regiment, Eleventh Brigade, Twenty-Third Infantry Division, operating under orders during Task Force Barker and under the command of Lt. Col. Frank A. Barker, were ordered to pursue and kill members of the Forty-Eighth Battalion of the NLF (National Liberation Front, aka Viet Cong), burn the villages and food, and poison the wells.

This travesty occurred just six weeks after the well-timed, well-planned, and well-coordinated countrywide attacks by the enemy during the two-day "ceasefire" agreement during the Vietnamese Lunar New Year, also known as Tet (Têt Nguyên Dán, the Feast of the First Morning of the First Day), which occurred on January 30, 1968. It was during this period that the US Embassy was attacked and captured in Saigon, the Imperial City of Hué was destroyed, and Khe Sanh was under constant siege for two months. The offensive was ineffective in that the VC were beaten back and defeated with heavy loss of life, but effective in its objective of turning public sentiment in the US against the war.

The commander of Charlie Company, Second Lieutenant William Calley, along with twenty-five other soldiers, was charged with war crimes. After a four-month trial, on May 29, 1971, Lieutenant Calley was the only soldier convicted of premeditated murder for ordering the shootings and was sentenced to life in prison at hard labor. Two days after sentencing, then President Richard Milhous Nixon reduced his sentence pending appeal, and Lieutenant Calley served three and a half years of house arrest at Fort Benning. Lieutenant Calley became the American scapegoat for the whole war; unfortunately, the Pinkville Incident, as it was later called, was highly suspect of being an isolated incident.

Accounts related to me by several vets who had returned after the war indicated that it happened more routinely than those watching the war on the six o'clock news back home would have liked to believe. Also there was no hard proof in many instances, just accusations, stories, and divided opinions on what actually occurred. Times were tense here and back home, most American GIs were draftees who would rather be anywhere but here, racial tensions pervaded the ranks, and we were all scared shitless. It was difficult to identify the enemy who wore no uniform; unless, of course, they were shooting at you. The smiling farmer in the rice paddy during the day could easily be lobbing mortars at you at o-dark-thirty. There was a war going on in Southeast Asia, tens of thousands were being killed, and the body counts from "search and destroy" missions were broadcast in living color on living room TVs across the country in what was aptly named by Michael Arlen as the "Living Room War," where parents and families could see their sons killed on the six o'clock news.

The singular focus for defining victory in Viet Nam by our government was the body count, and civilians including women and children were counted as enemy kills on their "kill boards." Competitions were held between combat units to see who could kill the most VC. High body counts equated to rapid promotions, extra days out of the field, and of course, beer and barbeques. Vietnamese farmers were randomly killed for running from helicopters or US troops, and villagers suspected of being VC sympathizers. The early credo during US "search and destroy" missions was simple. If the dead body was Vietnamese, they were VC. Many villages were bombed, strafed, and napalmed from the air before advancing troops entered (more on that later!). A "kill anything that moves" mentality became the order of some commanders.

This sick philosophy of industrial-scale slaughter translated into an estimated 2,000,000 civilians killed, 5,300,000 injured, and 11,000,000 Vietnamese refugees forced into slums and refugee camps in their own country. Whistleblowers who reported such atrocities to Army Chief of Staff General William Westmoreland pleaded for investigations; however, their pleas fell on deaf ears, and General Westmoreland thwarted any hopeful inquiries and buried the reports, but not before the Pentagon received and supported their heinous allegations.

A classic example of wholesale murder became apparent in late 1968 during my memorable tour there. During Operation Speedy Express, the notorious Butcher of the Delta, Army General Julian Ewell, commander of the Ninth Infantry Division, launched a large-scale massacre in the densely populous Mekong Delta packed with civilians. At the end of the operation, the number of VC killed was 11,000 but less than 750 weapons were captured!

A few weeks after the Tet Offensive in early February 1968, persuasive, mainstream, straight-shooting "Uncle" Walter Cronkite extricated himself from his anchor position with CBS Evening News and made a personal visit to Vietnam with assurances America was winning the war. In a conversation while there with General Creighton W. Abrams Jr., he was told 200,000 *more* American troops were needed for the war effort.

After hastily leaving the Imperial City of Hué during heavy fighting in a helicopter, depressingly accompanied by twelve dead Marines in black body bags, Mr. Cronkite returned to the US and later aired his famous pivotal speech about the war on February 27 when CBS aired "Report from Vietnam: Who, What, Where, When, Why?" In the first *two weeks* of February before the program aired, a record number 959 Americans were killed. As for Vietnamese KIAs, just assume a conservative kill ratio of 10:1 and do the simple math. Let's just round up to 10,000 for ease on our overtaxed neurons. Who will ever know for sure...

In the closing comments from his New York desk, a weary Cronkite acknowledged what he was about to say was "subjective" and his personally held opinion.

> *It seems now more certain than ever that the bloody experience of Viet Nam is to end in a stalemate.... It is increasingly clear to this reporter that the only rational way out then will be to negotiate, not as victors, but as an honorable people who lived up to their pledge to defend democracy, and did the best they could. This is Walter Cronkite. Good Night.*

When I landed at Da Nang air base, American troop numbers was approaching 550,000 and climbing. During the *entire* Vietnam War from 1955 to 1975, over 58,000 GIs were killed. In 1968, the bloodiest year of the conflict, 16,899 Americans were killed. I don't even want to do the math for the enemy. How and why in the hell did I survive over there with all the risk-taking, cavalier, immortal acts of youthful foolhardiness I committed walking alone or with a few friends in unknown hostile territory when others did not? God must have had a higher purpose for me to fulfill later in life!

The Cronkite moment was a pivotal speech that swayed public opinion, and despite losing the "numbers game" by an unspeakable margin, the Tet Offensive changed the eventual course of the war and completely undermined the credibility of the administration of Lyndon Baines Johnson. Not two months later, on April 16, President Johnson opined, "I shall not seek, and I will not accept, the nomination of my party for another term as your President."

It was not until seven years later on April 30, 1975, that "Peace with Honor," a term coined by President R. Milhous Nixon, was achieved under the administration of Gerald Ford, who stepped in and subsequently pardoned his crooked impeached predecessor after resigning in disgrace on August 9, 1974. The last Americans were airlifted from Saigon as South Viet Nam fell to the communist forces!

On a typical hot, humid morning after a few hours' sleep (I worked the night shift, 2300–0700), I would hitch a ride on a southbound convoy on Highway 1, just outside Da Nang, heading to Chu Lai. I sat on top of the back of a deuce-and-a-half truck, sunglasses on, hair blowing in the wind, carefree, keeping lookout on both sides of the road for suspicious activity. Somehow, I just knew that I was not going to die in this country; God had other plans for me. I was not brave, just young, proud, and stupid.

We stopped briefly at Hái Vân Pass, a twenty-one-kilometer grueling road with dangerous switchbacks and hairpin turns. This rugged pass, the highest pass in Viet Nam rising 500 meters above sea level, is part of the 1,100-kilometer-long Truong Son Range, and Hái Vân translates to "Sea Clouds," as it often is covered in clouds, but on a clear day, one can see the port city of Da Nang to the north with stunning views of the South China Sea. Its geography is obviously of great military strategic significance.

The altitude complimented with a gentle ocean breeze, afforded a slight break from the stifling temperatures at sea level. I bought a baguette, a loaf of hard bread, and a warm beer during our break. The small black specks in the bread that I thought were seeds or spices actually turned out to be small insects; oh well, add a little protein to the mix.

I asked to be dropped off at a remote small fishing village about thirty klicks (kilometers) south of Da Nang. I had visited this hamlet before to spend the day with the locals and pass out chewing gum and hard candy to the children and took pictures that I would process and return to them at a later date. The Vietnamese were kind, humble people, and the children were beautiful with their dark eyes and black hair. It was easy to fall in love with all of them. After sharing a meal of rice and fish, I bid them farewell, bowing with hands in "Namaste" prayer position. I had shot all my film already, and it was getting late in the afternoon, time to hightail it back to Da Nang before dark. Suddenly, the DJ on the oldies-but-goodies station KWTF interrupted without warning while he spun the 45 rpm record "Napalm Sticks to Kids," and in my subconscious mind, began pounding out the creepy lyrics:

We shoot the sick, the young, the lame
We do our best to kill and main
Because the kills all count the same
Napalm sticks to kids

Flying low across the trees
Pilots doing what they please
Dropping frags on refugees
Napalm sticks to kids

Flying low and looking mean
See that family by the stream
Drop some nape and hear them scream
Napalm sticks to kids

A group of gooks in the grass
But all the fighting long since passed
Crispy youngster in a mass
Napalm sticks to kids

Gather kids as you fly over town
By tossing candy on the ground
Then grease 'em while they gather 'round
Napalm sticks to kids

Flying at low altitude and coming from the south between a shrouded low mountain pass, suddenly, seemingly out of nowhere and without warning, a deafening, camouflage-painted F-4 Phantom jet streaked over at low altitude and dropped napalm bombs on the village where I had stood not five minutes earlier. In the blink of an eye, most or all the seemingly peaceful inhabitants of this hamlet were vaporized. One napalm bomb (jellied gasoline) can cover over 2,500 square yards and burns at 1,500 degrees Fahrenheit!

Ox cart rolling down the road
Peasants with a heavy load
They're all VC when the bombs explode
Napalm sticks to kids

Cobras flying in the sun
Killing gooks is macho fun
If one's pregnant it's two for one
Napalm sticks to kids

There's a gook down on her knees
Launching flechettes into the breeze
Her arms were nailed to the trees
Napalm sticks to kids

They're in good shape for the shape they're in
But, God, how I wonder how they can win
With napalm running down their skin
Napalm sticks to kids

Luck and timing definitely were working in my favor that day, but not for all the locals of the village. I was walking east toward Highway 1 to return north over Hái Vân Pass and back to Da Nang with a group of children following me from a distance, when the napalm exploded, sending orange flame and black smoke seemingly hundreds of feet high covering most of the village. Had I lingered but a few minutes longer, I would have been a toasted MIA (missing in action), never to have been found. Only a handful of friends knew of my general whereabouts, and traveling solo was retrospectively both stupid and dangerous. I do not believe that this village was a "free fire" area, as I had been there all day and had seen no activity suggesting overt VC or NVA activity; otherwise, I would have been killed or captured! I watched in horror as I saw the beautiful three-year-old girl in the black dress with lavender flowers I had just photographed not an hour before, running through fire and smoke, her body covered with jellied-gasoline, napalm, taking only a few steps before she collapsed, incinerated...*game over!*

CIA with guns for hire
Montagnards around a fire
Napalm makes the fire higher
Napalm sticks to kids

A baby sucking on a mother's tit
Children cowering in a pit
Dow Chemical doesn't give a shit
Napalm sticks to kids

Eighteen kids in a no fire zone
Books under their arms as they go home
The last in line goes home alone
Napalm sticks to kids

Fear and rage overcame the smell of gasoline and the carnage and smell of burning human flesh. Napalm really does stick to kids! To this day, I do not believe this was a sanctioned action, but yet another senseless civilian "collateral damage" of a soft target, much like the aforementioned atrocities. The population of that village, maybe two hundred Vietnamese, suddenly became a tally count for some commander to add to his "kill board." The senseless murder of friendly villagers further reinforced my growing antiwar sentiment. Two plus two equaled five. Nothing added up; nothing made sense to me anymore. I never returned to that village for fear of retribution and for fear of sensing the loss of those I had previously photographed and become friends with. Besides, there probably was little left of the village but a charred black stain with rotting corpses surrounded by a lush jungle. I still have the picture of the beautiful young girl with the lavender-flowered dress in an old photo album, and her innocent face etched in my mind as a reminder of how unfair and insane war really is. It was dangerous to share feelings of being against the war effort when wearing the uniform and supposedly fighting an enemy in a foreign country. However, a small group of six or seven of us in my unit felt the same way and were openly outspoken to our superiors of our feelings. This behavior definitely did not set well with them. I continued to do my job, but my attitude of war had definitely changed from my earlier years of watching John Wayne movies as a kid.

When I received my orders to rotate back to the States the following August, I thought back to the first day I had arrived in this godforsaken third world hellhole. I found myself with a wad of sweat-soaked Piasters in the front pocket of my fatigues as I was staging for my airplane ride back to the world. I took them out of the pocket and looked around for the nearest FNG who had just gotten off the airplane. There was a PFC with starched fatigues, spit-shined boots, a fresh crew cut, and clay-like pudgy white skin. He looked at me with awe and disbelief, for reasons I could not clearly understand at first. Then it clicked! Had I looked in a mirror, it would have become obvious. My skin was drawn across the bones of my hollow face; I had lost 65 pounds from my muscular 210 to a cachectic 145 pounds; my fatigues hung on me like a Hawaiian muumuu; the boots on my feet were unshined, scuffed, and covered with red clay; my eyes were sunken, distant, suspicious, and hypervigilant. I had become that GI I had seen thirteen months ago on this same tarmac: gaunt, distrustful, hollow, bitter, angry, sad, and confused. I was going home to face the wrath of the American youth that I so spiritually supported in their efforts to bring a halt to an insane war. Somehow I was suddenly more fearful of returning home than I was of staying in a war zone!

"Hey, you want some free money?" I asked the PFC.

CHAPTER 6

What's That Sound?

Theirs is not to make reply,
Theirs is not to reason why,
Theirs is but to do and die.

—Alfred Lord Tennyson

The VC and their 122 mm rockets had other plans for my imminent departure. As we were waiting in staging to board our plane, rocket attacks on Da Nang Air Base postponed our flight for three to four hours. Since my "home" was only a mile or so away from staging, I skipped out and went back to my hooch to party and say my final goodbyes again to my friends.

When I arrived later back at the staging area, I was notified they had repaired the runway damage sooner than expected, and my flight had already left. Unfortunately, I would have to wait until the following morning to catch a flight. I felt really sick, not so much over missing my flight. I felt *really* sick! I came down with an acute onset of high fever and a horrible cough, which became a thick productive green cough in a matter of hours.

No way in hell was I going to tell anyone or go to the *bác-si*. I could weather this one out until I got stateside. My connecting flight the next morning went without a hitch; I merely slept in my old bed one more night, praying for no mortar or rocket attacks. Just my luck, I could have been on my way back home to the good ol' US of A, only to get blown away on my—unnecessary—last night in country because I missed my flight! My prayers were answered, and the VC and the NVA left us alone that August night. The plane, the most beautiful sight in all of Viet Nam, a shiny Continental 707, was idling on the tarmac waiting to take us home. It must have been a weird sight to see over a hundred GIs boarding a commercial airliner in our jungle camos, some Marines having come right out of the bush, not wanting to spend one more second in this godforsaken land.

We spent another week layover in Okinawa doing the usual standing around, waiting around in line that the military is renowned for, getting processed, inspected, neglected, dejected, and rejected, until at last, we were placed on another Continental commercial airliner destined, finally, for the USA. During my stay in Okinawa, I continued to get sicker each day until I was one pasty, wasted, coughing infectious host agent. I probably contaminated the whole airliner with the air that is recycled over and over in the cabin area. I was now so sick I could hardly walk straight since I still resisted temptations to see a doctor and possibly be hospitalized. I just wanted to get home to the awaiting throngs of Americans lining the streets waiting to shower us with confetti and their affections for saving the world from Communism—*not!* I actually did not expect any such offering of thanks after reality set in my second day in country. But I did want to come home anyway.

The growing pneumonia in my chest was temporarily suppressed in flight by the free drinks offered to the returning GIs by the airline on the trip from Okinawa to California. We GIs were intermingled with tourists and businessmen who made a stopover in Okinawa from Hong Kong, so we had our first contact with nonmilitary and nonenemy for the first time in several months.

We landed at Los Angeles International Airport (LAX) in early afternoon and were debriefed by a senior noncom before being officially released to go our separate ways. I gathered my duffel bag at the baggage claim area downstairs and was again terrified at the looks received by the foreign people: hostile, distrustful, deceitful. I was wearing the uniform of the US Marine Corps, and I was being humiliated by antiwar protesters! The obscenities, shouts of "baby killer," and looks of disdain and contempt we were greeted with were only superseded by the paper bags full of excrement and fake red blood that were hurled in our direction by antiwar demonstrators.

I felt like yelling out "I'm on your side," but it wouldn't have mattered as long as I wore the uniform. I was the enemy again, only this time it was in my own country!

I found the nearest bathroom, dug into my duffel bag, and fetched my only "civvies," civilian clothes, which I had procured in my week-long stay in Okinawa: bright-yellow nylon pullover shirt (complete with green alligator on left breast) and coordinating Kelly green and yellow plaid pants with white background (not my first choice in blending in in Southern California). I looked like Rodney Dangerfield in the movie *Caddyshack*, and I also got *no respect*!

The whole ensemble was topped off with a cap and sunglasses, and I now was ready to see America through a different set of eyes. And this was the best Okinawa military PX had to offer, I might add. What can I say, the choice of styles in Okinawa were severely limited; better to look like a shorthaired computer geek in Southern California than a baby killer!

The first order of business was to call Larry O, a Marine born and raised in the LA area who had rotated back to the world about ten days before me. About an hour later, Larry picked me up outside LAX where the monotone voice repetitiously droned "This area is reserved for loading and unloading passengers only." He quickly whisked me off down side streets in his VW microbus, off the normal freeway access, to the Sunset Strip area while simultaneously handing me a familiar-tasting hand-rolled-in-banana-flavored-paper joint of Vietnamese-grown marijuana, which, coincidentally, found its way back home concealed inside a ceramic Taiwanese elephant he mailed, courtesy of the USMC, back to the USA.

Believe me, the cultural shock of returning to the United States was almost as shocking as being uprooted and shipped overnight mail to a third world country engaged in a civil war. Coming from near complete sensory deprivation in Viet Nam as compared to the technological society of bright neon lights, noises, colors, and smells of Los Angeles, it was truly a shock to the senses.

Larry gave me a change of clothes. A pair of sandals, worn Levi blue jeans, and a Mr. Natural T-shirt replaced the geeky Dangerfield clothes. I almost blended in with the young people walking the streets except for the length of my hair, which was long by Marine Corps standards, but short by the counterculture that seemed to be every-where. Larry offered me a hit of "purple haze" LSD before the sun embraced the horizon over California while the Jimi Hendrix songs "Stone Free" and "Purple Haze" blared over the eight-track stereo in his multicolored VW Microbus.

Purple haze all in my brain
Lately things just don't seem the same
Actin' funny but I don't know why
'Scuse me while I kiss the sky!

Twenty minutes later, the ground started to move. An hour later, I could see sound, hear colors, smell touch, and taste emotions. It was intensified even more when I closed my eyes. The mind-ex-panding experience continued on into the night and into the early morning hours, enhanced several times with the synergistic effects of frequent puffs o' pot. For those not fortunate to have remembered the '60s (both those too young and those too stoned!), it was a colorful, chaotic, confusing, carefree, psychedelic, free-lovin', rebellious era, which was directly responsible for changing the whole direction of political dogma in the United States.

Our leaders were not Tricky Dick Nixon and Spiro "the Zero" Agnew, but Bob Dylan, the Beatles, the Rolling Stones, Led Zeppelin, and Arlo Guthrie. The political turbulence and social upheaval, accentuated by the assassinations of Robert Kennedy (June 5, 1968) and Martin Luther King (April 4, 1968), America's first moon walk (July 20, 1969), the Woodstock Music Festival (August 15, 1969), the riots at the Chicago Democratic National Convention (August 1968) pretty much all occurred during my all-expenses-paid vacation to Southeast Asia.

These events eventually led to the withdrawal of troops from Viet Nam, "peace with honor," the long-overdue return of some but not all of our Viet Nam POWs, and the eventual resignation of our thirty-sixth president of the United States, one Richard Milhous Nixon, on August 9, 1974.

After a short leave and visit with my family in Kansas City during which I was treated at Olathe Naval Base for my pneumonia, I was stationed-again-at MCRD, San Diego. My very first day on base, I was arrested by the MPs not once, not twice, but three times for "unmilitary-like conduct," which included: (1) walking across a marked crosswalk and casting a nefarious stare at a waiting MP jeep, (2) having hair too long, and (3) being out of uniform (wearing a green T-shirt under my khaki summer uniform, which was all I had after my return from the Nam). All three charges were summarily dismissed by the duty officer of the day, after harassment, threats of violence, and detention by the MPs. On reporting to duty the following day, my company sergeant major made me get not one, not two, but three haircuts before he was satisfied that I had met the standard of the Corps. I knew right then and there it was time to get the hell out of the Marines before I got in more trouble than I had already gotten into.

The aircraft carrier *Constellation* was coincidentally in the San Diego harbor getting refitted, refueled, and restocked for a return to the South China Sea, to bomb more innocent babies in Viet Nam no doubt, the same time I was stationed in San Diego. Since I had just returned from the Nam, and since I had established a pattern of recalcitrant behavior (my fit-reps had gone from 3.9 to 4.0 in the beginning to a dismal 2.5-ish!), what better person to assign to baton-whip the antiwar demonstrators! No chance in hell!

Suddenly, my mind's eye channel surfed back to station KWTF (Kilo-Whiskey-Tango-Foxtrot), bringing the best hits of the sixties. This time it was Buffalo Springfield, a heterogeneous collection of Steve Stills, Neil Young, Richie Furay, Dewey Martin, Bruce Palmer, and Jim Messina. The song "For What It's Worth" sounded a warning to the Movement, with ominous undertones.

There's something happening here
But it just ain't exactly clear.
There's a man with a gun over there
Telling me I got to beware!

I think it's time we stop children,
What's that sound?
Everybody look what's going 'round.

Joan Baez, folk-rock icon, and her husband David Harris, "draft dodger" recently released from prison for same, staged a concert and rally, which I attended, to mobilize support for a flotilla of small boats to blockade the return of the *Connie* to Viet Nam. Meanwhile, my CO, a now-crippled fighter pilot captain shot down over South Viet Nam months earlier and no longer pilot-worthy, gave me the news. I would be assigned to an armed, baton-wielding, counterinsurgent force of Marines with the task of repelling the antiwar demonstrators who were preparing to protest and block the *Constellation*'s return to Viet Nam.

There's battle lines being drawn.
Nobody's right if everybody's wrong!
Young people speaking their minds
Are getting' so much resistance from behind.

This was the straw that broke this Marine's back! I could not in my heart turn my anger, my frustrations, and my weapon against my own people, Americans, especially because at the time, I sympathized with and supported the antiwar movement 110 percent. But neither could I directly disobey another order without suffering the consequences, and I was already in deep shit! My duty as a Marine was antithetical with my deepest religious, spiritual, and philosophical beliefs!

It all seemed so right and justified in the beginning; taking another life under the guise of government-sanctioned killing just did not give me inner peace. I was truly between a rock and a hard spot, only this time I was on friendly soil. I was one confused twenty-year-old, still not able to legally drink, only recently able to vote, but old enough to die for my country!

After much deliberation, I decided to visit the local hardware store and purchase a large pane of glass. After I drove home, and after serious introspection (and several shots of tequila!), I put my right hand through the glass, bled in the sink a few minutes, then wrapped my hand in a towel and went to visit the local emergency department.

> *What a field day for the heat.*
> *A thousand people in the street.*
> *Singin' songs and carryin' signs.*
> *Mostly say hooray for our side.*

My right hand required stitches in several places, bulky dressings for over a week, and light duty, precluding my scheduled duty assignment bashing American antiwar protesters. Instead, I attended incognito on the opposite side of the soldiers in my denim jeans, sandals, and Mr. Natural T-shirt and carried a protest sign.

The *Constellation* left as scheduled to conduct more bombing missions in the Gulf of Tonkin, but the message was clear: the people of America were sick and tired of sending its children to die in an unjust war run by politicians. Interesting, isn't it, that twenty-eight years later, former secretary of defense and sec-def during the Viet Nam "police action" Robert McNamara published his hard-back guilt novel, a formal apology for what had happened during his tenure. It was time to take some definitive action!

Since being labeled recalcitrant by my CO, I decided to seek the most immediate discharge I could arrange, with no thought of the consequences except staying out of Leavenworth. First, I paid a visit to an expensive private psychiatrist in La Jolla and spilled my guts to him on my experiences of the past two years, withholding critical information about unforgivable experiences I was loath to discuss with anyone. He recommended immediate discharge as I was suffering from extreme paranoia and on the verge of a "psychotic reaction" (not the song)!

Paranoia strikes deep.
Into your life it will creep.
Starts when you're always afraid.
Step out of line, the man come
And take you away!

This recommendation was taken to a sympathetic young military psychiatrist, a navy lieutenant (O-3) at MCRD, who interviewed me, made me take several written "examinations," had me draw several pictures, and recommended immediate discharge based upon a completely different diagnosis. He did not include the private psychiatrist's recommendation, and I'm unsure what information I confided to him about what I had experienced in Viet Nam ended up in his evaluation. I placed my future in the hands of that officer, and I truly believe he was one of the few doctors/officers at that time in history that understood what psychotrauma returning veterans experienced, and did not want to add insult to injury by imprisoning or stigmatizing us with some label that would stick with us forever.

There was no debriefing, desensitization, or mental health services provided during the Viet Nam *conflict*, but I was *conflicted* and didn't know what to do. It was not until several years later that the diagnosis of PTSD (post-traumatic stress disorder) was acknowledged and recognized, but the symptoms were there without a doubt. No way was I close to psychotic behavior; sure, I was messed up in my head mentally and spiritually, but I don't believe any of us returned from the Nam mentally and physically intact! He recommended and I received an honorable discharge.

Two weeks were spent dawdling in Casual Company, and on April 14, 1970 (two years, eight months, twenty-eight days after I raised my right hand), I was once again a civilian. Thanks to the understanding and sympathetic navy psychiatrist, I was given an honorable discharge. Upon receiving my separation papers, I promptly changed right in the hallway into a pair of blue jeans and a T-shirt and left my khaki uniform on the floor, walked out of Casual Company, and drove off the base, flashing a "V" peace sign salute to the startled MP at the entrance to MCRD-SD. I didn't even bother to gather my other uniforms, including my dress blues, which to this day I regret.

Thus ended my tenure in the United States Marine Corps; however, in retrospect, I still reflect back on the *good*, the *bad*, and the *ugly* parts, and it will be a part of my life forever. It is sad that I, as well as many thousands of other vets, had the misfortune of entering the armed forces at such a tumultuous time in American history, fighting an unpopular war that was doomed to failure before it had begun. I am convinced we could have won the war if the military, not the politicians, had been given tactical authority. I truly love and have always loved my country and would enter harm's way again for her today if the need arose. My sense of patriotism grows stronger every day and is stronger now than it has ever been.

For the next three years, I lived in and around San Diego. It took several months to readjust to the backfires of cars, firecrackers, gunfire, and other loud noises. They were usually welcomed with a quick dive to the ground and a quizzical look from bystanders who couldn't understand why one would dive for cover when a car backfired in the distance. Nightmares, flashbacks, sleep disturbances, and feelings of anger, rage, resentment, betrayal, and abandonment pervaded my psyche…

> *What's that sound?*
> *Everybody look what's goin' down!*

One of the saddest commentaries of the war and greatest injustices to the returning Viet Nam vets was the lack of recognition by the armed forces of psychotrauma, now recognized as post-traumatic stress disorder (PTSD). It was a decade later before recognition and treatment was made available to us. In 2012, 349 active duty soldiers committed suicide, eclipsing the number of GIs killed in action in Iraq and Afghanistan combined. Twenty-two American veterans take their life every day. After much prompting by fellow veteran friends, I finally gave in and filed for military disability in 2002 and was denied my petitions for PTSD after my VA-assigned social worker, a

Navy corpsman assigned to a Marine combat unit, agreed that I had PTSD as a result of my Viet Nam experiences.

Nowadays, school children are offered immediate on-site counseling when one of their classmates misses two days of school with the flu, given their own private safe space, and provided with an emotional support animal. My, how the pendulum has swung; America always goes beyond the extreme of normal.

Most vets were cast adrift to wander aimlessly without any help. Some have never really come back yet; just look at the homeless population in America today, and a large percentage (10-12%) of them will likely be vets who haven't fully recovered from the mental scars of war. In my Rosedale High graduating class of '67 in Kansas City, as many Viet Nam vets died from postwar self-destructive behavior and suicide as those that died from wounds from the enemy. My good friend and neighbor whom I grew up with, played baseball with, TP'd coaches' houses with, played hide-'n-seek with, Tommy B., came back from his tour and placed the barrel of his shotgun in his mouth to end his suffering. Lonnie P. decided a less messy way would be more appropriate; he shot up some junk (heroin) after setting his home on fire and self-immolated like many Vietnamese monks did, only he didn't feel the jellied napalm cling to his skin as it did to them, their screams muffled by inhaling superheated gases. He died with the needle in his arm, his pain masked by the effects of heroin. That's sad, so very, very sad!

Fortunately for me—and I give my parents a lot of credit for teaching me right from wrong and having the inner strength to overcome and conquer adversity—I slowly and without any government assistance learned to readjust and cope in society and slowly put most of my past experiences behind me, never speaking about it, hiding my feelings deep inside. I took advantage of the last government assistance offered and entered college utilizing the GI Bill like I should have done three years earlier, with scholarships, if I only had more sense and listened to my brother. At least I had survived my military experience physically intact; at least I thought I had until 1999! The mental and spiritual sides would take several more years to recover.

Twenty years ago, I had a close encounter with similarities to my near-death escape in the hidden wall fifty years ago, stuck between floors in a dark crowded elevator with no power. The vivid flashbacks of my near escape with death came back to haunt and torment my body and psyche, consuming me completely. My body trembled, shook, and ached, crouched in the fetal position in the corner while waiting for power to be restored. It took hours to gain physical and emotional composure of myself after that misadventure. It brought back deeply repressed memories I truly don't know how long it will take to overcome. Probably never.

> *There's something happening here*
> *But it just ain't exactly clear!*

CHAPTER 7

Waiting to Exhale

Strength is born in the deep silence of long-suffering hearts, not amid joy.

—Felicia Hemans

The next several years, living in and around San Diego, were a blur, a growth experience, and a time to heal. Even though Mary Jane visited me on nearly a daily basis, but unlike President Clinton, I *did* inhale, I continued my education slowly, taking advantage of the GI Bill, a whopping $125 per month, going to night school while working during the day, and taking day classes as my work schedule would allow.

I had decided on photography as my college major, since I was introduced to my first really good camera in the Nam when I purchased a Minolta SRT-101. My Minolta was surreptitiously removed from my '67 GTO (God, I wish I still had that car!) when I was in Casual Company awaiting discharge, and to this day I believe it was taken by the USMC intelligencia because I was covertly, though obviously not covertly enough, taking telephoto photos of boot camp recruits. Suspicion fell upon foul play because my camera was the only thing taken from the car despite having several other valuable items in the car which were untouched. The thief could have just taken the film.

After that setback, my collection of Nikons with several lenses and gadgets amassed in no time. It became apparent to my photography professor that I possessed a talent for composition and artistic ability. The darkroom became my obsession, experimenting with black and white, following in the footsteps of another of my idols, Ansel Adams.

One of his most favorite areas to photograph was Yosemite, a place I have always been drawn since my first visit there as a small child on a family vacation. Although my photographs are nowhere near rivaling Ansel Adams's photos, I spent several hundred days hiking, exploring, and photographing Yosemite and have scaled close to fifty mountain peaks, mostly in the high country in and around Tuolumne Meadows.

My favorite climb is still Mount Lyell, named after Charles Lyell, a nineteenth-century geologist, the highest peak in the park at 13,114 feet. The thirteen-mile approach to Mount Lyell from Tuolumne Meadows meanders for over nine miles from the Lyell Fork of the Tuolumne River and then ascends rapidly. One has to traverse the Lyell Glacier at its base and then climb to the summit up a steep face to the summit. It commands one of the most spectacular views of the Sierras and looks down on Mount Ansel Adams to the south. It holds special meaning for a few reasons: Lyell is my stepson Eric's middle name, and it was my solace during a severely traumatic experience later in life, which greatly affected my life.

Photography, I soon discovered, was a highly competitive occupation for which I was not yet mentally prepared to conquer. This awareness prompted a slight hiatus from college, with only six units remaining to obtain my degree in photography. Another career opportunity had stimulated my interest, which would ultimately lead me to an amazing career journey spanning four decades.

In 1973 I began working for the San Diego County Fire Department in a small rural community called Harbison Canyon. The department was comprised mostly of volunteers, but under a CETA grant, we were lucky enough to hire six full-time firefighters. It was during this time that I took my first advanced first-aid and CPR classes. I established the first American Cross First Aid station in the area, and then we began regularly responding to medical aid calls in our response area, which was about twenty to thirty minutes from the nearest acute care hospital. There was one particular call

I remember where two people were seriously injured from a motor vehicle accident (MVA). I will never forget the feelings of frustration and helplessness I experienced by not being able to help these two young people; I wanted to do more, and the only way to do that was to learn more. One must remember that the concept of advanced life support on ambulances was just in its infant stage, and the first paramedic classes were being established.

After this incident, I promptly enrolled in an Emergency Medical Technician 1A (EMT) class at Grossmont College. It didn't take long for me to realize that I was really good at this stuff, not only the classroom component, but the hands-on patient care aspect as well. The more I learned, the more I realized how little I really knew, and my hunger for medicine became insatiable. Now I was faced with a critical decision and was truly at a crossroads where I needed to decide whether to enter into a nursing career or paramedicine.

After consulting with several professionals in both fields, the nursing field won out, not because of the better hours, holidays, and weekends off, but rather because it offered a profession where I could work anywhere in the world and specialize in numerous areas. The fire department offered me a position in their El Cajon office to work in the education and training office: better pay, job security, and a career in fire service. A few days later, a call came from American Forest Products, a logging company in North Fork, California, only a half hour's drive from Yosemite National Park, offering me a position that I had applied for on one of my visits to the park earlier that year. I discussed the options with my new wife, PJ (Patricia Jo), and two days later, we packed up our meager household items and moved to North Fork, close to where I had always wanted to live.

The following year PJ and I bought a beautiful adobe home in Oakhurst, designed and built by the late great, notable builder Ken Kern, just ten miles south of Yosemite's park entrance and forty-five miles north of Fresno, the nearest city with a hospital, shopping center, and a college that taught nursing. For the next few years, I attended night school while working several jobs simultaneously and completed my nursing prerequisite courses.

Jobs in small mountain communities are scarce, but I had no trouble finding work that would allow me to attend college. I started working part-time for Sierra Ambulance Service as an EMT; part-time as an EMT in the ER at St. Agnes Hospital in Fresno; an EMT in the Emergi-Care at Sierra Meadows Convalescent Hospital in Oakhurst; EMT for Martin's Ambulance (no relation) in Madera forty-five miles away; a nurse tech at Valley Children's Hospital in Fresno; pounding nails as a carpenter, and in my *spare time*, cutting and selling firewood to the locals.

Just to put things in perspective as far as me becoming a shit magnet for tragedy and death in my long-distinguished career, let me digress to my very first ambulance call as an EMT for Martin's Ambulance. I *could* drive the ambulance, but I had no geographic knowledge of the flatlands and I preferred to be an ambulance attendant and focus on that aspect of direct patient care, not driving an ambulance.

My partner Doug Turpin was ten years my senior and a patient, professional coworker. Navigation from the passenger seat with lights and sirens distracting your every thought presented itself with its own set of challenges. The dispatch call reported an infant with trouble breathing about eight to ten miles southwest of Madera in rural farm country with a myriad of dead-end roads and T-intersections.

We were close when we saw a frantic man waving at us and signaling we were needed. Only one major obstacle: we were on the other side of a roadway that was separated by a median with a fence between the lanes, and the next turnaround to physically drive the ambulance near the house was about a half mile ahead. Doug and I looked at each other and neither said a word. I jumped out of the ambulance and said I would meet him when he navigated the road maze back to the location. Precious minutes could potentially be lost waiting to drive the loop back to the house.

With the impetuousness of youth and my desire to do no harm, I leapt over the wire fence and played a short game of frogger, dodging a few cars crossing the road. The disconcerted man met me outside his fenced yard with fear and panic in his wild, tearful eyes; he was screaming incoherent word salad.

Suddenly the front screen door flung open widely and a wailing woman much younger than myself appeared carrying a swaddled bundle in her arms, and she ran up to me and placed the sweet-smelling bundle of love in my arms, screaming very coherently, "Help me, help me, my baby's not breathing!"

Keep in mind, I was in the FNG role again, but I was trained well and exuded calm and self-confidence just as I did in a previous life. I knew in my heart that this profession was chosen for me. Upon opening the small blanket, I exposed what I later discovered to be a healthy full-term normal spontaneous vaginal delivery (NSVD) three-week-old breastfed female neonate with no perinatal complications who, despite being African American, was indeed apneic and her lips were cyanotic (purplish tinged) on her dark skin. Extremities were cool, no pulse. Holding the swaddled girl like a football cradled on my left arm, I began CPR while standing on the curbside, awaiting my partner Doug and the false security of the approaching ambulance.

After a few cycles of CPR, the expected response to positive pressure ventilation and an abdomen distended with air caused the partially digested breast milk in her tiny tummy to reverse course and spew upstream into my mouth. Unfortunately, this was *not* to be the most unpleasant exposure and taste to attack and take up temporary residence within my oral cavity over the years. Of course, in my impulsive decision to take the fast track to my patient, I had neglected to bring oxygen, suction, and airway equipment—like I expected to get a neonatal code blue on my first call!

I expectorated the less-than-pleasant acrid bolus, swept her tiny mouth with my pinky finger, and resumed CPR, oblivious to the repetitive exposure of milky emesis (it's sure better than beer and burrito puke). An eternity passed for all of us, and suddenly Doug was by my side to assist and drive us fifteen minutes to the hospital. Keep in mind, you millennials; this was years before GPS, smart phones, and mutual aid with fire and police on ambulance responses: no helping hands! Universal precautions and personal protection equipment (PPE) like masks and gloves were reserved for James Bond villains, employees at the CDC and the OR, but were virtually nonexistent elsewhere.

It was emotionally devastating and physically fatiguing carrying even an eight-pound bundle of love in one's arm while performing CPR (unfortunately and predictably futile!), especially unbelted in the back of a speeding, careening ambulance with Mom in the captain's chair wailing and watching my every move.

Cause of death (COD) on autopsy was determined to be a relatively new medical diagnosis based upon specific criteria named sudden infant death syndrome (SIDS). Only five years prior I had taken life, escaped death, and returned home with a renewed sense of purpose, to give others a second chance at life, and my first venture in my new vocation abruptly returned me to GO without collecting $200.

If only I would have stolen the crystal ball of the Wicked Witch of the West (www.www.oz) instead of a breeding pair of flying monkeys during my brief visit to Oz, I could have previewed my future in medicine and EMS and known that my career would be fraught with some of the greatest challenges in my entire lifetime. Thankfully for me, I have always embraced challenge.

When the time came to attend nursing school full-time, money became much scarcer. We were so broke that I could barely pay attention; so for the first two semesters I hitchhiked the fifty miles to college both ways or took the short-lived daily bus from Oakhurst to Fresno.

The following year, we were able to buy a kickstart Suzuki 400 motorcycle for my transportation. It was definitely cheap transportation but not well suited for winter driving in the Sierras. They still don't make tire chains for motorcycles. My multitalented seamstress wife made me a complete rust-red Gore-Tex outfit with pants, gaiters, Pendleton wool-insulated jacket with hood, and mittens. At least I was waterproof, but try as I did, I could never wear enough clothes to keep warm, with temperatures creeping down into the teens; add a windchill factor traveling at 50–60 mph without a windshield, and you can imagine how cold it got.

It took over fifteen minutes to dress into my many layered winter gear and then cover my body in Gore-Tex. When dressed, I looked and felt like the Pillsbury doughboy with a bad case of sunburn. Then I had to pack two changes of clothes: my white nursing uniform and street clothes to wear during class on campus. Not to mention all my textbooks, notebooks, lunch, etc., all of which I crammed into a backpack, which I carried all day wherever I went. Despite adverse road conditions, I never once went down, having driven on black ice, heavy rains, and yes, snow. There were several times when I came home from Fresno in the late evening that I would have to wait patiently on the south side of Deadwood Mountain between Coarsegold and Oakhurst and follow a Cal Trans snowplow over the pass to get home.

The only image that allowed me to maintain my sanity was the promise my wife and I made: when I graduated, we would buy a new car and more importantly, a California Cooperage redwood hot tub. Some nights I would come home literally chilled to the bone. Every bone in my body would ache for over an hour until I warmed up in our heated waterbed or fell asleep from sheer fatigue. Driving those long miles at night all alone on my scooter, I would frequently flash on images of soaking in my hot tub. True to our promise and dreams, I was sitting in our new hot tub a week after graduation, with a brand-new red Honda Accord in the driveway. Thank God for credit and a good job guarantee!

Right after graduation, I began working in the ER at Valley Children's Hospital where I was already working as a nurse tech, which offered a tremendous opportunity to learn and take care of pediatric patients. Most nurses feel uncomfortable working with kids, and I will always cherish the experiences, training, and knowledge I obtained there. The doctors, nurses, and staff were all great to work with. Dealing with the tragedy and death associated with the job was hard, and even then, there was no mechanism for treating the psychotrauma the medical staff encountered on a daily basis. You just dealt with it.

My dream nearly realized, to work as a mobile intensive care nurse (MICN) and work on a helicopter as a flight nurse, I transferred full-time to St. Agnes Hospital three miles to the north after two years of caring for children. In 1982, I completed the MICN class, just in time for the departure of the air ambulance based out of St. Agnes. A setback to be sure, but I was not going to give up.

I still continued to work for Sierra Ambulance in Oakhurst, since 1975, and when I became a nurse, I could still only function at the level of an EMT-1 on the ambulance. I had also become more active in the company, having served as a member of the board of directors for several years. In 1982 I was elected to serve as president of the board. During my tenure, I helped to obtain a grant to build a permanent home for our ambulances, a two-bay garage, which later included offices and sleeping quarters.

Prior to this our ambulance was housed in a dilapidated unlit, noninsulated, unheated garage at the lumber mill. I worked to obtain grants to send some of our employees to paramedic school in Fresno. Since I was an experienced EMT and an emergency nurse, I petitioned the County of Fresno Emergency Medical Services (EMS) to challenge the paramedic course. There was a policy in place, but no one had ever tested it before me.

A few months later after written and didactic tests and hundreds of hours as a ride-along paramedic trainee, I became the first nurse in the state of California, to anyone's knowledge, to challenge and pass the paramedic exam. I and another Ron, Ron Cohan, a dear lifelong friend and now CHP commander, were the first full-time paid paramedics for Sierra Ambulance, and we became the first ambulance company in Madera County to provide round-the-clock twenty-four-hour paramedic coverage.

After serving as president of the board of directors, I was assigned to the position of operations manager, accountable for the day-to-day operations of the ever-expanding company. In addition to running calls and functioning as a full-time paramedic, it was my job to ensure there was adequate staffing; maintain inventory; help with training and education; figure payroll; hire and discipline employees (not a big problem with good leadership!); give employee performance evaluations; process accounts for billing; and serve as representative to the county EMS agencies.

As chairman of the Madera County Emergency Medical Care Committee (EMCC), it was my goal to secure exclusivity of operating areas for the two existing ambulance companies. Within the year, with the help of several others including County Counsel, we negotiated exclusive operating areas (EOAs) for our ambulance companies, which prevented encroachment by any A-B-C Ambulance company from setting up shop in our area and lowballing us out of business.

Another goal was to purchase two "disaster kits," one for the valley area and one for the mountain area. The disaster kits were portable, self-contained trailers stocked with enough advanced life support (ALS) supplies to treat at least twenty-five multicasualty victims. Their portability allowed for rapid transport of the supplies to any local disaster. There were IV supplies, backboards, cervical collars, two H-cylinder oxygen tanks with manifolds to supply several patients simultaneously, dressings, splints, blah-blah-blah, you get the message. The two trailers were stocked and placed in strategic areas within the county before my term expired.

The greatest value in serving on these committees was my ability to meet and work with high-ranking officials from several related professions. The members were comprised of the undersheriff of the sheriff's office, a captain from the California Highway Patrol (CHiPs!), chiefs from the California Division of Forestry (CDF, now Cal Fire) and the Madera City Fire Department, a lieutenant or captain from the police department, the medical director of the EMS agency, managers from the two ambulance companies, a representative of the EMS agency, and a member of the community at large. I had the opportunity to address the board of supervisors and speak with the media, judges and attorneys, and several influential businessmen in the community.

It was imperative, however, to maintain decorum and "play the game" by the bureaucratic rules, which I found to be painstakingly slow, burdensome, and for the most part unnecessary in my opinion. I preferred to get right down to the nitty-gritty, cut through the bullshit, and get the job done. To get something accomplished, I feel a committee should consist of only three members, two of whom are dead! However, as I learned, the game nevertheless had to be played out by the established rules, like it or not. They were there long before me, and they were not going to change the established rules of the game despite my desire to revert to my normal impetuous, recalcitrant impiety. Despite these obstacles, I learned that I possessed a unique talent to effect positive change playing by *their* rules.

When I took charge as operations manager, the company was eking by and there was no ALS or paramedic ambulance in the county. Our response times, with volunteers responding to the ambulance from their private residences, sometimes exceeded thirty minutes, and then it was nearly an hour drive, code 3, to the nearest hospital in Fresno. We transitioned from all volunteers to a professional full-time paramedic ambulance service within two years; our response time out the door from time of dispatch was less than ninety seconds, or someone had to have a damn good reason when they got back from the call (don't flush the toilet, please). The company logo, the standard white ambulance with orange stripe, and our ice-cream-vendor uniform were all revamped to more contemporary standards. We became one of the most respected ambulance companies in the region by the care we provided to our patients, our professionalism, and our attitudes. Despite all the changes, some expensive, some controversial, our company became more financially sound. We evolved from the dark ages to a professional paramedic company in just a few years!

Sierra Ambulance became one of the first ambulance companies in the US to require stringent physical agility standards prior to gaining employment. We were unique in our area in the fact that we covered a huge geographical area, which included hundreds of thousands of acres of national forest, rivers, streams, mountain ranges, lakes, and weather extremes unlike most of California.

There were times when we had to carry patients in a Stokes litter literally miles to the nearest trailhead where a vehicle could access the patient. Sometimes we literally spent the night in the backcountry with our patients. We hiked to them, climbed to them, swam to them, and sometimes flew to them via helicopter. Ergo, the company's rationale for rigid physical fitness standards. They were fashioned after the CDF physical agility testing standards since they had met the legal challenges of the feminist extremists of the time and had won in the court system. No one questioned the fitness standards, and we unfortunately lost a few long-time, loyal employees, but the company and the patients benefited in the long run.

Fortunately for those of us law-abiding citizens who had the desire to carry a concealed weapon, we had a sheriff who granted CCW permits to good people. I had a CCW permit for over ten years until I moved out of the county and had no luck obtaining one since again until moving to Montana in 2002, even though my life had been seriously threatened several times by really bad people. Some of our medics carried a concealed weapon on duty, since we encountered hostile situations without the aid of law enforcement backup. The safety standard now is for an ambulance to "stage" in the area and wait for the cops to secure the scene before entering. We entered homes with domestic violence, "unknown problem" calls, shootings, stabbings, and the occasional disturbance on Native American tribal lands, with only your EMT partner as backup. Scary shit! No way would I do something so stupid now. Well, probably not. Fortunately, I never reached for my gun, despite several opportunities when it might have been justified and I felt my life was in imminent danger.

A seemingly calm and sedated 275-pound prisoner was being transferred in the prone position from the Bass Lake Sheriff's substation to a Fresno hospital for "medical clearance," booking, and a free pass to the gray-bar hotel. He was high on God-knows-what, and he chose an inopportune time to awaken fifteen minutes into the trip and break out of his "soft" restraints, rip the bolted-down captain's seat out of its attachment, and commence to make good on his aforementioned promise to guarantee I would not see the sun rise.

My partner, dedicated-but-near-deaf even with hearing aids, did not hear my screams for help or see the mayhem occurring in back, maintained course for Fresno while listening to his country radio station up front. Fortunately, I got off a distress call on my portable radio and called in an 11-99 (I'm in deep shit, need assistance stat!). Lucky for me, my dispatcher recognized the distress call and summoned help immediately; in a few minutes and several bruises later fending off his blows, Harold was surprised when he came around a corner and encountered several sheriff's cars and a CHP car blocking both lanes of the road in the middle of Highway 41 in Coarsegold with red lights flashing and officers standing in the road with their guns drawn, pointed directly at the ambulance.

Harold stopped, rolled down his window, and asked, "What's the problem, Officers?" Doh!

I bailed out the back door as soon as the ambulance started slowing and directed the closest gun to the back of the ambulance. Drugged-out Shit-for-Brains (SFB) was secured facedown on the gurney by several cheery, polite deputies with black batons who double handcuffed him to the gurney, wrists and ankles. Officer Goody escorted me and SFB the remainder of the trip to Valley Medical Center with Mace and six gun, where it took six strong males and 10 of vitamin H (10 mg haloperidol IM, an antipsychotic) just to transfer him, still cuffed, to their hospital gurney. He sure as hell wasn't just smoking pot. Most likely PCP (phencyclidine), coke (not the cola variety), crank/meth, or "D," all of the above. I could have shot the SFB son of a bitch and turned it into a really good trauma call!

Just one other honorable mentions case, and then I'll move on. It's a rather pitiful one, but life is full of hard luck cases. Jack was known locally as a somewhat disturbed recluse known to experience occasional fits of perceived superhuman powers; he tested his theory by wandering down the middle of Highway 41 and jumping in front of cars. A year or so prior to my second encounter with Jack, I had transported him, intubated, code 3 to the trauma center in Fresno when his theory failed. A carload of tourists from Sweden en route to Yosemite had the misfortune of meeting Jack on a blind corner, sending him headfirst onto the asphalt, unconscious. Jack survived to retest his theory.

I was off duty, driving through Coarsegold a year later when Jack, sans red cape, blue tights, and red boots, tested my evasive maneuvering skills. Missing him by mere inches, I pulled over to the side of the road, radioed dispatch for sheriff's backup, and set out to ruin Jack's encore performance. Unfortunately, in order to apprehend Jack, I placed my own life in extreme danger. Some great thinker once said, "It is human to think wisely and act foolishly." My intentions were indeed noble, although my actions somewhat foolish. Something inside me has always prevented me from *not* getting involved when I experience injustice or see someone's life in danger, and it has nearly gotten me killed several times. Most people run away from danger; some run toward it. I tend to embrace the latter persuasion.

Jack was about my height, six feet, but leaner and my elder by nearly a score. In his excited state, he was very agile, too agile, in fact, because he had failed to kiss any bumpers yet. Attempts to coax him from the roadside proved unsuccessful, and I quickly realized that either (1) I needed to physically remove him from danger, or (2) I treat his severe injuries when he became successful in his current venture. I decided on option 1 and, after causing several cars to skid out of our way, caught up with Jack and pushed him to the side of the road.

At this point, Jack became the paltry pugnacious pugilist, caught me completely off guard, and stained my shirt with my own blood after crushing my nose with his right fist. Knowing Jack's past history (a Korean War veteran and POW, probably a direct correlate resulting in his current mental state!), I tried to subdue him without "hurting him." Jack was getting the upper hand, and we were just on the shoulder of the highway with cars and logging trucks flying by at 50 mph plus. One slip, and it is Road Pizza times two, hold the anchovies! I got behind Jack and got him in one of my Marine chokeholds (without exercising the options of breaking his neck or crushing the trachea), subdued him, and lowered him to the ground. Finally things were getting under control. Not!

Seconds later, I felt a dull thud at the base of my neck. Two young large male newcomers who had just witnessed the last thirty seconds of the encounter from the adjacent restaurant, thinking I was beating up on some old man, decided to exact judgment on my head. Before I could recover or explain, Jack was back on his feet and prepared to challenge the oncoming logging truck. My only course of action was to tackle him and knock Jack back before the Big Mac smacked Jack, and take my chances with the two bullies. Guns speak louder than words, but I again resisted the temptation and placed my faith in common sense and negotiation.

This time, the two bullies listened to my twenty-words-or-less-explanation, and I identified myself and showed them the radio on my hip (a lot of good that did, but this was before everyone owned a personal cellular phone!) and told them that the cops were on their way. The bullies-turned-good-guys apologized and assisted me in keeping Jack under wraps until Officer Goody showed up. Jack was taken for psychiatric evaluation, and I drove myself to Oakhurst for medical evaluation. Just more bruises, a couple of nasty abrasions, and a bloody broken nose. I decided not to press charges if the judge could either guarantee additional psychiatric help for Jack or issue him his own red cape, blue tights, and red boots. Jack got help, my nose is permanently crooked, and I still can't breathe normally through my right nostril.

Restless and still not content, I joined the Sheriff's Technical Search and Rescue Team (SAR) as a special deputy. As a special deputy, I was not a full-fledged sheriff (no badge, no gun), but it was still way cool, man. At the time I joined SAR, it was partially funded by the county, and the orange-shirted team was a tight group of very talented individuals with a strong desire to train and learn. We had new state-of-the-art equipment for the times to affect a rescue for just about any situation we might encounter. Most of us became proficient technical rock climbers, certified avalanche specialists, experts in snowshoe and cross-country skiing, winter survivalists, and a small group of us became dive team specialists in swift-water rescue. We worked hard, partied harder (off duty, of course!), and became a tremendously cohesive unit responsible for some awesome rescues.

Unfortunately, our water "rescues" became body recoveries due to the vast geographic area of response and the time it took to gather resources and personnel. It was hard work diving in murky lakes and rivers where you could hardly see your hand in front of your mask. It was merely a pattern search using sense of touch instead of sight. The only reward for recovering the bloated corpse was getting out of my wetsuit that was custom fitted when I got out of the Marines when I weighed 145 pounds (!) that was now straining around a body weighing close to 200. Like any organization or government, it is only as good as its leader. When funding dried up for our SAR team (another county budget cut for "nonessential" services), so did the talent, myself included. Fortunately it has been successfully resuscitated and is now a very professional, well-equipped, diverse, and exceptional unit again. The training I received was exceptional, and the experience was one I will never forget.

In 1989 I divorced my wife of fourteen great years for the usual irreconcilable differences, leaving my then six-year-old son, Forrest, in her able hands to raise without my daily direct influence. It was one of the hardest decisions I would ever make, and I missed a big part of his life growing up on a daily basis. PJ and I worked out shared custody, and I paid her our own negotiated child support payments without missing or being late for the next thirteen years. We are still close friends, and the divorce was one we negotiated between ourselves without making two lawyers richer. Our sole lawyer fee for the divorce cost around $450.

The following year, on top of the mountain at Kirkwood Ski resort, I proposed to and married my wife of over thirty years, Karen. We were having such a great day skiing I nearly had to restrain her on a flat spot of snow long enough to get down on my knees, complete with skis on, and ask her for her hand in marriage. I only had to ask once. Karen had two children from her previous marriage, Eric (born 1980) and Katy (born 1983). My son Forrest (born 1983) and her two kids have meshed well and get along just like one family from the same biological parents. They are all beautiful, handsome children with high intelligence, common sense, athletic and artistic talent, and thank God, haven't yet done some of the things Karen and I did when we were their ages!

That year we moved to Fresno and rented a home in the Tower District, a nice older part of town, and I took up residency at Valley Medical Center ER, the county hospital and level 1 regional trauma center in Fresno. It was truly the wildest, busiest, harshest, most dangerous place to work and absolutely the best place to learn, gain knowledge and experience, and personally partake in the tragedy of urban trauma and violence. ER employees were paid an additional stipend of $125 for "hazard pay," much like the $75 per month we received for "combat pay" in Viet Nam.

It was not uncommon to run two or three "major traumas" in the same trauma resuscitation room or perform two open chest thoracotomies simultaneously with the nightly assemblage of penetrating trauma and carnage darkening our doors. Average major traumas for one twelve-hour night shift was eight to ten, not to mention multiple drug overdoses, cardiac arrests, heart attacks, PCP-induced psychotics, demonic possessions, homeless people just looking for a warm bed and a sandwich, IV drug abuse (IVDA) infected abscesses, alcoholic noncompliant epileptics who drank and never took their meds, renal failures, liver failures, heart failures, and the multitude of poor seeking treatment for minor chronic ailments, all utilizing the emergency department as their primary access for medical care. Some patients who I triaged on Friday night would still be there waiting to be seen by a doctor when I came back to work the following night! In comparison, working one year at VMC is equivalent to working ten years at most hospitals in terms of patient acuity and volume.

It was a tough decision to move from the mountains to the valley after fifteen years for Karen and me, but the commute was killing us. We both commuted over one hundred miles a day in separate cars, me working at the hospital and Karen attending college to pursue her nursing degree. We decided it more prudent to live closer to our objectives. Fresno got old very quick, and I put in my "ten years" at VMC.

My heart was still yearning to fulfill my dream and fly in helicopters, so we packed our bags and moved to Modesto, home of Memorial Medical Center and Medi-Flight of Northern California, an older, established, and highly reputable helicopter air ambulance service. We both drove up to Modesto one summer day to survey the area and check out the hospital. I met with Dan Leong, the ER director, and discussed my intentions to consider working there and was hired on the spot. Karen, who had only come along for the ride, was offered a job working in the ER the same day as an ER clerk/Medi-Flight dispatcher. Things were indeed looking up.

CHAPTER 8

Home at Last

The secret of success in life is for a man to be
ready for his opportunity when it comes.

—Benjamin Disraeli

We rented a brand-new four-bedroom house on Orangeburg Avenue less than two miles from the hospital in a nice neighborhood that would be our roots for the next year. I worked hard in the ER and established myself quickly as a leader and future flight nurse. A core of about five or six flight nurses worked there then, and the turnover rate was low. Fortunately, however, one nurse quit to return to school to pursue her career as a nurse practitioner (RNP) and physician's assistant (PA) at UC Davis in Sacramento. Open door, opportunity has knocked.

The interview was nonthreatening but intense. All these years of preparing had come to fruition, and my future now rested in the hands of the five-person (shazbaak, that sounds so politically correct!) interview panel: the chief flight nurse, chief flight paramedic, chief pilot, medical director, and program director. I blew my own horn that day and sang praises of all the great things I had done. I even mentioned how I came to love flying in helicopters when in Viet Nam twenty-plus years ago.

One of the hardest aspects of the job was the ability to maintain a weight of two hundred pounds in full flight gear that was a job requirement. Karen prepared Weight Watchers meals, hounded me constantly, pumped me full of vitamins and herbs (still does!), and we worked out religiously at Club Super Fit just a few blocks away. I lost over twenty pounds over the course of several months to make pre-hire weight.

The ten-kilo weight loss was not in vain. A week later I was offered the job of part-time flight nurse by the program director. I was in! The door slammed behind me. Now I could really go to work!

Six months later, another flight nurse injured her back getting out of the helicopter when she missed the step on our newly designed left skid, forcing her into early retirement. I stepped in to her full-time position. The first six months were spent learning the ropes, training and retraining, developing strong safety habits, honing new skills, and observing areas that could potentially benefit from my experience and expertise. Medi-Flight had been around for eleven years in 1989 and was a strong, respected entity; however, there was a growing need for expanded policy development and a broader scope of practice and standardized procedures for the nurses in a rapidly evolving profession. I recognized it as a malleable, high-potential energy form that only needed some fine-tuning and careful sculpting to make it the best in the west!

This was my calling, and I was determined to become the best flight nurse I could be. Helping others and saving lives have been my all-consuming passion, with no thought of recognition or reward. We together would go on to risk our lives as many times as we helped save lives, and the delight of resuscitating someone who has crossed death's door and been given new breath is a feeling of personal satisfaction that cannot be matched, a priceless emotion that helped nurture and support my career for over three decades.

CHAPTER 9

On Death and Dying

Men are seldom more commonplace than in supreme occasions.

—Samuel Butler

Manuel Gonzales awoke with the first light of day. The sound of crowing roosters and the aroma of coffee his wife Maria had made on their makeshift cook stove in their humble seasonal casa adjacent to the fertile San Joaquin Valley orchards reminded him of his home in Oaxaca, Mexico, where he had fled five years ago with his wife and three children to find a better life as a farmworker in California.

Manuel was a migrant farmworker who moved with the seasons and with the crops. He made a meager living and sent part of his earnings back to his family in Mexico. Today would be like any other day in the fields, except today was payday, a day to let off some steam after work and drink the afternoon away in a beer-induced stupor with his friends Miguel, Arturo, and Diego.

He ate breakfast with Maria, took the prepared lunch she had made him, hopped in his unregistered white '74 Chevy van, and headed down the uneven dirt road to pick up his coworkers for a hot day in the grape orchards. The summers in the valley were fairly predictable in the summer months: sunny, clear, hot, and dry. Today promised to be a scorcher, because the last three days had been over one hundred degrees Fahrenheit.

Today, after pruning and irrigating, Manuel and his cohorts decided to take an early lunch, stop by the Western Market for a few cases of beer, and maybe even catch a siesta in the hot of the day while the fields were being irrigated. They wouldn't be missed for a few hours on such a large farm anyway.

Toby Henderson couldn't sleep most of the night. His dad, Robert, who worked two jobs to support his rapidly growing family of seven, had promised to meet Toby, his four siblings, and his pregnant wife, Carla, at Chuck E. Cheese's pizza parlor for his seventh birthday after he got off work. He had planned to leave after lunch, a manager's prerogative on occasion, and surprise Toby early.

Despite working nearly seventy hours a week at his two jobs, Robert Henderson placed God and family high on his priority list. Devout German Baptists, they attended church at least two days each week. Robert had met and wed Carla right out of high school and settled on the west side to raise a family. Carla valued her life as wife, homemaker, mother, and provider and taught her children the laws of God, the difference between good and evil, right and wrong, and taught them to be accountable for their behaviors. Robert supported her, loved his children as all parents love their creations, and brought home enough money to maintain a comfortable lifestyle. He worked forty hours a week as department manager of Montgomery Wards, starting there as a salesclerk right out of high school. He worked after hours and on weekends delivering animal feed to the local farmers.

Because they lived in a rural area, there was no one Robert could commute with to work each day at Wards, so he opted today to drive his motorcycle, a 1976 Honda 750 cc, to work in Modesto. He wore a nice pair of work slacks, a short-sleeve shirt with narrow striped tie, a light tan khaki jacket, and a full-face helmet. It would be a great day to ride the scooter to work, he told his wife.

Tony Silviera Jr. was a Portuguese farmer who grew up on the same land he tended with his father and his family for over thirty years. His parents and sister died in an airplane crash five years earlier, and Tony and his wife Rachael had inherited the 1,500-acre almond ranch and all its headaches. Despite the headaches and stress of running a large ranch, the Silviera family was well-off by most standards.

Rachael wore a 1.5 carat wedding ring on her left hand and drove a new 1990 GMC Suburban when she carted their three children to school functions. Tony drove the '88 Jeep Cherokee or the '90 Ford F-350 4×4 crew cab on the ranch, and he shared driving duty with Rachael in the BMW 325 when she would let him have it.

The Silviera Ranch operated smoothly with Tony and his brother-in-law managing the business. Little Tony Jr. always wanted to be a fireman when he grew up, but Tony Sr. always needed his son to work on the farm and help establish the family estate. His only time away from the ranch came when he attended college at Fresno State, getting his BS in agriculture. Tony's chance came after his family died. The Westley Volunteer Fire Department seemed just the thing to satisfy his childhood dreams, so he joined as an on-call volunteer firefighter. His wife complained about the training sessions every Thursday night and the abrupt departures at all hours to respond to emergencies, but she softened a bit when volunteers saved their barn and several horses when an electrical short nearly burned it to the ground two years ago. It was an altruistic endeavor that returned to the community more than it realized.

Being a volunteer firefighter means being on duty twenty-four hours a day, every day of the year. Wherever you went, a pager was permanently affixed to your hip. Most carried and/or had installed in their vehicle(s) a radio scanner for monitoring all the local frequencies of fire, ambulance, and law enforcement. When a call was dispatched, the response was dependent on several variables, and if you were out of position, it was easier to drive your private vehicle to the scene of the emergency, since the truck or squad would respond when there were ample bodies to staff it. Therefore, Tony, like most of the WVFD volunteer staff, carried his boots, turnouts, and helmet wherever he went.

Rachael had already taken the kids to school and had driven home to prepare lunch in the nude for Tony. They had not found enough time to be intimate on a regular basis with the demands of three kids and the ranch, so she decided to seduce him when he returned for lunch with a slab of bread, some aged sliced cheese, and a bottle of Robert Mondavi '86 Cabernet Sauvignon. A few well-placed sprays of Rapture perfume and a translucent red negligee draped over her creamy white shoulders with thong panties and skimpy bra, and she was ready; the bread was not the only object to be spread during lunch.

Adam and I had completed our aircraft checkout, counted the narcs, washed the aircraft before it got too damned hot, and were thinking about lunch, in between those every six-to-eight-second-intervals-when-men-think-about-sex. It was already 97 degrees at 1130, the humidity was 30%, and the usual Delta breeze out of the northwest was nonexistent. If that wasn't bad enough, we were in N84MH, which had no air conditioner. Our flight suits were cotton/polyester blend (Nomex was not a management-approved option yet!) and didn't breathe much as a result. Air temperatures inside the aircraft could exceed 120 degrees on hot days, and dehydration was a serious problem we all took seriously. Priorities on hot days were (1) drink lots of fluids, (2) try to keep an empty bladder, and (3) drink more water until you had to pee again.

Memorial Hospital was *the* place to go when you were FUBAR (fucked up beyond all recognition) back in those days. We were an American College of Surgeons (ACS) accredited level II trauma center with an excellent trauma program, administrative support from the board of directors, and championed by our wonderful CEO David Benn, and our influence spread for hundreds of miles in all directions as a direct result of our own hospital-based flight program. Never in my entire career spanning nearly forty years now have I ever worked with such a talented, cohesive, professional group of doctors, nurses, and technicians. Our hospital motto, "Trauma takes teamwork," was a living, breathing organism always striving for excellence, and I was one of many who were blessed and fortunate enough to be one of the standard bearers.

We completed all our obligatory daily aircraft-related chores, so we decided to take a stroll through the hospital, closely adjacent to the helipad, maintenance hangar, pilot's quarters, 911 dispatch center, and our crew work offices and breakroom. At least it was air-conditioned inside, and it was 102 degrees on the helipad now. Adam and I stopped in the Ivy Cafeteria for a large to-go drink, and then we headed to the ER to see if they needed any extra help. It also allowed us the opportunity to check the "duty roster" to see who was on call for trauma, neurosurgery, anesthesia, ortho, etc. We all had our favorites and those we wished would take a long extended vacation. Two of my favorite ER docs were working today, and Dr. Morgan, our director of trauma services, was on call for surgery. The usual array of great ER nurses was sharing a rare moment chatting away at the nurse's station. It was shaping up to be a slow day in the ER today.

Things were about to change dramatically.

The faded white 1974 Chevy van left a snaking trail of dust for nearly a half mile through the grape orchard frontage road as Arturo subbed as driver for Manuel, who was in back slamming down Budweisers with Miguel and Diego. An hour earlier, Manuel had carried two cases of Bud over his shoulder back to the van, with assorted munchies in his other hand. Since pulling out of the Western Market parking lot for the short drive back to their lunch spot in the orchards, the oppressive sere heat was relieved by the icy-cold beers they were chugging. Their day was almost over, and payday Friday was just another reason to party. Arturo was twenty, the youngest of the four men, and "learned" to drive while working the fields of the San Joaquin Valley driving small machinery. He was familiar with Manuel's van, but being unlicensed, he usually only drove the orchard roads. Major roads and freeways were frightening experiences he avoided whenever possible.

Today would be one of those exceptions to Arturo's realized fears. As a favor to Manuel in back with his amigos, he had agreed to drive since he had only had six beers and the others were far ahead of him in ounces consumed. Getting back to their ranch required them to drive about two miles on Highway 132, a two-lane east-west state highway that connects Modesto to several small agricultural towns before meeting up with Interstate 5 intersecting the state from north to south. Mariachi music blared through the radio speakers, the van's windows were wide-open, and the odor of stale beer permeated the interior, supplanted only by the reek of cigarette smoke and sweat.

Arturo was heading east at 65 mph, wiping the sweat from his brow and squinting through the windshield into the scorching sun. His mouth was parched, and he wanted another beer. In his relaxed alcohol-induced state, his sensorium was obviously blunted, but his loss of inhibition even made him feel less afraid of driving on high-speed highways. He reached back and shagged a now lukewarm Budweiser, and as he returned his attention forward again, his left hand had jerked the steering wheel ever so slightly to the left, crossing the freshly painted double yellow stripe of the asphalt pavement.

The diesel engine turned over slowly and then started as sooty black smoke belched from the pipe exhaust of the John Deere tractor on the Silviera Ranch. Tony Jr. removed the negative-grounded clamp from the JD, then the red clamp off its battery before disconnecting the battery charger cables from his F-350 battery poles. Sweat ran down his forehead from under his straw hat, his once-clean white T-shirt now clinging to his hairy muscular chest, and his hands were in need of a long scrub with 20 Mule Team Borax before the anticipatory preprandial "nooner" with Rachael. It was hard to schedule alone time with his wife, what with work, kids, and now dead batteries. He was already twenty minutes late, and his Garmin screen on the pickup dash said it was 3.6 miles home.

"Damn it all to hell, why did fate choose *today* to have a dead battery?" he muttered to himself, since his employee was already on the JD driving away to the south. "What else could happen to screw with my head today?" He slammed the Ford's lift gate closed and was securing the jumper cables in the storage compartment when he felt his left hip vibrate, followed by the all-too-familiar ear-piercing screeches and familiar voice who unknowingly answered his previous thought. Five minutes away, Rachael nibbled on the watercress salad, wondering dreamily where her Tony was.

One of the greatest perks to being a hospital-based flight program, at least in my opinion, was the ability to hone our skills in the hospital setting, mostly in the ER, but elsewhere throughout the hospital as well. Since we could be called to the helipad at any time to conduct a mission, as flight nurses we were not allowed to take patient assignments, "escort" or transport patients. We got requests through dispatch several times daily to start difficult IVs on inpatients. We were on the paging groups for all code blues (cardiac arrest) and all medical and trauma alerts. The ER docs would request us for all intubations, RSI procedures (more on that acronym later!), chest tube insertions, or patients requiring arterial lines for pressor drug administration/ICU admission. We responded whenever we were available and not engaged on a flight mission and offered our skills, expertise, and an extra hand. This on-the-job training was excellent, because we were observed by the ER doc and/or trauma surgeons who initially trained us as probies. Before I became chief flight nurse, we could intubate like a lot of EMS first responders, but other than providing a really fast-flying ambulance armed with ACLS skills, our list of advanced procedures was virtually nonexistent.

My goal was to raise the bar to a higher level in the number and complexity of nursing standardized procedures we flight nurses could perform. Whether we landed in the middle of Interstate 5 and closed it down for thirty minutes during rush hour or landed at a tiny remote hospital or clinic, we were called upon to perform complex surgical procedures under the most inauspicious conditions. Some of what we did would cause some doctors to bow and mutter "We're not worthy!" in their awed subconscious.

This endeavor involved the five *P*s: (1) patience, (2) persistence, (3) policy and procedures, (4) practice, and (5) proven proficiency. That's actually seven *P*s. It typically took six to nine months to write the policy and then distribute it to several multidisciplinary committees for approval, and then finally train our staff to perform to near perfection every time. After two years of meetings, one year of research, and one oral presentation at an international aeromedical conference by yours truly, our quiver was now filled with several nursing standardized procedures that would prove to save many more lives in the years to come.

Every attention to detail had to be catered to, since the California Board of Registered Nursing was very explicit in how standardized procedures, aka advanced nursing practice, were to be administered.

Once the P&Ps were approved, our performance in the field setting was scrutinized by those same committees who were assembled to review and approve them initially. Whenever an RSI procedure was performed on a flight mission, as many as eight committees scrutinized our documentation and outcomes. To err is human, but to be a flight nurse was to never fail. It has never been in my nature to accept quitting or defeat. There are no do-overs in life. Not long after implementation, I learned that I erred, ergo, I *was* human.

In order to ease the burden of the PC police and help put their minds at rest, we practiced advanced procedures in animal labs before performing these dangerous procedures on humans! We had to keep our activities on the down-low, because if the public knew we were performing procedures on anesthetized hours-old male Guernsey calves (aka veal) under the most humane (cow-mane?) conditions, we would have been in the crosshairs of PETA and every other animal rights group. It was deeply personal for me knowing I might one day *save* a life by slicing someone's throat. Thankfully for Elsie and Elmer, sophisticated programmable interactive lifelike mannequins have supplanted those baby big-eyed bovines; nevertheless, at the time they helped us save countless human lives.

It made my first surgical cricothyroidotomy (cric) on a human just a *little* easier as I held my Mini-Mag flashlight between my teeth as my light source at zero-dark-thirty during a heavy December 23 rainstorm, crouched in a drainage ditch with a severely injured MVC patient who had a bloody, occluded airway and a LeForte III facial fracture! I spoke with him a few weeks later just after New Year's when I saw him in the Ivy Cafeteria walking the halls with IV stand in tow at midnight on a night shift. He walked out of our hospital under his own power weeks later after several reconstructive surgeries with, among others, a 4 cm scar in his neck with no neurologic deficit. It was the first time in over twenty years that I had sliced another man's neck!

My second cric occurred less than twenty-four hours from the first with a dreadful outcome. The Church of Christ held their Christmas Eve afternoon service in the town of Ceres just off Ninth Street, a main throughway running north-south bisecting the small town just south of Modesto. When the service ended, young children filled with visions of sugarplums and Santa's imminent arrival ran out the doors helter-skelter to run off some of their pent-up energy from sitting quietly in their pews for the last hour.

Young Jason, a six-year-old towhead closely resembling our youngest seven-year-old son Forrest, ran across Ninth Street directly into the path of a speeding car who did not even have time to brake before impact. Dave Toal, our pilot and director of air operations, landed us in the middle of Ninth Street surrounded by a menagerie of curious onlookers on all sides.

The paramedics were unable to intubate or gain IV access. CPR was continuing in earnest. Every one of Jason's long bones was severely fractured and angulated from the impact and flying several feet and landing on the cement road, unconscious and unresponsive. When I knelt at Jason's side and was getting report from the EMS on scene, Gayle Mason showed up looking over my left shoulder like a summoned angel from above. "Well, Hair Ball [her humorous sobriquet for me!], you've got your hands full, don't you?" Gayle had just been relieved by me a half hour earlier after she worked the 0300–1500 shift. The call was dispatched just after shift change, as the sun was racing for an early winter departure on the horizon while she was driving home and by happenstance drove upon this tragic site. Her emergency nursing experience combined with her decades of military nursing practice as a colonel in the US Army Reserves made me revere her with a sense of esteem and respect. Gayle had likely performed many of these procedures whereas I had just done my first with my knees knocking the night before.

By now, the gaggle of gathering gawkers was drawing nearer while Dave idled just north of us with Ceres F. D. providing aircraft security. The decision was made to perform a surgical cricothyroidotomy versus a needle cricothyroidotomy normally performed for a child of his age. Gayle agreed, gathering the kit while my paramedic partner worked on gaining IV or intraosseous (IO) access. CPR was continuing during this whole process; airway control and breathing for Jason were compromised by his misshapen facial anatomy and blood oozing everywhere.

In my heart and through years of experience I realized that Jason's multiple injuries were incompatible with life; survival from blunt trauma cardiac arrest in the field setting is *extremely* rare. Nevertheless, everyone continued the full-court press in full view for all to see. The fat lady had not sung yet! A 2 cm horizontal incision across Jason's cricothyroid membrane was created with a number 11 scalpel blade; the opening was widened temporarily with a Trousseau tracheal dilator, and a 6.0 mm cuffed endotracheal tube was inserted and secured after performing the proper placement confirmation techniques. Airway now secured, the A of the ABCs was now addressed. The B and C would continue en route to the trauma resuscitation room. No IV access could be obtained and no IO was attempted since all his extremities were fractured. The final outcome was a Christmas Eve nightmare for everyone involved. A fountain of tears followed, as well as a CISD (critical incident stress debriefing). Fortunately, the frequency of this procedure only was necessitated a few times each year. I had sorrowfully met my quota in less than twenty-four hours!

Our quiver of standardized procedures now included rapid sequence intubation (RSI), chest tube insertion, central line insertion, arterial line insertion, and surgical cricothyroidotomy. We were on our way to bigger and better things.

"Hey, Ron, let's head back to quarters. It's not busy and we're just distracting the staff," said Adam over his shoulder. He was flirting with Yvonne, one of the cute blond RNs who would later bear his children after they married a few years later. I was/am happily married, so I didn't discriminate; I flirted with *all* the staff.

"I'm right behind you, man. I just gotta micturate first." Kids pee, dogs urinate, drunks piss, and nurses micturate. Same-o, same-o. Our oldest son, Eric, was working as an ER tech today, and my wife Karen was working in the ICU on the second floor. I planned on making my ICU rounds before long to visit her.

"Medi-Flight 1, Flight Com. You have a request for a scene flight in the Westley area for a motor vehicle crash [MVC] with injuries," our dispatcher's voice said matter-of-factly over the radio. Our dispatchers had been educated to not release detailed information over the airwaves, since our pilot is paged simultaneously with the nurse, paramedic, and hospital security. Any information that could emotionally influence the pilot's decision to accept or decline a mission was sanitized and Martin-ized. Coincidentally, even though I don't believe in coincidence, *and* it is totally irrelevant trivia, Martin Enterprises Inc., the largest dry-cleaning company in America, "One-Hour Martinizing" was founded the same year I was born, 1949.

"Damn, I know I should have peed when I had the chance!" I uttered to no one in particular. Our average liftoff time from time of dispatch to skids up averaged just over three minutes. The pilot's sleeping quarters (the only hospital employees who get paid to sleep at work; FAA regulations trump hospital rules) were separated from the fenced helipad by a fifty-foot-wide driveway that surrounded the hospital structures. Our helipad was designed to officially land two helicopters, but a third could be accommodated under the right circumstances.

During that three-to-four-minute pre-liftoff time, the pilot had to check weather (we were fortunate to have our on-site weather station, an AWOS, or Automated Weather Operating System, purchased with donations), file a flight plan with dispatch, figure the aircraft weight and balance, spool up the two turbine engines (that takes two minutes), program the GPS with scene coordinates, eyeball the laminated folding map, then go over the preflight checklist with the three-man crew once we were all secured prior to liftoff.

The medical crew had to sprint from the ER to the helipad while squeezing what information we could from Mom (dispatch) over a protected frequency, gather the medication bag from the locked refrigerator in quarters, and secure all equipment on board, while the other crew member stood fire watch off the nose at ten o'clock and two o'clock to the pilot while he started each engine sequentially. Once the pilot gave the thumbs-up signal to the fire watch, that person did a walk around the aircraft, ensuring all doors were secure, checked to ensure oxygen tanks were turned off, then disconnected the APU (no, not Homer's 7-Eleven Quick Stop owner!), or auxiliary power unit, unchalked it and pushed it safely to a corner of the helipad, and chalked it again so it didn't roll into the helicopter during takeoff, then climbed aboard, fastened seat belt, plugged into the commo link, and participated in the preflight checklist. The attitude inside the cockpit was regimented, consistent, professional, and absolutely necessary for crew member safety, priority one even before patient safety in my eyes. I also do not believe "the customer is always right." Elaboration on that tenet will become clearer on several encounters of my tale.

I had fire watch on this flight, so I took the port side seat (left, ye landlubbers). As our pilot, Geoff, pulled pitch, we rose to a ten-foot hover, and then he pedaled the aircraft left where we taxied out to a large grass field, our safety approach area for takeoffs and landings. From there, we rose vertically about 150–200 feet while simultaneously hovering backward slightly so he had the whole field ahead of us before we neared the closest building. The helicopter's nose dipped slightly, and he powered forward, picking up forward speed and altitude quickly. It was a fifteen-minute flight by air to I-5, close to an hour in busy traffic. Adam and I pulled maps, and I contacted Mom on guard frequency for ground contact.

"Engine 42 will be Air Ops on Red channel," replied dispatch.

"Medi-Flight 1 copies Air Ops on Red," I replied. Our Wolfsburg radio had radio input presets for thirty frequencies, each channel with capability to program both transmit and receive frequencies, as they were typically different. Most of our frequently utilized frequencies were preprogrammed. If they were not, we were tasked with pulling a three-ring binder out, locating the agency's frequency, then programming that into an open channel—even more stress. Fortunately, today we were on our most well-used frequency.

I switched from guard to County Red channel. "Air Ops, this is Medi-Flight 1, ready for LZ information. ETA five minutes."

"Medi-Flight 1…this…is…Air…Ops. Oh my god, you gotta hurry, it's real bad down here!" he bellowed, an eerie sense of fear and apprehension in his voice. We gathered landing zone information while the pilot circled the LZ overhead, checking for power lines, towers, etc. Whatever awaited us below would soon become apparent in ninety seconds.

Robert Henderson was well-liked and respected by his coworkers. He was fair, open-minded, and pitched in to help when the floor was busy. He possessed leadership qualities one can't easily learn at a weekend management conference.

Today, he was all about his son, Toby. He waved goodbye to his staff, secured his helmet strap after starting his Honda motorcycle, then drove off west toward home at ten minutes past two o'clock. The hot, dry air was a shock to the previous comfort of the air-conditioned building he had just left, but soon his thoughts wandered to his family, and he continued his thirty-minute drive home in relative comfort.

Now just five minutes from home, his thoughts wandered to his five children and his pregnant wife. He was truly blessed to have such a wonderful family. Suddenly his attention was redirected to the speeding white van approaching from the west that he noticed weaving across the centerline. He slowed and eased his bike over to the right to make more space between them. What he could not anticipate was the Chevy van suddenly careening across the double yellow at 75 mph directly on a collision course with him, the left bumper and front fender making direct initial contact with his left pelvic area. Then he dreamed he could fly.

"Flight Com, Medi-Flight 1, ground contact established and on short final for landing," I replied over guard channel to dispatch.

"Copy, Medi-Flight 1."

"Below 40 door?" I asked Pilot Geoff.

"Go ahead, you numbskull!" was his affable retort.

Below forty knots, the crewmember was allowed to open the left side door to gain better rearward visibility of the tail rotor and to check for obstacles in the LZ. This moment is definitely not a good time to fall to your death because you forgot to fasten your seat belt. It was also the first breath of refreshing hot air that felt invigorating after being in a small, enclosed aircraft with no air-conditioning!

We saw the east-west power lines, and the LZ was Highway 132, a paved two-lane highway. I could see traffic stopped as the CHP had blocked off and closed the major access road, cars and trucks idling for miles in both directions. I would be tasked with performing my job flawlessly and expediently, as the CHiPs are tolerant but get testy should we tarry too long when we land in the middle of their highways.

The scene below was littered with shiny flashing emergency vehicles—fire trucks, CHP vehicles, sheriff cars, ambulances, tow trucks, and volunteer firefighter vehicles parked haphazardly alongside the road. A single motorcycle, or parts thereof, seemed to be the area of first-responder focus. As soon as we landed, I flipped the Wolfsburg radio back to guard so I could talk to the pilot with patient weight and destination. I hopped out and made a beeline for the LZO, or landing zone officer, while Adam prepped the aircraft for patient transport.

Air Ops LZ Officer, volunteer fireman and full-time farmer Bill Caruthers, whom I had spoken with just minutes before, was still freaked out but felt better we were there. We had almost attained deity status with many of the agencies we interfaced with because we were angels without wings who swooped out of the sky and brought the dead back to life.

"Your patient is the driver of the motorcycle. He's my neighbor, man, you gotta help him!" he pleaded. He was close to tears but retained his professional decorum.

"I'm on it. You keep an eye on the aircraft and watch for any signals the pilot may direct your way!" I yelled over the turbine engines.

The SPF (that's sphincter pucker factor) was high, and I hadn't even gotten to my patient yet. The scene was scattered over an area of about fifty meters. I noted a group of Hispanics near a white van who were standing next to an ambulance and speaking with CHP officers several hundred feet away. Another ambulance idled closer in the middle of the closed roadway, and I noticed a flurry of activity on the pavement adjacent to it. I quickly walked over to the ambulance, rivulets of sweat already running down my face and soaking my flight suit.

The medics were frantically working on my patient, trying to start IVs unsuccessfully in both arms. My initial five-second across-the-room assessment told me we were in deep doo-doo. I recognized the familiar face of the paramedic attending the patient.

"What have you got, Bob?" I asked.

"Robert Henderson, twenty-seven-year-old male, helmeted driver of the motorcycle down the road. Struck by a full-sized van at high speed. The obvious amputated left leg, open fracture of right tib-fib. Multiple abrasions and lacerations, altered mental status, and probably internal injuries. Haven't got a BP yet, but pulse is rapid and thready, respirations thirty-six per minute. We've C-spined him, splinted his right leg, started O2 at fifteen liters by nonrebreather. No luck with an IV yet, he's really peripherally shutdown," Bob rattled off quickly while still feverishly focusing on Robert. "Oh, he weighs 165 pounds, and we would like him to go to Memorial."

"Is that weight with or without his missing leg, and just where is his leg?" I asked.

"With both legs, and I think it's scattered over a hundred feet of highway," replied Bob.

"Geoff, Ron here! Patient weight is 165 pounds and we're going back home. Adam, prep for two IVs and emergent intubation. We've got a traumatic amputation at the hip comin' hot your way in about five."

"Copy and copy," said Geoff. Most of our communication was nonverbal. A glance or a nod was usually mutual acknowledgment of prioritization, and I'm sure Adam and Geoff got my transmission, glanced at each other, and knew what was ahead. Nothing said, just coordinated, orchestrated actions on autopilot.

That being done in a span of maybe sixty seconds, I turned my full attention to my new patient. I dropped down onto both knees on the scorching asphalt next to Robert's chest and looked into his eyes while simultaneously holding his right hand in both of mine.

"Mr. Henderson, my name is Ron. I'm a flight nurse who is going to help you and take care of you. Can you tell me where you hurt?"

"Everywhere, but mostly my left leg and abdomen."

This seemingly simple maneuver gave me a wealth of information on Robert's status. He was conscious and alert, his eyes opened to my voice, and he answered my questions appropriately. A GCS of 14, not bad considering Robert's injuries, but experience telling me that compensated shock would deteriorate rapidly to decompensated shock. While holding his right hand, I got a feel of skin temperature (cool, diaphoretic), capillary refill (delayed), and pulse (140, thready). I also formed that special bond in the nurse-patient relationship by touching, reassuring, caring, and trust building.

"I'm going to perform a quick exam, and then we are going to carry you over to the helicopter and take you to Memorial Hospital. The doctors are standing by awaiting your arrival right now." All patients get a primary and secondary survey. The primary survey is the basic ABCs—airway, breathing, circulation. The secondary survey is a complete head-to-toe examination performed by looking, listening (auscultating), feeling. The focus is on life-threatening injuries, and these must be addressed before moving on. Your primary doctor may perform an exam in his office and take thirty minutes covering all the bases. In the field setting of trauma, I could perform a rapid accurate examination in about ninety seconds or less.

ABCs intact for now, breathing supplemented with high-flow oxygen, dressings already applied with no overt external hemorrhage. Helmet already removed by EMS and C-spined, facial bones intact. No missing teeth. Neck in cervical collar, trachea midline. Chest rise symmetrical, ecchymosis right lower chest. Crepitus to the right lower chest wall, subcutaneous emphysema palpated, diminished breath sounds right lower lung. Abdomen firm, tense, with peritoneal signs. Pelvis—*missing* on the left with loops of intestine protruding from the gaping hole where minutes ago his leg was attached. Open fracture of right tibia and fibula, fixation splint applied with four-by-fours applied over the open fractures. Distal pulse present, weak. Both arms had closed wrist/forearm fractures, not a big deal when looking at the big picture. No time to waste even with arm splints; broken arms weren't going to kill him. I grabbed all the multitrauma dressings in the combined trauma bags lying on the highway and stuffed them into the dark, bloody pelvic opening, pushing the dangling loops of his large intestine back in slightly.

"Let's get out of Dodge. The rest we'll do en route," I said. "I need four people to carry the gurney. Make sure that your chinstraps are secured on your helmets. Keep your heads low under the blades, we're loading hot. We'll load feet first from the left side of the helicopter." We, well *actually* the four firemen, carried Robert, two on each side of the long backboard. I needed to be hands-free to assist my patient while simultaneously carrying from one to three equipment bags. I continued speaking with Robert en route to the helicopter, gathering pertinent information. He related how his day was to have unfolded with Toby's birthday, his family, his pregnant wife. I told him he might not get the chance to talk to his family for a while and asked him if he had anything he wanted me to relay to them. I have listened to more death-bed declarations than hookers at a DNC political convention, and I knew already that this was going to be another one. If he would have asked, "Am I going to die?" I would not lie to him, but fortunately he didn't ask even though I believe he knew his injuries were likely nonsurvivable.

"Tell Toby I'm sorry I can't make Chuck E. Cheese's. Tell my wife and kids I love them very much, and I promise to sell the Honda." That's a knowing death-bed affirmation if I ever heard one, and I have. He was so calm it was hauntingly unnerving. My inner self lamented inwardly while outwardly I was in full control.

"I promise that will be my priority after I make you better! I might have to put a tube in your throat to help you breathe before we land."

"Shit, shit, shit!" I said over ICS frequency (intercom communication between flight crew) when I plugged into the radio while loading the patient on board. I had completely forgotten about Robert's missing body part(s). "Air Ops, Medi-Flight 1," I said after switching frequencies.

"Go ahead, Medi-Flight 1. This is Air Ops."

"Air Ops, we need to have someone retrieve the patient's left leg for transport with him."

"Air Ops, this is Westley Fire Department, Firefighter Silviera. Copy last transmission, I'm on it," Tony Jr. replied over the radio. From several hundred feet away from our helicopter, rotors now at full rpm's creating a more forceful downwind turbulence, I could make out a couple of firemen gathering objects from the road and then running toward us.

Tony Silviera Jr. had delivered hundreds of calves during his lifetime, but nothing had prepared him for his task at hand. He had never seen human carnage or a dead human being before, mostly just brush fires since becoming a rural firefighter. While his fellow firemen gathered up large chunks of flesh, bone, and muscle of Mr. Henderson's thigh and lower leg, Tony scooped up the thirty-six-inch-long forty-pound piece of lifeless lower leg, cradled it in his arms like he was holding an infant in his arms, and ran like a fire was licking at his heels as he headed eastbound on Highway 132 toward us.

I had jumped in on the right side of the aircraft, and Adam took fire watch for liftoff on the left side where the patient was loaded. We were already at a feverish pitch inside, checking for further bleeding; attaching leads for cardiac monitoring, pulse oximetry, and NIBP (noninvasive blood pressure); prepping for IV starts; reassessing; etc.

When Tony and his partner neared Air Ops, they made eye contact with our pilot. Geoff signaled for them to come to the starboard (right) side to load the left leg. Our Eurocopter Twin Star is a small helicopter with just enough space (well, most of the time) to perform the mission. I have flown with a four-pound preemie with tetralogy of Fallot (a rare cyanotic congenital heart disease of the newborn) and a six-hundred-pound man who crashed his 250 cc motorcycle in the wilderness, yet somehow loading Robert's whole left leg onboard seemed like another ghostly patient. It was truly an eerie experience, with Geoff pushing his seat forward and leaning so we could load the bloody leg through the much smaller right door opening. The only place for it was on the short bench seat that faced inward toward the patient on the right wall, the same seat the crew member occupied during flight. If we would have loaded it from the left side, however, the dripping leg would have been passed right over the face of our supine patient, and there was not enough room to place it on the floor between us anyway. The infamous James Bond 007 villain Max Zorin once said, "Intuitive improvisation is the secret of genius." It seemed to work for me in this particular circumstance.

When the leg transfer was complete, I looked down at the saucer-sized eyes of young firefighter Silviera, and he gazed into mine. It amazes me that sometimes a glance into someone's eyes can reveal numerous feelings and emotions and expose that person's soul for a fleeting moment. I could sense his feelings of fear, helplessness, horror, and despair. No way that I could have known then that he had sacrificed a beautiful afternoon of lovemaking to perform this heroic, thankless, nonremunerated job he had just performed. It somehow formed a bond, a common link, between us from that moment forward. We had just shared a moment of abject horror that would leave an indelible mark on our lives forever, and no matter how this all turned out, we were of the same spirit on that day. He missed his lunch date with Rachael. I missed lunch and dinner.

I bid my thanks to the crew and to Air Ops as we lifted off the scene after we went through the preflight checklist once again. I quickly gave Adam a sit-rep on the patient over ICS so he would know what we faced besides the glaringly obvious. The intensity and harsh realities of caring for multisystems trauma patients is minimized only by years of experience, tenacity of spirit and compassion, and adhering to the cookbook recipes provided by the ENA (Emergency Nurses Association) and the ACS (American College of Surgeons). Trauma Nursing Core Course and Advanced Trauma Life Support, respectively, are intensive two-day didactic and hands-on (with the aforementioned lifelike mannequins) clinical courses that prepare doctors and nurses for systematically assessing, planning, and intervening in critical life and death situations.

These courses, along with a coordinated trauma team approach, a supportive hospital administration, and a well-developed trauma program that begins in the prehospital setting through ER-surgery-ICU-rehab continuum of care, have made one's chances of surviving a major traumatic event much better.

But, buyer beware! Your odds of survival all depend on where you decide to impale your car on a bridge abutment! Not all hospitals treat you the same, despite what plaques they hang on their walls. I have worked in levels I, II, III, and IV trauma centers, some excellent and some that I had to leave after working there. All level I and II trauma centers in the US are accredited by the American College of Surgeons Committee on Trauma (ACS COT) and provide the highest levels of trauma services, always have trauma surgeons, anesthesia, and neurosurgery immediately available 24/7/365. Levels III and IV are generally more rural facilities but still can do a great job of stabilizing before transporting the patient to a higher level of care. One of my proudest accomplishments was working at a remote hospital in Livingston, Montana, and bringing them out of the wilderness to twenty-first-century trauma care in less than two years. Through mostly my personal efforts, but with full support of hospital administration and *most* staff, we became the *first* level IV trauma center in the state of Montana. Those efforts were rewarded by a huge reduction in morbidity and mortality, a renewed sense of pride in the staff, and a plaque on the wall that really had meaning. But that is on the distant horizon of my career, and I ramble once again.

"Memorial Medical Center, Medi-Flight 1 with STAT trauma!" I hoarsely squeaked over the med-net frequency, stress and dehydration testing my fortitude. The interior cabin temperature was probably 120+ degrees in our little flying breadbox as it was 105 degrees outside. Our flight altitude was usually 1,000–1,500 feet above ground level (AGL), so not much cooling assistance there. Sweat was rolling off Adam and me like someone had poured a Big Gulp on our heads. It burned the eyes and made it harder to see between blinks.

I had just started a 16-gauge IV of normal saline in Robert's outstretched deformed right arm while sitting in front of his bloody left leg lying on my bench seat, trying not to think about his angulated and broken radius and ulna or the blood soaking into my flight suit. My butt was wet too, from sitting in a pool of blood, not sweat or…Robert was also diaphoretic, albeit from a different mechanism, so taping the IV was not done in the usual neat fashion. A quick circumferential double wrap of his arm with the tape followed by a quick wrap of Kling gauze tied off in a bow knot was the most expeditious; not neat, but functional. Adam, sitting at Robert's head looking over his torso, had started a 14-gauge "upside down" in his left forearm, a daunting aeromedical procedure performed due to lack of space. We attached the two prepared 1,000 mL bags of 0.9% normal saline attached with blood tubing on pressure infusion pumps and opened the clamps to run wide-open while I ignored the hospital's return call over the radio. Now with a free bloody-gloved hand, I went back to the task of my radio report.

"Memorial, Medi-Flight 1, MICN Martin with Paramedic Christianson. We are en route to you with a twenty-seven-year-old seventy-five-kilo male driver of a motorcycle versus auto at freeway speed. He was wearing a helmet, no leathers. His injuries are obvious amputation of the entire lower leg at the left hip, open tib-fib fracture of the right lower leg. Right chest trauma with possible multiple rib fractures and underlying lung injury—suspect hemothorax. Abdomen is tense with ecchymosis over the right upper quadrant and positive peritoneal signs. Numerous lacerations and abrasions, closed fractures of both wrists. Vitals are as follows…Stand by, Memorial."

"Hey, Adam, I think you better get ready to intubate him. I think he's going to stop breathing any second," I spoke over ICS.

"How do you know?" Adam replied.

"I just do, trust me. He's going to go apneic, look at how he's breathing now!" Decompensated traumatic shock had progressed rapidly.

Experience is the best teacher, and it has taught me to be proactive and anticipate events before they occur, thus reducing or mitigating future deleterious consequences. The number of people I have watched die as they take their last breaths as a biped carbon unit on planet Earth were by now in quadruple digits, and I can almost *smell death* before it occurs. It is that sixth sense that gifted persons are both blessed and cursed with.

Adam did not question me further; he grabbed the airway bag, pulled out the laryngoscope handle, a number 3 MacIntosh curved blade, 10 mL syringe, two 8.0 mm ET tubes, and a packet of lubricant jelly. He went through the usual preintubation checks while I went back "live" on the med-net. Everyone in scanner land waited with baited breath for me to continue. Anyone with a scanner could listen in to every word we said, so one had to constantly be vigilant to not let slip vulgar language or patient identity, violating the sacred HIPPA scrolls.

"Memorial, Medi-Flight 1 continuing. Vital signs on scene were a GCS [Glasgow coma score] of 14, weak pulse at 140, respirations 36 and labored, and delayed capillary refill. Vital signs as of five ago..." I glanced over my right shoulder at the Propaq monitor screen to check his vitals that I preset to auto every two minutes. "Pulse 175, we've lost peripheral pulses and I can't palpate a right femoral pulse. BP is 56/40, pulse oximetry on fifteen liters per NRBM is only 85%. His respiratory rate was in the forties, but he's getting brady on us now, and I believe we're going to have to emergently intubate. His GCS has deteriorated dramatically in the past few minutes. Our patient is in full C-spine precautions, O2 at fifteen liters per non-rebreather mask, we have two large-bore IVs established on pressure bags with 1,500 mL infused thus far. His right leg is splinted with good distal CMS. We will need additional help on the helipad to transport his left extremity. ETA ten minutes for a hot off-load. Any questions or orders?"

"Medi-Flight 1, Memorial Hospital MICN Williams. I copy your report of a hypotensive major trauma victim from a motorcycle versus auto. Copy vitals and treatment. Let us know of any changes if you have time. If not, we will see you in ten. A level I trauma alert has been activated, and the surgeon is awaiting your arrival in trauma 2."

Back to work. My gut was right. Before I had completed my radio transmission, Robert had gone apneic and Adam was already inserting the 3 Mac curved blade into Robert's hypopharynx. Out of habit, I took the 8.0 mm ET tube, inflated 10 mL of air into the cuff to check for air leak, applied lubricant to the tip, and handed it to Adam. He visualized the vocal cords and inserted the tube effortlessly into his now flaccid airway, while I had our Yankauer suction poised for secretion control. Stylet removed, I inflated the cuff to secure the trachea from passive aspiration of fluid and secretions while Adam secured the tube to his face with an adhesive ET tube holder at 24 cm at the lip. Meanwhile, I hastily applied an end tidal CO_2 monitor (ETCO2) to check for exhaled carbon dioxide.

The next critical step was the daunting task of auscultating for breath sounds with two Lycoming 800 HP turbine engines screaming four feet above our heads. I removed my flight helmet, placed the stethoscope in my ears, and listened over the abdomen while Adam breathed for the patient with an ambu-bag attached to the ET tube and hooked up to 100% oxygen. No air sounds over the abdomen—good. Next, I listened over both lung fields and heard what I had heard on scene. Nearly symmetrical chest rise, lung sounds decreased over the right lung. After six breaths with the ETCO2 sensor attached, if the ET tube is in the trachea, the colorimetric sensor will turn from purple to yellow indicating proper placement. No color change, i.e. remaining purple, indicates tube placement in the esophagus, a potentially fatal error and sentinel event. It usually also means you're going to get puked on posthaste!

Adam nailed it on the first attempt. Flight crew intubation and standardized procedures we performed were unmatched by any other professionals I have worked with in my whole career. We trained like Special Forces and performed specialized maneuvers under the most inauspicious circumstances imaginable, with no backup. Compare that to the "controlled" situation of most ER procedures conducted with bright lights, easy patient accessibility, lots of extra hands, and a host of backup specialists, and one can imagine how tough our jobs really were.

Airway now secured and Robert's ventilations assisted by Adam, I reassessed him, listened to breath sounds again, and checked IVs and vitals. I grabbed two more liters of NS and replaced the nearly empty IV bags with fresh ones. What he really needed was blood, something we didn't routinely carry on every scene flight. So we infused an isotonic volume expander while simultaneously hemodiluting his remaining blood that was leaking from many unplugged holes. Despite our best efforts, things were SNAFU with my FUBAR patient. His condition continued to decline; vitals were in the tank. *What else is left to do?* I asked myself.

Sometimes you just have to go with your gut. We had been positive-pressure ventilating our patient with a major chest injury. Forcing air into a lung with a hole allows inspired air to enter the pleural space between the visceral and parietal pleura, increasing intrapleural pressure. Trapped air fills this invaginated pleural space with air that compresses the injured lung and, left untreated, will continue to compress the heart, the major vessels of the mediastinum, and the other unaffected lung.

With positive-pressure ventilation, this process can occur within minutes causing cardiovascular collapse, hypotension, tachycardia, hypoxemia, shortness of breath, chest pain, and death. Since our patient already had all the above symptoms *before* we intubated him, logic follows that the likelihood of him developing a tension pneumothorax was high.

John Wayne once opined, "A man's gotta do what a man's gotta do." With nothing to lose and everything to gain, I glanced over at Adam and he looked back and just nodded. Something is to be said for working repeatedly with the same crew, no matter what profession one works in; we worked together as one, mostly communicating with just a look because we knew what the other was thinking without speaking aloud.

Our flight suits had more pockets than we could fill with necessities. On both thighs were Velcro closure slots to accommodate IV needles. I kept two 10-gauge by three-inch-long IV catheters (that's huge!) for emergent needle thoracostomies rather than scrounging through the airway bag for one while my patient was gasping for breath. Since Robert's chest was already bare (clip, strip, and flip; all clothes come off in major trauma patients!), all that was needed preinsertion was a quick skin prep. Next, I removed the needle holder, located the second and third ribs, and quickly stuck the 10-gauge needle perpendicular to the chest wall, guiding the needle over the superior margin of the third rib in the second intercostal space at the midclavicular line. Once I felt the "give" as the needle entered the pleural space, I continued to advance the catheter over the needle while listening for air to exit the needle hub. Now the air trapped in the pleural space compressing on his right lung had a means of escape, albeit a temporary measure. He would get a chest tube as soon as we landed.

Unfortunately, Mr. Henderson's condition remained critical, but at least he was not deteriorating further.

"Can you fly this bird any faster?" I jokingly asked Geoff.

"Why, you knucklehead! If you throw Adam's fat ass out the door, we could gain five knots." We were all part of the 199'er club, but Adam weighed 270 pounds before working on Medi-Flight. Every three months we were required to weigh in with full flight gear (sans helmet and jacket) at less than 200 pounds. Most of the male crew members were around six feet tall and not spring chickens, so each employed whatever drastic measures it required to make weight. A few days of fasting, fluid restriction, laxatives, diuretics, or saunas before weigh-in, we all seemed to just make it until the next quarter. Hence, we were 199 lb. or less at least four days out of the year!

We were three minutes out from landing. I sure didn't want to be doing chest compressions when we landed. "Just hang in there, Robert!" We had just enough time to get off one more radio update to Memorial before landing, so they were aware of the emergent intubation and needle thoracostomy procedures we had already completed.

"Flight Com, Medi-Flight 1 has landed!" I moaned, exhausted and relieved. Dispatch knew we had landed since a huge picture window looked right out on to the helipad. The transport crew waited anxiously behind the plexiglass blast shield until we were "skids down" for safety reasons and because the rotor wash generated 50 mph winds on landings and takeoffs.

Critically ill and injured patients are almost always off-loaded "hot," meaning with the engines running and rotors spinning. It is inherently more dangerous than a "cold" off-load, but it takes two to three minutes for the pilot to cool down both turbine engines before shutting them down, then slowing the rotors with a hand-controlled rotor brake. That three-minute delay can mean life or death when time is measured in seconds for these patients. Further, no one who had not gone through our helipad safety training program was allowed to proceed or near the aircraft while the blades were moving.

As soon as our pilot gave them the okay signal, they scurried over to the left side of the aircraft and assisted Adam in transferring our patient onto the ER gurney. Then they quickly whisked him away, all the while keeping their heads lowered while under the spinning rotors. That being done, an inexperienced young ER nurse came over to the right-side door, and I passed the forty-pound leg into his waiting arms. I could see the nurse change color when he took custody of the limb, but he persevered and made it all the way to the ER. It was my privilege to hire Balvir as a flight nurse years later.

The course from the helicopter to the ER was long, circuitous, and offered little in the way of patient privacy. We had to traverse about 150 feet of outdoor sidewalk and then enter the hospital from the rear, then proceed down a long corridor another 150 feet that opened into the hospital's main hallway access for patient, staff, visitors, family, etc. for about 50 feet until we finally reached the back doors of the ER. Once inside, it was maybe 50 feet down the hall to the trauma rooms. Oftentimes, when visitors were fortunate or unfortunate enough to be in the hallway when we brought a trauma patient down the hallway, leaving a blood path in our wake, they would have some pretty vivid stories to tell when they got home.

As soon as I passed the left leg off, I sprinted with what reserve energy I could muster to the ER to catch up with my patient so I could give a complete report to the trauma team. I caught them in the main hallway; security had done a good job this time of keeping gawkers from getting too close. By now I was overheated and dehydrated, and my flight suit was so wet it appeared like I had just climbed out of a swimming pool filled with tomato juice!

The trauma room is a sacred place. Despite the appearance of chaos, at least it is organized chaos. Every player has his or her role to play and a particular place to stand when the patient arrived. The ER doctor and/or trauma surgeon stand at the head with the respiratory therapist(s) for overall command and airway control. Two trauma nurses, one stationed on each side of the patient: one places monitoring equipment on the patient and gets initial vitals, while another one starts or manages IVs and facilitates phlebotomy for blood sampling. Next, one places a nasogastric tube through either the nose or mouth depending on injuries, while the other places a Foley catheter into the urethra attached to a thermometer probe to monitor the patient's core temperature. Lab and radiology stand nearby to handle the blood specimens and shoot quick portable x-rays. The pharmacist stands in a corner with emergency drugs for rapid accessibility and to act as a resource. Our patient representatives, mostly specially trained nurses, are responsible for greeting the families when they arrive and keep them informed during the resuscitation. Then there are social services, pastoral care, and the specialty physicians—orthopedics, neurosurgery, and anesthesia.

Don't forget the trauma case manager (one of my moonlight jobs) who is attached at the hip, so to speak (well, not with this patient) from the time the patient arrives on hospital property and escorts the patient to procedures (x-ray, CT), surgery, recovery, ICU, rehab, and finally discharge. They are the patient advocate and know more about the patient than anyone. Finally there is the trauma program manager who oversees the hospital's trauma program. Trish Carlson was our TPM and was strict in her management approach, but she was very approachable and fair in dealing with issues. It was because of her staunch dedication that we had such a great trauma program at Memorial during these times.

Again, our hospital trauma program motto was "Trauma takes teamwork," and we truly worked as a team, from the doctors to the housekeepers. We all recognized each individual's importance and that without one, the others could not function to their full capabilities. With all the players in one trauma room, if you weren't invited, it was best to stay home. The rooms had colored tape that mapped out territories; where the trauma gurney was placed for optimal patient access and the two-inch red tape that defined the limits of uninvited guests. If one dared cross the red tape when Ms. Carlson was watching, that person was quickly confronted and politely escorted out.

When Robert, the transport team, and I arrived in the trauma room, one could hear a pin drop; it was so silent. There were no raised voices, lest it became a shouting match that led to confusion and greater risk of errors. The first thirty seconds I rattled off my quick patient report using the MIVT acronym: mechanism-injuries-vitals-treatment. From there the trauma surgeon Dr. Morgan performed his rapid trauma exam while simultaneously calling out his findings for the ER tech/scribe in the corner (oh, I forgot about her!) and ordering trauma panel tests that were already in progress. Everyone did their assigned tasks with very little talking; communication was mostly nonverbal via visual cues and nods of acknowledgment.

Admissions had registered our trauma patient by utilizing our prepackaged alphanumeric trauma packets since history had demonstrated we treated a lot of John and Jane Does with unknown identities sometimes for days on end. Robert's "Bravo Six" designator would follow him all the way through the admission through discharge process. As soon as information was forwarded from the CHP and EMS agencies, Bravo Six then became Robert Henderson. Our patient representative Mike was on the phone contacting family members the minute he received that information.

After the portable x-rays of the chest-abdomen-pelvis were completed, the trauma surgeon placed a 40F throracostomy tube (chest tube) between the fourth and fifth right ribs at the midaxillary line. The nurse standing next to him on the patient's right side was quickly greeted by a gush of blood all down her barrier gown and running onto her shoes and socks; the surgeon forgot to place tube clamps on the distal open end of the chest tube. ER rule number 12: don't wear $400 hiking shoes to work unless you like red shoes. The nurse barely flinched, shook her leg like my dog when she shakes after a bath, then proceeded to hang the fifth and sixth bag of uncrossmatched O-negative blood through the blood warmer without saying a word. Meanwhile, trauma nurse two hung a 2 g IV piggyback of the cephalosporin antibiotic Ancef and gave a tetanus shot in his left deltoid muscle while handling a call from the lab, giving critical values on Bravo Six's blood test results. We were only at T + 10 minutes into the trauma resuscitation.

I wanted to stick around and help, but my first priority was to get cleaned up, hydrated, and prepared for the next flight. A quick stop at the Ivy for two giant glasses of iced water, and I was on my way to help Adam clean up.

Geoff had us refueled and plugged back in to the APU. Adam had pulled out the gurney mount from the floor and was hosing blood out of the patient compartment with a garden hose. Since we both worked with bloody gloves for over fifteen minutes during the flight, everything we touched was bloodstained, so we had to do a thorough decon wipe-down with soap and water followed by 10% bleach solution. Then off to our supply room storage to restock all the supplies we had used. This particular bloody flight took nearly an hour to sanitize the helicopter before it was again mission-ready. Fortunately, we had two helicopters staffed.

No job is complete until the paperwork is done, and our computerized charting software interfaced with the dispatch module, so times, location, etc. logged during the flight interfaced well and transferred over to the patient's chart. Ditto for all our vital signs documented on the Propaq monitor. The bulk of the chart was patient information, most of which I kept in my head or from the scribbles on the strip of three-inch tape we stuck on the front of our pants leg just above the knee. When one sits, it's easy to write data bits on your lap; it just looks upside down when you walk. The software churns out a five- to eight-page detailed document of everything that occurred from patient contact until arrival in the ER.

Now rehydrated and in a clean, dry flight suit, I decided to postpone paperwork and check up on Mr. Henderson. Taking the long walk to the ER in the oppressive heat quickly sapped my remaining strength. As I entered the main hallway, visitors and staff walked in small groups talking quietly. I nodded with a grim look and said hi to a large family with equally grim and careworn expressions sitting quietly on a couch with two older adults, a younger pregnant woman, and five young children.

As I walked down the ER hallway, I suddenly became sick to my stomach; I knew the inevitable had already occurred. There was a dark, silent pall that my sixth sense detected the moment I drew my first breath. I was too late. We were all too late. Mr. Robert Henderson, proud German Baptist, father of five children, husband of Carla, and son of Hubert and Irene, had died from his injuries.

It took several years of experiencing death, tragedy, and mayhem every day at work before I could accept the death of those I could not save and praise God for those I could save. Often, despite heroic measures and everything happening timely and correctly, people will die. Some are as clear and vivid as if it happened yesterday; others cloudier, but none forgotten. Kids' tragic deaths have always affected me horribly; fortunately, the emotional breakdown has always occurred after the event. I'm still the consummate professional while working; I just need my time to cry later. Some patients like Mr. Henderson break my heart.

Since I've discussed emotional breakdown and crying often in my accounts, it seems appropriate to interject here and to explain this powerful feeling in clearer perspective. As a child growing up in the '50s, social mores portrayed the male as the defender, the strong, silent type, emotionally detached and incapable of crying. From a very young age, I was raised being told, "Boys don't cry!" So, no one ever saw me cry. Obviously, I had received bad counsel. But there was a high price to be paid for holding in my tears for decades. It was not until I was thirty-six years old before the dam broke loose.

I was in attendance at a CISD (critical incident stress debriefing) after caring for a two-year-old child who was fatally injured when a relative accidentally backed over him with a car in their driveway in Bass Lake when I worked for Sierra Ambulance. He was the same age as my son Forrest. There was a circle of about twenty EMS peers sitting in the room contributing their thoughts and feelings regarding the tragedy.

When it came time for me to replay the incident from my perspective, I broke down in an audacious display with a long tearful refrain in full view for all to see. It was the first time anyone had seen me cry. And I did not feel self-conscious, foolish, or embarrassed as I thought I would all those years. Instead, I felt *free!* The release of years of pent-up feelings sent a flood of near-orgasmic warmth and a sense of pleasant calm washed over me. I soon discovered that crying was not a weakness as I had been taught, but rather a sign of strength and a tremendous emotional release of unexpressed negative energy. Crying has since become a powerful ally allowing me to more easily maintain homeostasis after times of extreme emotional crisis.

While Adam and I were outside cleaning 84MH, efforts in the trauma resuscitation were proving futile. Not long after I left, ten minutes into the resuscitation, Mr. Henderson continued to deteriorate. He had only a few milliliters of urine in the urinometer and 500 mL of blood collected in the PleuroVac drainage system from his right chest tube. Blood was oozing from his IV sites, ET tube, nose, everywhere. Disseminated intravascular coagulation (DIC) had already started, a horrible cascade of blood clot formation and bleeding, and often fatal sequelae of multisystems trauma (MST). The lab was shuttling bags of O-negative packed red blood cells and fresh frozen plasma (FFP) like a manic UPS delivery man on meth, and the nurses were pouring them in just as fast.

At T + 14 minutes into the resuscitation, just as the trauma surgeon and trauma case manager were preparing to head toward surgery, Robert's pulse began slowing precipitously, until the monitor showed a wide complex QRS ideoventricular rhythm that deteriorated to asystole—flat line. Game over. Not even enough time to go to the OR and patch up the internal leak(s). Robert Henderson did not survive past the trauma room in the ER!

It was my sincerest hope that Robert would have been able to deliver his death bed affirmation to his wife personally. Unfortunately, that burden now fell on my weary shoulders. It clicked now in my head, the family I sensitively acknowledged in the main hallway were Hubert, Irene, Carla, Toby, Isaac, Sara, Michael, Eli, and Young Mr. Abraham in utero, due to make his grand appearance in only two weeks' time.

Every year at the annual Medi-Flight Christmas Party, we presented gag awards to each other for some rare quirk or accomplishment, whatever. My "harem" of beautiful flight nurses (men and women!) gave me an engraved plaque for being Mr. Androgynous. "To Ron Martin—the Nurse Most In Touch with His Feminine Side." I was once a male trapped inside a woman's body; then I was born. It still hangs proudly in my home to this day. Today, I really needed that incentive to get me through the next hours. It has never been my strong suit to speak with families of the deceased directly following sudden death; however, that task falls in the nurse's lap quite often, and this time I felt I had a promise and an obligation to fulfill.

The Hendersons had not left the private nook with the couches where I last saw them. They were all impeccably dressed in their conservative traditional religious attire, and the children all very well behaved. I walked over and introduced myself, explained what my role in this tragic event was, and told them they could ask me anything and I would answer their questions. They all stood, and Carla walked up to me first and hugged me while the miracle in the belly of Mrs. Henderson, Young Mr. Abraham, and mine shared a magical mystical connection. Toby stood by his mom, placed one hand on his mom's waist, and hugged my leg with the other. This was not the birthday surprise Toby had expected today. Tears flowed like it was monsoon season in Southeast Asia. We all needed that! More hugs and stories were shared, and I was welcomed into the fold, at least temporarily, of this wonderful, loving family who just lost their father/husband/son.

We spoke for over an hour, and I answered all their questions truthfully, being brutally honest. They appreciated that I did not sugarcoat something that was not. Despite my somewhat macabre desire to attend funerals of those who have died, I gave that up long ago. Too many attempts ended up with me losing it standing in the waiting line and then leaving early. I mourn their souls, and their screams still haunt me in the darkest chasms of my mind, awakening me suddenly on random nights.

It was now 1700, two hours until my shift ended. It was time to complete the patient's chart before I could call it a night and go home. Hungry. Tired. Angry. Frustrated. Sad. There were so many emotions to deal with and sort out. And still one more of the hundreds of senseless drunk-driving fatalities I've experienced for me to try and process. One act of poor judgment set in motion a cascade of horrific events that immediately affected the lives of hundreds. Ten minutes after I bid the Henderson family goodbye, we got a call from dispatch to respond to a three-car accident with two reported fatalities and four criticals in southern Merced County forty-eight miles away. A multicasualty incident, or MCI, was called and multiple air ambulances were responding. I missed lunch and had not eaten dinner yet. It was going to be another eighteen-hour shift.

At least I had an empty bladder. *Semper fi!*

CHAPTER 10

Gang Rape

A man who can keep a secret may be wise, but he is not half as wise as one who has no secrets to keep.

—Edgar Winton Howe

Saturday, August 20, 1993

As if I couldn't get my fill working full-time as chief flight nurse for Medi-Flight and per diem as trauma case manager as well as helping teach BLS and ACLS at Memorial Hospital with the esteemed educator extraordinaire Elaine Paradis, RN, I moonlighted most weekends at St. Dominic's Hospital in Manteca about twenty miles northwest of Modesto. I worked night shift in the ER from 2300 to 0700. The doctors were mellow, and at night it was usually not terribly busy since it was a new hospital in a small yet flourishing bedroom community for Bay Area commuters.

The hospital is situated on the western fringes of town just off Highway 120. The ER is rightfully situated near the front of the hospital, and there is an adjoining long hallway that connects to the inpatient beds. There is always one ER doc, one RN, and one patient registration clerk staffed in the ER, so the nurse is tasked with doing everything from triage to discharge or admission. When it is busy, the nurse gets his ass kicked.

This particular Saturday was an exception to that rule. It was calm and the department was empty at 0400 but for the staff: Louise

(Weezy) was seated up front in registration, and Dr. Baldy was sleeping in the adjacent doctor's lounge, while I sat in a chair at the nurses' station trying to stay awake.

Just a little past 4:00 a.m., I heard Weezy talking to someone, but something didn't sound right. The pitch of her voice was higher with a large dose of fear mixed in. I stood, stretched, and rounded the corner to the registration desk and saw Weezy shaking and her skin white as newly fallen snow. Meet Sam Montalvo!

As soon as I appeared, twenty-eight-year-old Sam Montalvo, well-known by the local LEOs as a known meth dealer and local slime ball that I didn't know before this inauspicious moment, easily jumped over the low registration counter after stupidly pumping the gun, ejecting an unspent round on the waiting room floor, just like all the idiots do on TV for dramatic effect. He immediately pushed the barrel of the pump-action 12-gauge shotgun he was toting into my sternum. Doom on Ronnie!

Static squealed and scratched in my head as someone turned the dial on the AM transistor radio and finally tuned into KWTF. Since it was night shift, the graveyard DJ must have put on an eight-hour tape and vacated the station property. The tape stuck on one particular track, and it repeated over and over in my head.

> *Well, come one all of you, big strong men,*
> *Uncle Sam needs your help again.*
> *He's got himself in a terrible jam*
> *Way down yonder in Viet Nam*
> *So put down your books and pick up a gun,*
> *We're gonna have a whole lotta fun.*

Sam was aptly dressed for a meth-headed tweaker in the summertime. One pair of grease-stained, stinky, filthy blue jeans, no shirt, no shoes, no socks, and one loaded 12-gauge shotgun with a pocketful of shells. His sweaty, unctuous skin was rancid, his hair unwashed and uncombed for God knows how long, his eyes sunken, wide, dilated, and wild like Charles Manson's. He looked just like a psychotic on a four-day meth binge who was having paranoid delusions. Doh, no shit, he *was* a crazy psychotic son-of-a-bitch tweaker on a four-day meth binge who was having paranoid delusions. For a brief minute, I tried all my de-escalation measures to try and calm him, drop his gun, and accept my offer of surrender and psychological assistance.

Didn't work for a second! He was way beyond the outer limits at this point, and no reasoning techniques were going to be effective. His paranoia was his undoing.

"What's in your pack?" he asked.

> *And it's one, two, three,*
> *What are we fighting for?*
> *Don't ask me I don't give a damn,*
> *Next stop is Viet Nam.*
> *And it's five, six, seven,*
> *Open up the Pearly Gates,*
> *Well, there ain't no time to wonder why,*
> *Whoopee! We're all gonna die.*

"Just alcohol preps, scissors, gloves, stuff," I retorted as my blood began to boil. Nothing angers me more than someone pointing a gun at me, and this was not the first time!

"Let me look!" Sam took his right hand off the trigger, much to my relief, and began to grab at my fanny pack located on my front waist, gun barrel pressed firmly into my sternum. As soon as his finger left the trigger, I grabbed the muzzle of the shotgun and pushed it away from my chest. Louise was still standing next to me, looking stunned at the two of us. I told her to get out of there and run to the back and call 911. I didn't have to ask twice. She disappeared quicker than Hillary's acid-washed email servers, leaving Sam and me locked eye to eye.

"Let go of the gun!" I yelled, now more confident and really pissed, both of my hands gripping the shotgun. Negotiations were now officially over.

"I'm gonna kill you, asshole!" Now there's something I haven't heard spouting from a CMF (crazy motherfucker) in the ER before! Not!

Sam got off one good blow with the butt of the shotgun, striking me right in the stones. Normally, that pain would have caused me to drop and writhe on the floor like a worm on hot asphalt, but not tonight. My blood was aboil, and rage coursed through my veins like the madman standing opposite me.

> *Well, come on, generals, let's move fast;*
> *Your big chance has come at last.*
> *Now you can go out and get those reds*
> *'Cause the only good commie is the one that's dead*
> *Any you know that peace can only be won*
> *When we've blown 'em all to kingdom come.*

The struggle for the gun escalated, but at least I had managed to get the only other potential victim to safety, and I was not going to let go of the barrel. Finally, Sam managed to get his finger on the trigger during our struggle, and the shotgun went off at the nurses' station, missing me by mere inches, blowing tile off the floor, knocking a giant hole in the wall, and continuing on to penetrate the stainless steel blanket warmer on the other side of the wall.

At this critical juncture, I wrestled the gun from his hands and he ran for the (locked after 2300 hours) sliding ambulance entrance doors. He hit them at full stride, knocking them outward off their tracks. I was tempted to rack another shell in the chamber and reciprocate his kindness, but thought better of it, initially. Meanwhile, Louise had called 911, only to get hung up on. The repeat call to 911 brought the cavalry. Not much was happening at 4:00 a.m. in Manteca, so Manteca PD showed up along with the sheriff's canine unit just as I was pursuing my attacker, shotgun in hand, out the ambulance entrance. Where was hospital security? you ask. Good question.

Come on, mothers throughout the land
Pack your boys off to Viet Nam
Come on, fathers, and don't hesitate
To send your sons off before it's too late.
Any you be the first one on your block
To have your boy come home in a box

As soon as I saw the LEOs (law enforcement officers) pull up, I did the wise and prudent thing and placed the shotgun on the ground and began pointing toward the perp. No sooner had I done that, the sheriff opened his left passenger door and let Rin Tin Tin, a black Belgian Malinois, out to stretch his legs and have a late-night snack after giving him a silent voice command.

Ten seconds and twenty long strides later, Sam was in dog custody, and his legs became a milk bone treat for Mr. Tin Tin. He continued to gnaw on his leg until the deputy reluctantly gave the command to let go. I would have invited him to have seconds. Sam looked like Old Yeller of old, growling and frothing at the mouth like a rabid animal.

MPD took Sam into custody, cuffed him, and dragged his skanky ass off to jail. The deputy came inside, collected evidence (shotgun, spent shells, damaged property, etc.), and took my statement. I had to wake the doctor up, check myself in as an ER patient, take my own vitals, and then have the doc fondle the family jewels to ensure the boys were intact. I spent the rest of the shift with an ice pack stuffed in my pants to ease the swelling, just like some of the unconscious heroin ODs I'd encountered over the years who were dropped off in the ambulance entrance. As if the ice pack would restart their opiate-induced apnea when they stopped breathing!

Besides the LEOs statement, I had to complete a hospital incident report form, notify hospital security and then hospital administration. Our sole security guard, armed only with his wit, white shirt, blue tie, and impressive good looks, was far away in the inpatient tower with all the hospital employees except me, Louise, and Dr. Baldy in the ER. My ER doctor was totally unaware a shooting had occurred minutes before only twenty feet from his bed until I called and awakened him. Hospital administration did not show up; however, they immediately initiated their great spin and cover-up procedures. They instructed me not to speak to anyone from the press.

Suddenly, I was transported back in time, and KWTF came blaring in both ears in full stereophonic sound. I had just arrived in Sydney, Australia, for seven blissful days of R&R in December 1968. The well-meaning but clueless senior NCOs were presenting a "safety briefing" for GIs to obey while they were in Sydney. We had all just been in a combat zone twenty-four hours before, and they were giving a safety briefing for Sydney, Australia! As they began citing all the pubs, discos, and clubs to avoid due to their support of the antiwar movement, several of us were quickly jotting down the names and addresses for further reference.

> *And it's one, two, three,*
> *What are we fighting for?*
> *Don't ask me, I don't give a damn,*
> *Next stop is Viet Nam*
> *And it's five, six, seven,*
> *Open up the pearly gates,*
> *Well, there ain't no time to wonder why,*
> *Whoopee! We're all gonna die.*

So, I called the local newspapers and news stations, gave an interview, and basically erased as much spin as I could. In the meantime, administration had awakened several maintenance workers, and within the hour they were busy desecrating and destroying the crime scene, replacing new floor tiles, repairing the holes in the sheetrock, painting over the gaping wall holes, and sanitizing the entire crime scene before 0700 shift change. It was beyond belief that they failed to acknowledge a near-fatal event had occurred in the hospital to one of their own staff. I even had to complete my shift from the 0400 time of assault to 0700, caring for patients with an ice pack stuffed in my crotch below my fanny pack. This was to be the last shift I would work there for several months.

When I got off work that morning, I related the ordeal to Karen and our children. I told them I needed some man time alone to contemplate this brush with death. There was lots of PTO (paid time off) in my vacation bank, so I got coverage for my Medi-Flight shifts, packed my backpack, and the next day I drove to Tuolumne Meadows in Yosemite National Park for an extended hike in the high country.

Mount Lyell, the tallest mountain peak in Yosemite, stands at 13,114 feet (4,000 m) at the southeast end of the Cathedral Range. From the Tuolumne Meadows Ranger Station, access to the John Muir Trail led me south up the Tuolumne River Canyon to the head of the Lyell Canyon, about nine miles of slowly ascending altitude as I meandered along the river's edge. From there, the climb became steeper as Donahue Pass loomed ahead in the distance. The trail to Mount Lyell turned south before traversing the pass. The last four miles were quite strenuous as the terrain turned to large boulders, scree, talus, and finally the approach over the Lyell Glacier, largest in Yosemite but shrinking and paling in comparison with those in other countries I've seen.

Upper base camp made for a longer first-day approach, but it also made the final ascent the next day that much closer. The upper campsite was above tree line, probably around 10,000 feet, so I had to hike quite a distance to find a tree where I eventually tied up my food and anything that gave off a scent, except me, to keep the bears from eating it. I had left sea-level Modesto earlier that morning, driven for several hours, and then hiked almost ten miles uphill at high altitude before the sun began to drift toward the horizon in the west. I had not seen one other human since the first few miles of trail, but flowers and wildlife abounded all around me. There was no firewood to gather for a fire, but my freeze-dried lasagna and veggies heated on the propane burner and some Nutty Butters for dessert was a meal fit for royalty.

My endogenous catecholamines were still surging, and despite total body fatigue, sleep evaded me. I stretched my dense foam pad over the hard, rocky ground, rolled out my down sleeping bag, crawled in, and engaged in serious stargazing until sleep finally overcame one very stressed-out nurse.

The next morning, I had a light breakfast, packed my daypack, and began the ascent of the Lyell Glacier. In the summer months, the glacier takes on the appearance of a giant egg carton, with wide, deep cups cut out in the ice by the sun's glare. It made for slow going, and I felt relieved to finally cross the bergschrund, or crevasse, at the top of the glacier and finally stand on solid rock again. I followed the northwest approach that nears the saddle between another giant, Mount McClure, and then scrambled up the huge chunks of rock on a leisurely class 3 ascent to the summit, 13,114 feet ASL. Somewhere up here, I needed to find answers.

Most mountains in the US have a US Coast and Geodetic Survey marker embedded at the summits, and Mount Lyell was no exception. There next to the marker was a heavy metal box with a crude latch cover, and inside it was the also crude and crumpled ledger where successful ascenders entered their names and whatever thoughts the experience evoked. I remember signing the ledger but have no memory of what I wrote. However, this experience began my practice of keeping a daily journal to document, document, document. It must have been the nurses training coming out in me, I guess.

The day was perfect for sitting on top of a 13,000-foot mountain; just a few gathering mountain cumulus clouds, 80 degrees, 5 mph winds. I took a self-portrait of myself with a smug look on my face, and then spent several hours just sitting, looking out in all directions on top of the world, and meditating on the events of the past few days. Something positive must come from this shitstorm.

After three days of solitude, contemplation, meditation, and freeze-dried food, I was ready for a hot tub and a margarita and my beautiful wife wrapped around my waist. The descent from upper base camp was initially grueling on my knees going down the steep rock, but the return trip was pleasant and relaxing, and I took several rest stops along the river's edge just to watch the butterflies flit about and the bees work their magic pollinating the wildflowers in the meadow. The route roundtrip to the summit of Mount Lyell and back is 26 miles (40 km) and 4,500 vertical feet (1,400 m). I had logged another 5–7 miles hiking the summit twice and a quick jaunt west across the saddle to Mount McClure (12,900 feet).

Now back in the car and on the way back home, I felt refreshed and had a plan of action, but there was still a lot that needed to be done. I needed to talk to someone. The hospital offered the Employee Assistance Program (EAP) counseling that was free to all employees; however, this was a workers' compensation claim, so I was quite troubled when I received a billing statement after my first visit with the social worker. I met with social worker Bonnie Rabbit to discuss the shooting incident at St. Dominic's. She was kind, a good listener, and during our sessions, we established a connection to events that occurred to me in Viet Nam. She went on to say that she had been counseling several Viet Nam veterans and gave me a brochure on PTSD. That was the *first time* I had ever heard of PTSD; I'd been back from the Nam for almost twenty-five years and had experienced symptoms I had no clear explanation for, and now for the first time in my life, I knew I wasn't alone!

Unfortunately, I did not pursue my PTSD issues with Ms. Rabbit and ended the counseling sessions after a few weeks. Maybe I was afraid to let anybody get that close, afraid they wouldn't like me after they'd heard what I had done. I wasn't ready to share those nightmares yet. Besides, I still had the big showdown in the courtroom coming up.

One thing I knew for sure. I was not going back to work at St. Dominic's until they enhanced safety measures in the ER, and I had several suggestions. There were virtually no safety devices in place. I suggested (more like demanded!) to administration the following: (1) Install an impenetrable barrier between patient waiting room and registration; (2) install solid core locked door between waiting room and ER; (3) install "panic buttons" under counter areas of registration and ER nursing station with direct notification to local law enforcement; and (4) provide more hospital security. When these measures were implemented, I would consider coming back to work.

The hospital called a few weeks later and said the barrier was in place and the locked door was installed. I drove over to inspect their work. The registration desk was about thirty inches tall; then it was open to the eight-foot ceiling above. Maintenance had installed a single one-fourth-inch-thick piece of plexiglass approximately four feet high and six feet long into the opening and secured it with a few clips anchored into sheetrock with molly bolts. The only security it provided was from coughing patients. When I touched it, the plexiglass shuddered and rattled, very insecurely. One good push, and it would have pulled from its flimsy attachments. Sorry, call me again when you fix this! I stormed out, angry at how this quick fix was supposed to placate me. My next phone call would be awhile.

The long-awaited court date had finally come. This was all a new experience for me, as I have not accustomed myself to the inside of many courtrooms. I prefer to view them from a distance while watching *Perry Mason* reruns. I received a call from the prosecuting attorney the day before the trial and met with her the morning of the trial to discuss strategy. It sounded like I was going to get to testify and have my day in court. I could have never been more wrong.

The judge called the case before the court, Mr. Sam Montalvo was ushered into the courtroom from the jail entrance adorned in orange jumpsuit and arm and leg shackles. The four felony and other misdemeanor counts against him were read aloud: attempted murder, assault with a deadly weapon, felon in possession of a firearm, under the influence of illegal drugs, drug trafficking, possession of illegal drugs for sale, resisting arrest, and destruction of property. There was some shuffling of papers; then the judge called both attorneys to the bench. They spoke privately for a few minutes before the judge announced the three of them were going to retire to his chambers for private discussion.

They were gone for maybe ten minutes. When everyone had returned and settled into their chairs, the judge announced that he and the attorneys had reached a settlement while behind closed doors. Mr. Montalvo was to be released from jail today with time served, plead to three misdemeanor counts, do two hundred hours of public service, and attend counseling for his drug problem. Gavel down, court dismissed. Just like that, he was free to pick up where he left off. No testimony on my part, only betrayal and a gang rape from the criminal justice system whose job it is to prosecute and incarcerate guilty assholes, not let them walk free. For what it's worth, Mr. Montalvo's parents approached me after the trial outside the courthouse and apologized for their son's dastardly behavior.

The hospital's cover-up of the whole incident, lack of support during my ordeal, sending me medical bills for a workers' compensation claim, then the coup de grâce by the judicial system, it was all just too much to assimilate. Something needed to be done.

It was not until several weeks later that I returned to work, but it never was the same there, despite the renovations they reluctantly installed for employee safety. Since the statute of limitations had to have expired if there ever was a statute of limitations for what I did, I can freely state it now. Not feeling safe returning to work alone at night in a desolate ER and knowing Sam lived a half mile west of the hospital, I fulfilled Mr. Montalvo's earlier paranoid delusions of me carrying a gun in my fanny pack. Until I quit several months after the incident, every shift I worked there I carried my loaded concealed .380-caliber semiautomatic pistol right above my boy toy in the fanny pack around my waist along with my scissors, gloves, and alcohol preps.

Months after the incident, hospital CEO Richard "The Obsequious" called me into his office after hours for a private chat. After he closed the door behind us, he spoke of the "bravery and sacrifice" I had made to the hospital and presented me with a plaque from the board of trustees of St. Dominic's hospital that now resides in my garage workshop. It read as follows:

Meritorious Service
For
RON MARTIN, RN

WHEREAS, an individual suspected to be on drugs entered St. Dominic's Hospital at 4:00 AM on August 20, 1993 bearing a loaded shotgun, and
WHEREAS, said individual entered the Emergency Room by crawling over a counter and intimidating the clerk and nurse in a threatening manner, and

*WHEREAS, this individual could have cre-
ated great harm, and*

*WHEREAS, the R.N., at great personal risk,
reacted immediately to restrain and disarm the individual; the clerk assisted and alerted the authori-
ties, thereby preventing the individual from further
harming staff, patients, visitors, and*

*WHEREAS, because of his courage and quick
actions Ron Martin, R.N. protected and ensured
the health and safety of all present at St. Dominic's
Hospital during this crisis,*

*NOW THEREFORE BE IT RESOLVED,
that We the Board of Trustees of St. Dominic's
Hospital bestow our thanks and honor on Ron
Martin, R.N. for showing such courage and quick
thinking during these moments of extreme crisis and
high risk, and commend him for meritorious service,*

*Resolved and approved this 20th day of August
in the year of our Lord 1993.*

This was a well-meaning but poorly timed validation of my
actions, and if one would ask almost any employee who worked
there during that time, most would not even know the shooting ever
occurred. Hospital spin, Doctors! Over the months, I had done my
homework and research. I was ready to strike back.

The St. Dominic's shooting incident was a distant but still clear
memory, and it was time to make lemonade from the lemons piling
up in my inbox. Hospitals are strictly regulated by federal, state, and
local regulations as well as the major accrediting agency, JCAHO, the
Joint Commission on Accreditation of Hospital Organizations, now
ambiguously renamed for political correctness reasons, I suppose,
TJC, the *Joint* Commission. Sounds like they should be regulating
cannabis, not hospitals!

Managers are frequently faced with disgruntled employees who
vent and lay their problems on their desk, wishing for a quick remedy
to their perceived problem. I have always been one who listens to

staff concerns, but then ask them, "Have you talked to the individual who is causing the problem?" or "Have you considered any alternate solutions to the problem?" That gives the employee an opportunity to go back and find the answer for themselves, making both of our jobs easier. It helps empower them.

I did not wait for the hospitals to increase staff security; I became the *voice* of hospital staff security! After months of research, I enlisted the support of the ER medical director and medical director of Medi-Flight, Dr. Terence Sweeney, and a wonderful ER nurse, Rita "The Incorrigible" Corrigan. This trio became the ad hoc Northern California hospital safety and security consultants, beginning with our own hospital. Most of the hospital security measures one takes for granted today were influenced in some small measure as a result of my contributions nearly twenty-five years ago. We were invited to several hospitals to perform on-site surveys and make suggestions for security improvements.

Some of the upgrades made at our hospital and surrounding hospitals included (1) installation of a comprehensive hospital-wide video security system; (2) concrete barriers installed outside the ambulance entrance doors to prevent cars from driving through; (3) locked ambulance entrance doors with key code entry access; (4) employee badge with individual barcode access and all major hospital egress doors locked with barcoded IDs allowed admittance; 5) metal detector at the entrance to the ER waiting room with security guard; (6) under-the-counter "panic buttons" to allow easy access for employees to summon LEOs in registration, ER, and treatment rooms; (7) barcoding of all hospital equipment to enhance inventory and prevent expensive equipment from "growing legs" and being stolen; (8) increased security presence with uniforms, badges, enhanced training, and physical deterrents; and (9) staff training on dealing with hospital violence. The list is not all-inclusive, but you get the message. Lemonade was running over the top of the pitcher.

I made a difference. I still believe rape is a crime against humanity and those convicted should receive the death penalty or incarceration for life. I had been symbolically raped by hospital administration and the criminal justice system, more aptly named the *criminal's* justice system, and yet had not even been physically penetrated. My consciousness cannot even begin to fathom the physical, emotional, and psychological trauma a person experiences with sexual abuse and rape; but I have experienced betrayal, abandonment, deception, and duplicity. Strange bedfellows for institutions of caring and healing. If only this were the last time, maybe I could still make it to the finish line.

> *Well, there ain't no time to wonder why,*
> *Whoopee! We're all gonna die.*

CHAPTER 11

Dream Catcher

When you wish upon a star
Makes no difference who you are
If your heart is in your dream
No request it too extreme
When you wish upon a star
Your dreams come true.

—Jiminy Cricket

1999–2002

Our lives and careers continued to grow and prosper working at Memorial Medical Center (MMC) for over ten years now. Karen and I both loved our jobs working in ICU and Medi-Flight, respectively. During this period, our two oldest children graduated from Yosemite High School and entered college and Forrest was just finishing up. In early 1999 I saw my doctor for progressively worsening physical symptoms that raised concern on my radar. The hunt for the cause began with standard blood screening panels to identify any outliers. That trail led to more specific testing and then a referral to a gastro-enterologist for further studies. After even more blood tests and a liver biopsy, it was determined with certainty that I had been playing host to another uninvited guest for decades.

The hepatitis C virus (HCV) genotype 1 had been running amok, taking up permanent residence in my liver and had been living and spreading unchecked inside me long enough to cause serious liver scarring and create undesirable symptoms. The incidental blood exposures during my tour of duty thirty years prior carried the highest probabilities for blood-borne contact. My liver enzymes were very high when I returned from overseas, and I was refused thrice as a blood donor. My penance for allowing this unwanted parasite's free access to my liver consisted of daily doses of the anemia-inducing oral antiviral ribavirin and the immunosuppressive antiviral drug alpha-interferon 2a administered subcutaneously by injection in the abdomen every other day; treatment was for fifty-two weeks. The drug treatment cost thousands of dollars each month, and the hospital employee health plan thankfully paid for all but the co-pay for monthly refills.

The nearly unbearable symptoms began not long after the first injection and continued unabated throughout therapy. Thirty pounds were shed in the first month; vomiting, anorexia, and intractable body pain. Depression and despair. After a few months on the drug regimen, my lab values revealed a hemoglobin drop from around 16 g/dL to 8 g/dL, clinically explaining and validating my increased fatigue, dizziness, shortness of breath, and persistent near syncope. Despite my weakening condition, I still continued to work but surrendered the chief flight nurse position due to my declining health and switched full-time positions with another flight nurse, Peggy Williams, who helped make a seamless transition.

It took every ounce of effort to perform the simplest of tasks during my pharmacologic nightmare. Complex tasks executed at high altitude with added stress and anemia was a potential liability I had to ponder. The fog of pain was more distracting while at work, and I withdrew into my own world, unsure of the next moment. Each interferon injection while at work created increased angst; experience had taught me that an hour after administration, the drug's side effects would launch its legions of nefarious side effects, only to diminish just before the next scheduled shot in forty-eight hours.

It was 1100, four long hours into our 0700–1900 shift. My paramedic partner today, Cindy Bowling, and the second duty crew had graciously let me sit out the ceremonial daily hot soapy bath

our helicopters received. I was content to sit in dispatch and provide backup for incoming 911 calls. The pilot and crew briefing had
occurred at 0900; no specific flight issues, but our aircraft, Medi-
Flight II, had a scheduled maintenance due this morning, so we were
out of service until further notice and the other crew moved up to
first on rotation.

While sitting in the 911 dispatch center PSAP (public service
answering point), I heard the distinct familiar ring tone for Medi-
Flight's 1-800 emergency access line picked up by dispatch on the
second ring.

"Hello, Medi-Flight dispatch, this is Lou. How may I help you?"
answered our ever-so-professional seasoned dispatcher, Lou Menton.
Lead dispatcher Teri Norton filled out the duty roster for the day.

"I'm Cathy, a nurse at the Yosemite Clinic. Our doctor would
like to speak to your ER physician for an air ambulance transfer."

"No problem, Cathy. Let me get Dr. Phillips on the line for
your doctor."

One of the personal services MMC and Medi-Flight provided
was a one-stop shopping 1-800 phone line. Part of the acceptance criteria for transfer requires a doctor-to-doctor conversation to ensure
the necessity, appropriateness, and availability of a warm bed at the
end destination. As soon as the phone transfer was completed, Lou
returned to her usual unabashed proud role as perpetual unrelenting tormentor, spun her chair in my direction, and began a lengthy
impertinent tirade intended to give me insufferable grief way beyond
what Lucy van Pelt regularly doled out to Charlie Brown. Good grief!

"So, Ronnie Jim Gomer Dude, looks like the other crew gets to
go to Yosemite and you get to stay here where I can give you shit *all
day long*. Neener, neener, neener old man. Eat shit and die!" It was
a good feeling knowing that I was so loved; no punches were pulled
even during these darkest times of my illness. If Lou *didn't* give me
a hard time, it was very suspicious. I was senior to her and most of
the flight crew in chronological age only, so many of my monikers
contained references to my "advanced" age. Many unsolicited applications for AARP membership suspiciously arrived at my home even

though I was just nearing fifty. Sadly, with the advent of the progressive PC culture, ageism has prevailed over humorous repartee.

"Hold your skanky water, crone, or I'm going to open a can!" I snorted weakly yet playfully, offering a feeble defense.

"Say what?" Lou intoned

"Whoop Ass! A can of Whoop Ass! I'm gonna open a can of Whoop Ass and use it on you!" I retorted, weakly.

"Yeah right, Ronnie Jim. You couldn't whip me on my deathbed, and you're the only one who's going to get his ass whooped today!"

That momentary healthy exchange of trifling banter reflected, in our strange way, the love and respect we all shared for each other in ways the casual observer might seriously misinterpret. Without humor in this profession to lighten the moment, none of us could survive. The ongoing exchange of impudent banter was interrupted by multiple emergency lines lighting up nearly simultaneously. Several EMS frequencies on the scanner became active with fresh chatter. CHP had dispatched units to a report of an overturned semitruck with a fluid spill on Highway 33 in the Newman area in Stanislaus County; CDF was sending fire units with rescue and extrication equipment; and multiple ambulances were requested to this remote rural area. Based upon pre-hospital dispatch criteria, an air ambulance is always requested. Sure enough, within fifteen seconds of the various EMS tone-outs, the Medi-Flight 1-800 line rang.

Merced CHP dispatch center spoke with Lou requesting Medi-Flight to Newman. While gathering pertinent information, Teri toned out Medi-Flight I and security for the scene flight in Newman. I answered a nonemergency call line that lit up on the console; it was our favorite mechanic Brian Gardner (RIP, dear friend!) advising that the maintenance was complete and we were back in service. Hallelujah, the call gods were in my good graces.

Medi-Flight I had just lifted off the helipad and was hovering over the transition field, talking to Modesto Tower for a southwest-bound flight pattern, when our emergency line lit up the console. I hoped it was Yosemite Clinic calling back to request air ambulance transport now that transfer and admission had been arranged by Dr. Phillips in our ER.

"Medi-Flight, this is Lou, how can I help you?"

"Lou, hi again, this is Cathy from Yosemite Clinic calling back. The transfer has been arranged between the doctors. I need to speak to the nurse that's coming for our patient so I can give them report."

"Just one sec, the flight nurse is sitting next to me in dispatch, I'll patch you through." Lou turned to me with an incredulous smirk on her face while transferring the clinic to another phone line and reflexively extended her middle phalanx to remind me I was still "number 1." "Don't screw it up for us, old man. You owe me big-time for this one!" Our two most favorite flight destinations were Yosemite Valley next to the Ahwahnee Hotel, and San Francisco where we landed adjacent to the Bay at the Presidio next to the Golden Gate Bridge for obvious reasons. The views were indescribable!

As I exited the dispatch center, I waved goodbye to Lou and Teri. "I'll bring you back some pine cones to wipe your ass with while we're gone," I said, laughing happily all the way to the helipad. Good karma today—so far.

Patient information was gathered while our pilot, another Viet Nam Army helicopter pilot and UC Berkeley alumnus Jon Miller, checked weather for cross-country conditions. We had to fly to six or seven thousand feet AGL to cross the Sierra Nevada before landing in Ahwahnee Meadow in Yosemite Valley at 4,000 feet (1,219 meters), surrounded on all sides by sheer granite cliffs rising 3,500 feet, and the tallest waterfall in North America, the majestic Yosemite Falls plunging 2,425 feet as a backdrop to the northwest.

The flight was indescribably delicious and uneventful, and forty-five minutes later we landed safely in a lush green meadow adjacent to Northside Drive to a gathering crowd of inquisitive tourists with camera shutters clicking faster than a one-legged man in a butt-kicking competition. Suddenly but briefly, the appearance and landing of our helicopter outrivaled the majesty of our surroundings. A National Park Service ambulance met us when we shut down, and Cindy and I rode the short quarter-mile road to the clinic where staff and patient were anxiously awaiting our arrival.

Once inside, we were ushered into an exam room where we met with Nurse Cathy and Dr. Jones. Pleasantries were exchanged with complete patient status updates and a review of completed x-rays and lab results. Cindy introduced herself to our patient while she reattached him to our Propaq monitor for cardiac monitoring, heart rhythm, and pulse oximetry along with portable oxygen and checking IVs for patency and rate. She briefed him on basic inflight safety procedures as required; however, most of our patients are preoccupied with their injuries or unconscious, so many do not retain all the information.

Avid outdoorsman and mountain climber Sergei Romanov was a fifty-four-year-old Belarusian from the capital city of Minsk, a landlocked western SSR wedged between Poland, Russia, and the Baltic nations. During the huge migration of refugees after World War II, his family immigrated to America from Poland through Ellis Island in 1952, two years before its untimely closure. His lifelong dream of climbing the face of El Capitan came suddenly crashing down, quite literally, on the first pitch. A small piece of granite broke loose from above, striking him in the head. The helmet he was wearing saved his life, but not without serious consequence. He fell twenty feet, landing on loose talus and scree. His fall was reported quickly, and the park rangers conducted an arduous rescue with Stokes litter and body-length vacuum splint to the clinic.

Sergei was alert on our initial exam, but it was reported he had sustained a short loss of consciousness before arrival. He was anxious, nauseated, and in obvious pain. And, he had to pee. Cathy inserted a Foley catheter into his bladder with resultant heme-positive urine, indicative of potential renal injury. His portable chest x-ray revealed several posterior rib fractures on the right and left. Initial lab results were unremarkable but for an elevated white blood cell count. His skin, the largest organ in the body, was abraded and cut in innumerable areas. Closed fractures of both splinted ankles rounded out his obvious injuries. Yosemite Clinic had very limited services; the nearest CT scan was at the destination hospital, and a head CT would be a most desirable diagnostic tool to have today with Mr. Romanov.

The clinic had started one IV of normal saline, given a tetanus shot, and provided morphine and Reglan IV for his pain and nausea.

We transported Sergei in his prepackaged full-body vacuum splint for the ride back to Modesto after starting a second IV, maintaining his cervical spine and head from movement. Not long into the flight, his condition began to fluctuate from moments of mental clarity to periods of drowsiness, confusion, and stupor. Next began complaints of increasing headache and projectile vomiting. Preprimed suction cleared most of his secretions, but acidic bilious emesis now permeated the cabin. Thank dog I wasn't flying with Don today (rest in peace, dear friend)! After clearing his airway, additional doses of morphine and antiemetic were given IV. His oxygen saturation on fifteen liters was slowly decreasing, and his fluctuating level of consciousness was most disturbing.

The expression "GCS less than eight, time to intubate!" rang true for Mr. Romanov. Cindy and I both agreed to heed the need for speed and secure his airway quickly, as he was becoming unable to control his secretions or maintain his respiratory efforts. He was now at great risk for pulmonary aspiration and airway compromise, complicated by his fixed position in C-spine precautions, cervical collar, and vacuum splint flat on his back! We both believed Sergei was experiencing an acute EDH!

"Let's do an RSI *now*, Ron!" Cindy declared. "I've got yellow puke soaking in my shoes and socks!" Due to the limited space inside the aircraft cabin, the attendant on the left sits facing forward with both feet straddling the patient's head. It's not the optimal position for performing an emergent intubation but ideal for passive emesis collection.

A few years prior, Cindy and I were dispatched on a scene flight on a dark and rainy night, landing in a short alfalfa field adjacent to a rural road. Cindy exited the helicopter and walked the short distance to the barbed-wire fence separating the road and field in two to three inches of standing water. Just between the fence and the field was an invisible obstacle, an encircling irrigation ditch about eighteen inches deep used for watering their crops in the summer months.

When Cindy stepped in the unseen obstacle, she was submerged to her knees in water to compliment the pouring rain saturating the rest of her flight suit from above. When we loaded the patient and Cindy climbed aboard, I noticed her grossly swollen, misshapen legs that resembled Alice the Goon from E. C. Segar's Thimble Theater and Popeye cartoons. Her lower legs from the knees down had more than doubled in circumference and brought me to tearful laughter. As iterated previously, our flight suits were designed with more pockets and Velcro than we could possibly fill. This particular flight must have occurred on the peak day of her moon cycle, I presumed, because she had wisely prepared and stashed several tampons in both her lower leg pockets, inconspicuous and totally unobtrusive until they became saturated with water!

We both shared years in several memorable moments on exciting rescues. One of our shortest flights was also one of the most frightening. Our pilot Mike Antonelli (rest in peace, brother!), another ex-Army helicopter pilot who served in Viet Nam, had just lifted off from Memorial Hospital and had left the transition area, dipping the nose slightly while we gained forward speed and altitude. Instead of his usual relaxed exchange with Modesto Tower, his tone reflected one of somber frightening clarity.

"Modesto Tower, Lifeguard 84 Mike Hotel has just lifted off from the hospital two miles northwest of the airport. *Mayday, mayday, mayday!* Requesting emergency clearance to land at the airport."

"Lifeguard 84 Mike Hotel, Modesto Tower copies your mayday request. I'm clearing all traffic in the ATA and activating airport fire and rescue." Multiple transmissions ensued in these critical moments over the radio between Mike and the airport, while everyone in our dispatch center anxiously awaited any updates.

The cockpit instantly became eerily silent as our pilot busied himself with keeping the helicopter in control. Cindy and I looked at each other and immediately began instituting crash control procedures. Strict radio silence was initiated, even over the ICS, as it could distract Mike from his difficult task. This was not time to ask "What's going on?"

Instead, we ensured every piece of equipment on board was double-checked and secured tightly, most importantly ourselves! After everything was checked and double-checked, we assumed the crash position bending forward and hugging our ankles in absolute silence while probing each other's deepest thoughts with wide bewildered eyes (this was before our seat belt restraint system had shoulder harnesses installed).

Mike made a safe landing at Modesto Airport, surrounded by numerous emergency vehicles. Only after we landed did Cindy and I discover the problem. The Eurocopter TwinStar has two engines; on initial liftoff, the cockpit gauges indicated to the pilot an engine failure to engine one, effectively leaving only one engine operational to make an emergency landing. Any landing you can walk away from is a good landing in my opinion, and I experienced more than my share of close encounters in Viet Nam. Those crucial minutes of helplessness and unknown terror were rewarded with a safe landing and rejoicing in our good fortune. Our mechanic Brian later identified the problem as a power transfer imbalance or some such thing I did not fully understand. We would all live to fly again.

"I wish we could have done this while we were still at the clinic with more space. This is certainly quite a stark contrast to his condition just fifteen minutes ago. I'll get the meds drawn up, you grab the airway bag and intubation supplies."

RSI, or rapid sequence intubation or induction, involves using an array of drugs given intravenous rapidly, generally with rapid onset and short duration of action. Each drug given is based on mg/kg of body weight; fortunately for me, in another life I worked the carnival booth guessing people's weights, so my calculations were consistently within the acceptable therapeutic limits. I made miniaturized RSI charts laminated for all crew members; I kept my RSI drug calculation chart in my fanny pack next to my frayed copy of the *Thirteen Laws of the House of God*. It was a fairly straightforward cookbook recipe with allowance for modification based upon age, weight, and other critical factors or contraindications.

Cindy began hyperoxygenation with fifteen liters blow-by oxygen using our BVM. Lidocaine 1.5 mg/kg was given to blunt the effects of increased intracranial pressure that can occur during laryngoscopy. At T minus two minutes, the nonbarbiturate sedative/hypnotic and anesthetic induction agent etomidate, 0.2 mg/kg was given over thirty seconds while Cindy applied slight cricoid pressure over the neck through the front opening in his cervical collar to mitigate gastric insufflation and subsequent aspiration. The etomidate was quickly followed by 1.5–2.0 mg/kg of succinylcholine, a depolarizing neuromuscular blocking agent (NMBA) that causes rapid and complete skeletal muscle paralysis, resulting in transient visible muscle fasciculations just before flaccid paralysis and drug-induced respiratory arrest occurs (a variable to the procedure could include a small defasciculating dose of Norcuron/Zemuron before succinylcholine; however, it also expands the time continuum during emergent intubation). It is cardio-protective and does not affect the beating heart muscle. In essence, your once-breathing patient of two minutes ago is now unable to move, talk, blink, or breathe, an extremely frightening experience especially if one were still semiconscious like Sergei, so we had to remember the seven Ps of RSI: (1) preparation, (2) pre-oxygenation, (3) pretreatment, (4) paralysis, (5) positioning, (6) placement, and lastly, (7) post-intubation management.

At T minus zero minutes, with suction at the ready, Cindy visualized his vocal cords with a number 3 MacIntosh curved blade and inserted an 8.0 ET tube in our flaccid, nonbreathing patient with a healthy beating heart. After the usual airway confirmation checks were performed, his ET tube was secured, and Cindy was now tasked with breathing for him and controlling his CO_2 with the BVM. As soon as I got the chance, he received 5 mg of the benzodiazepine sedative Versed (midazolam), which has the wonderful side effect of amnesia so the patient has no recall of the incident. Fully aware of the short half-life of succinylcholine, precious moments remained before our patient would begin moving again. With the airway now totally protected and monitored under Cindy's attentive control, it was time for the last drug in the RSI countdown.

Norcuron 0.1 mg/kg (or Zemuron 1 mg/kg), a nondepolarizing NMBA, was given for longer-term muscular paralysis of thirty to forty-five minutes, which should allow us enough time to manage Sergei more effectively during the flight and allow the drugs to wear off about the time we arrived in the trauma room for the neurosurgeon to perform an evaluation and get a STAT CT scan. His blood pressure throughout the flight was adequate enough for me to give him more morphine for the silent screams of pain I could not hear.

His end tidal CO2 (ETCO2) was monitored by the mainstream in-line sensor attached to our Propaq monitor, placed between the ET tube and the BVM, which provided both real-time numeric and waveform results. With controlled ventilation we able were to maintain his ETCO2 values between the preferred 35–45 mm/Hg. His oxygen saturations improved post-intubation as well.

Meanwhile, the flight nurse was feeling the combined effects of stress, altitude, anemia, pharmaceuticals, and the effects of my weakened condition. Things began to get fuzzy around the edges. Cindy placed the radio call to Memorial Hospital while I took over ventilations. All the players were gathered together awaiting our imminent arrival in the trauma room.

Cindy accompanied Mr. Romanov from the helipad to the ER with the trauma team in tow while I remained behind to clean up, replace supplies used, and restock the meds we used during the flight from the hospital pharmacy. I was feeling pretty puny and pitiful and had no idea how much longer my body could endure this agonizing treatment and continue to work.

Mr. Romanov's CT scan showed an epidural hematoma (EDH), and he was taken directly to the OR where it was successfully treated by the neurosurgeon before moving him to the ICU for weeks of close monitoring and repair of his many fractures. He survived his short climb up El Capitan, though I felt his technical rock-climbing days were over or at least severely challenged. However, I didn't rule anything out. Ten years earlier on July 26, 1989, twenty-nine-year-old Mark Wellman became the first paraplegic to successfully climb the 3,500-foot granite monolith, his forty-second ascent and first time since being paralyzed from the waist down from a 100-foot fall in 1982.

On my next days off, one morning I arose from a bad night of restless sleep, stretched like a sore old dog, and walked outside our bedroom a few steps before reaching the thirteen stairs leading downstairs to the living room. The next thing I remembered was Karen kneeling close to me at the bottom of the stairs. She said I passed out and tumbled down the carpeted stairway, and it made sense to me at the time. Somehow my body had escaped serious injury, just a few rug burns. Not long after that tumble down the stairs, early in the morning our employee health nurse Liz Pearson witnessed me wobbling unsteadily down the presumptively empty long back hallway entrance to the hospital at 0700, just as I had begun to lean against the wall to prevent me from going to ground (see appendix, HOG Law 2). This audacious display on my part sent a clear message as to the urgency and necessity of my next decision.

My request for FMLA (Family Medical Leave Act of 1993) time off from work was requested and granted through Employee Health. This gave me the opportunity to stay at home and more safely and privately endure the horrible side effects during my continued therapy until such time I improved enough to return to work or…

Among the many holistic therapies she employed to help me heal, Karen introduced me to the spiritual practice of yoga. It sustained and nourished me, helping to guide me through seemingly endless days of darkness, pain, and despair. I began to wonder which would kill me first, my HCV or the pharmaceuticals I was taking to rid myself of this unwelcome invader. Absolutely no alcohol consumption was allowed for months before or during drug therapy. This was not a problem or great sacrifice, and I was fortunate enough to have the fortitude to quit at any given time and not miss alcohol.

Several months passed at home while my body slowly adjusted to the prolonged anemia and the host of other nefarious symptoms before I felt strong enough to return to work.

Through renewed spirituality, meditation, yoga, a wonderful loving wife, and a strong desire to live, I survived those several months of self-imposed hell without further incident. *Except* for eight dental caries, two broken teeth, oral herpes simplex virus (HSV / cold sores) for twelve months, a right branch vein occlusion in the fovea centralis of my right retina causing central vision loss, and one hospital admission from blood loss and acute colitis. Surrender was still not an option!

The months passed slowly after my unceremonious return to work. It became more obvious that the demands of the job exceeded my supply side. Finally, the treatment ended with promising results; the virus had been "undetectable," stopped in its tracks for nearly a year. The important lab markers were three- and six-month posttherapy to determine lasting efficacy. The long-awaited test results were not unexpected but nevertheless not good tidings. The combination antiviral therapy was ineffective: Big Pharma 1, Patient 0. My viral load quickly rebounded on the quantitative HCV RNA PCR test to several million IU/L, and my body continued to experience even more intense unpleasant symptoms.

We both had the greatest jobs ever working at Memorial Hospital and worked with the absolute best in their respective professions. Our youngest son, Forrest, had just graduated from Yosemite High and was headed to Great Lakes Navy Training Center in Illinois and then off to SEAL BUD/S training at Coronado Island, California. Karen and I were both tired of living for thirteen years in "the city," Modesto, and we both longed for more peace, solitude, space, and *less stress*.

Besides the terror-filled yet innocuous mayday flight in the past, two other critical incidents occurred after my return to work that made me question my own mortality. Medi-Flight was dispatched on a cross-country mission to Bear Valley Resort Ski Area, elevation 8,500 feet, for a severely injured skier in the Stanislaus National Forest in Alpine County. We were forced to cancel en route due to high winds, snow, and reduced visibility. On our return leg home with the beloved Mr. Frangos once again at the helm, Geoff was forced to perform some serious treetop flying at slow, almost hover speed, as a heavy ground fog and clouds had formed and now completely shrouded the San Joaquin Valley during our absence flying in the snowy mountain whiteout. Six eyes were silently transfixed scanning in all directions outside, trying to locate any landmark on the ground to help effect a safe emergency landing.

Geoff briefly changed his focus from outside to his cock-pit gauges while we were in the foothills a few miles northeast of Oakdale. I was the first to see the giant chopper-stopper obstacle that was right off our nose a few hundred feet ahead, same altitude. I got off a quick terse warning over the ICS. "Power lines, twelve o'clock!" Geoff pulled pitch and banked right, missing the high-tension power lines by mere seconds. Eventually we landed safely, a long, spooky dry run. My SPF was so high I don't think I pooped for a week!

Late one starry night we received a request to rendezvous with Tuolumne County Ambulance (TCA) at Pine Mountain Lake Airport (PMLA) three miles northeast of Groveland for a sixty-year-old man experiencing a heart attack. Chief Pilot John Dias checked weather for the sixty-five-mile moonlit cross-country mission and gave his medical crew a "thumbs-up" and a clear sky forecast. Mr. Murphy stowed away just before liftoff. Thirty minutes later we landed at Pine Mountain Lake Airport, shut down, and waited. And waited and waited.

Due to unforeseen complications, the ground ambulance transport from the patient's home to our rendezvous point at the airport took over an hour after we had landed, and the ambient temperature had dropped dramatically. My partner, long-time chief flight paramedic Cliff Larrabee, and I received our patient from TCA, promptly packaged him for transport, and cleared the scene in record time. Strangely, the moon was no longer visible above. The area surrounding the airport and the surrounding hills were clear, and lights twinkled from the sparse mountain homes scattered below. The cowardly stowaway Mr. Murphy quickly bailed out. We hovered over the departure end, and John dipped the nose of 95MH slightly as he accelerated down the runway to gain forward speed and altitude more easily. John busied himself on the aviation radio frequency notifying any local air traffic of our position since the airport tower was not manned at night. Within seconds of his previous transmission, we had transitioned from the tarmac at 2,932 feet to maybe 300 feet AGL and were immediately cloaked in a heavy wet fog denser than Joy Behar's skull.

"Okay, guys, I'm going IFR!" was all John had time to squawk over the ICS. Cliff and I were quite busy attending and medicating our acute MI patient who had no clue as to the dire predicament we found ourselves engaged in, but we also became austere adherents to the French mime Marcel Marceau and practiced "the art of silence" for our communications while John tried to figure a way out of the soup.

The total radio silence was unbroken, *except* for the *beep-beep-beep* of the pilot's cockpit gauge, the radar altimeter (RA). The RA measures the helicopter's height in altitude above terrain immediately beneath the aircraft, inspiring pilot confidence in knowing just how much room there *might* be to maneuver before sudden impact. It did just the opposite for Cliff and me, and the obnoxious RA alarm did not inspire my confidence, but rather signaled a brief three-second warning before the big flash and bright white light.

We tried our best to stay focused on patient care to distract our intrusive thoughts. The terrain surrounding the airport contained many other taller mountains, and we were now flying blind in a fish bowl surrounded by tree-and-granite-covered mountains for nearly five minutes with the RA echoing in our headphones, while John calmly and professionally navigated up front. Medi-Flight was not an accredited IFR (instrument flight rules) program, but our very experienced pilots, all military veterans mostly from the Viet Nam era, were all certified in IFR, thankfully.

Just when I felt I could not take another *beep-beep-beep* from the RA gauge, John finally guided us through the fog, and we lifted suddenly to a bright moonlit sky with stars above, a foggy blanket of white clouds below, *and* a colossal radio tower rising high above the fog layer with a menacing red warning beacon flashing atop its highest point well above our current altitude and directly off our nose at our twelve o'clock position about a mile away. That's less than thirty seconds' distance at a forward speed of 120 knots!

The sight of that imposing tower was a sobering event for the three of us that sent a collective shock wave of "what-ifs," and I silently prayed for all our lives being spared to serve a higher good. A lengthy debriefing and discussion of the account was held into the wee hours of the morning. It became a sober reminder of the fragility of life we all too often took for granted, especially serving in the role of rescuer and caregiver, while expending little or no thought for our own personal safety or becoming a victim through our altruistic desires to help our fellow human being. I became even more determined after those two near misses to ensure I would live long enough to spoil my grandchildren growing up.

Discussion about moving to Montana came up, and we determined that we both shared the dream of living in Bozeman, Montana, in our younger years before we knew each other. Decision made, in early 2002 we took a much-needed vacation in our camper to southwest Montana to explore property and hopefully find a respectable home.

Our homegrown realtor and soon-to-be good friend Michelle Goodwine showed us several homes both within and outside our price range. It quickly became evident in our search that the city of Bozeman had become gentrified and appeared similar to any other big city in California. Big money had long since arrived, and it had lost its small college town appeal. Fortunately, just about twenty miles east over Bozeman Pass sat the small town of Livingston, which was more suited to our tastes. Dubbed the "Fly Fishing Capital of the World," it was the site of the 1991 hit movie *A River Runs Through It*, and its low-key atmosphere offered a private and relatively undisturbed haven for many movie celebrities. With a population just over seven thousand, it was a major western railroad town located right on the Yellowstone River, and the northern gateway to Yellowstone National Park via Paradise Valley just an hour drive to the south.

We put an offer on a small five-acre ranch adjacent to a 1,500-acre cattle ranch five miles north of town on a gravel road at five thousand feet elevation, fenced and cross fenced, including a large barn and tack room overlooking the Yellowstone River and the famous Sleeping Giant mountain feature to the south in the ten-thousand-to-thirteen-thousand-foot high Absaroka Range of the Rockies. The range extends south for 150 miles into Wyoming, forming the eastern boundary of Yellowstone and the western edge of the Bighorn

Basin. Our generous offer was accepted the day before our return trip home. It was time to put our home for the last twelve years on the market and to say farewell to great jobs and great friends. Bison and wolves and bears—oh *my*!

CHAPTER 12

Big Sky

Oh, give me a home where the buffalo roam,
Where the deer and the antelope play,
Where seldom is heard a discouraging word,
And the skies are not cloudy all day.

—Gene Autry

Our home was put on the market within days of our return. It took nearly a decade for our home to appreciate despite all the improvements, as the housing market took a nosedive in the early '90s and we were upside-down on our mortgage for several years. The hardest part was giving our thirty days' notice, contingent upon selling our home, to our employer and coworkers, who were like extended family.

Things began moving very quickly. We sold Karen's first learner bike, an 883 Harley Sportster to make room for the one hundredth anniversary edition 2003 Harley Road King I secretly preordered months earlier for her as a surprise. While cruising McHenry Boulevard one afternoon, we passed by a stunning red 1994 Harley Custom Softail in showroom condition with low miles and thousands of dollars in aftermarket custom accessories with a For Sale sign on the windshield. Two days later, it found its way inside our garage; I canceled her Road King much to another buyer's glee, who eagerly snatched it up before the ink dried. We then sold our cab-over Lance camper and bought a thirty-seven-foot Forest River Toy Trailer to accommodate our two Harleys during our travels.

Our home was very desirable and turn-key move-in ready. It received several viewings, and a realtor showing our home to another couple ended up submitting an offer that was countered and accepted in just a few weeks. Best friends Sharon and Ricky Moore, both ER/ICU nurses we worked, traveled, skied, and played with since day one at MMC (Sharon self-appointed herself as the nurse to orient me and long-time friend Alicks Ekstrum when we were first hired!) hosted a blowout going-away party punctuated by long hugs and teary eyes as we bid farewell to dear friends before the next adventure.

I would be remiss if I did not mention those excellent flight nurses who made my tenure as chief flight nurse so easy and enjoyable. It was my honor to work with such compassionate, talented people. My sincerest love and appreciation go out to Kathy, Rick, Elaine, Alicks, Peggy, Renita, Sharon, Roxanne, P-Wave, Brian, Bill, Cathy, KB, Vickster, and Balvir, with apologies to any I may have forgotten. Accolades to our flight medics, dispatchers, mechanics, and the greatest pilots who always brought us home safely!

The move had to be well-coordinated because we made the decision to take an assignment as traveling nurses for a year while exploring the New England states and the East Coast. We would live in our trailer and see the sights on the Harleys on our days off. Karen followed me in our Mustang while I drove our fully loaded traveling home over the Sierras and the Rockies with a stuffed United Van Lines truck trailing us by a few days.

We moved into our new ranch home five miles north of Livingston and immersed ourselves in the local history for a month, then sealed and weatherproofed our home for the long winter while we were away traveling. A grueling two-thousand-mile drive to East Canaan, Connecticut, still awaited us for our first travel nurse assignment on July 5.

Spending late summer and fall in New England riding our Harleys from Maine to Maryland was an incredible experience. Suffice it to say Karen and I had many memorable experiences during our nursing travels. I won't bother bringing out the carousel slide projector.

Our early unannounced return to Montana in midwinter after exploring the East Coast was blessed with hundreds of huge dried tumbleweed skeletons surrounding our airtight and unmolested home. No frozen pipes, no dust, not even a cobweb was found inside our home.

Karen was speeding westbound on I-90 just approaching Livingston, Montana, two miles ahead on the afternoon of July 4, 1991, with our three young children and black Lab in the back and me riding shotgun. The family three-week vacation had taken a sudden turn in the early morning of day two when I veered off the highway shoulder about one hundred miles west of Salt Lake City, Utah, rolling three times at 65 mph. Our Suburban landed on top of our tow-behind travel trailer in the wide median between the divided freeway lanes. The car and trailer were totaled, and all of us were injured, but mostly minor cuts and bruises, with one exception. Yes, seat belts do save lives. I was struck in the back of my head by the portable TV/VCR located in the console before it exited the front windshield requiring several stitches in my head, a whopping headache, and another concussion; Karen drove the rest of the vacation.

The ominous reflection of flashing red lights in the rearview mirror signaled it was time to ease up on the accelerator and pull off the road. The Montana highway patrolman walked up to the driver's side of our car, his vehicle's emergency flashers still activated. Karen rolled down her window. The kids were surprisingly speechless.

"License and registration, please?" the officer kindly asked.

Karen complied and he walked back to his vehicle to check the documents and check for outstanding warrants, I presumed. After a few minutes he returned.

"Excuse me, but could you and your husband please step out of the car and come around to the back of the vehicle?" There was no trepidation or concern in his voice and the strap to the holster on his service weapon was not unsnapped, so we politely complied with his request. And we had done nothing wrong with the possible exception of Karen exceeding the posted 75 mph speed limit, even while other cars passed us driving even faster.

The three of us spoke for five to ten minutes, with semis zipping by at Mach speed, before we collectively agreed to follow the officer's lead and let the kids add even more suspense and drama to their vacation memories. The MHP vehicle pulled in front of us with his emergency lights still flashing, and we followed behind from a safe distance to the next off-ramp to downtown Livingston. The kids were freaking out at this point.

"Mom, are you under arrest?" the back seat trio all asked.

"Yes, kids. Mom has to follow the officer into town where we can talk more." She had a hard time keeping a straight face.

"Are you going to jail?" "Will we get to visit you?" "I have to pee!" "Will Dad have to go to jail with you?" "Who's going to take care of us?" "I'm hungry!" And on and on it went, nonstop.

Thankfully, just a few short blocks off the freeway exit, he pulled into a large open field adjacent to a restaurant on Park Street where the patrol car directed us to park in circular fashion with two other cars sporting out-of-state licenses and large families in tow. Minutes later, from a secluded location, a troop of ten to twelve horse-mounted players dressed in frontier attire of early Native American Indians and frontiersmen surrounded the three cars, racing in circles, howling, and firing their six-shooters in the air. Squeals of delight and relief could be heard over the din from the kids in the cars when they collectively realized this was a gag and their parents were not going to jail!

Each Fourth of July, a selected officer from the Livingston PD, the Park County Sheriff, and the Montana Highway Patrol each pull over one vehicle with out-of-state tags and families, likely vacationers like us. We were from California, driving a Dodge van licensed in Oregon that we rented in Salt Lake City, Utah, two weeks earlier, so we aptly met their inclusion criteria. While the kids were in the back seat pondering their current predicament, the officer asked us if we would like to be honored guests on July 4 at their sixty-fifth annual PRCA Livingston Roundup Rodeo. Front-row tickets to the rodeo and fireworks plus a complimentary hotel room, dinner, and breakfast. Fortunately, we were not driving much farther before stopping for the night, so we eagerly agreed. The three families all sat next to each other later that night at the rodeo, and our names were all announced over the loud speaker as being this year's annual "hold-up families." That kind gesture touched all our hearts; we had a fabulous time visiting this quaint mountainous high-plains town, and unknowingly at the time, that kindness would figure into our decision to move back there eleven years later.

A few days later, a reporter from the *Livingston Enterprise* visited us at our ranch, took pictures, and interviewed each of us at length. The next edition featured our in-depth story taking the top half of the front page, even with a nice five-by-seven photo of us sitting on our deck, looking at the Sleeping Giant of the Absaroka Range. We did not have trouble finding jobs. Our phone was ringing with job offers before we even actively applied.

Livingston Health Care (LHC), previously Livingston Memorial Hospital, was a small, rural critical access hospital (CAH) located 115 miles west of the nearest level II trauma center in Billings. Karen started work in the ICU, and I found work in the ER and helping out in the GI lab initially until securing a full-time position in the ER. For the first year, I kept my ears open and my mouth closed, learning the system and the doctors, and plotting my itinerary for potential future endeavors.

The abrupt yet long overdue departure of the micromanaging director of nurses gave a promise of hope, and a popular refrain from "Munchkinland" in the *Wizard of Oz* echoed in the hospital hallways as the door hit her on the way out. Marsha Vanderhoff, RN, competently filled the position and recognized the flame burning inside me to effect some real change with proper support. We had talked on many occasions, and she knew of my experience and background. My offer was graciously received by Marsha and our CEO Sam Pleshar; now I only had to impress and convince the members of the board of directors that spending money up front can both save human lives and generate income. I was quite familiar with trauma systems development and trauma center designation criteria.

My PowerPoint proposal to the board presented a detailed overview of the requirements for acquiring trauma center designation for LHC through training, education, outreach, policies and procedures, *and* the full financial and philosophic commitment of hospital administration. A monumental task, but with a jumpstart from the top tier of administration on my side, my job would be easier.

The biggest obstacle was the reticence and resistance encountered by a few (well, mostly just one misanthrope, who believed I made all this up in my head and tried unsuccessfully to discredit me) of the family practice physicians. Some of them tried to work shifts in the ER during the daylight hours while still attempting to see their private patients in their office, so my doctor would sometimes disappear unexpectedly and later be discovered in his office dangerously double dipping. And of course, our lone young surgeon and father of small children who did not relish getting out of bed at 0300 to care for trauma patients; however, they all warmed to the program over time. I promised results within two years; a lot of education, training, and practice were first necessary to lay the foundation for raising the trauma standard. I became LHC's first ever trauma program manager.

With further persuasion, Marsha allowed me to modify my job description to include the position of education coordinator for the hospital. Coordination with our partner hospital, Deaconess Billings Clinic (DBC, a level II trauma center), allowed me to become an affiliate faculty member with their education department. Monthly continuing education (CE) was provided for all the physicians and pharmacists with physician guest speakers from DBC. In addition to teaching BLS, ACLS, and PALS, I became an instructor's instructor that allowed me to train others how to teach the classes, giving me a core group of instructors to assist in our full monthly classes.

Every nurse who worked at LHC was trained and certified in BLS, ACLS, PALS, and NRP at a minimum. All the ER nurses received additional training in TNCC (Trauma Nursing Core Course) and ENPC (Emergency Nurse Pediatric Course). After that training was completed, I arranged to have each ER nurse and our new Livingston Fire Department Paramedics attend and audit the physician-mandated ATLS (Advanced Trauma Life Support) class developed by the American College of Surgeons. With determination and persistence, every doctor who worked in our ER and our surgeon was trained in ATLS. The LHC education department was generating revenues; my classes attracted HCPs (health care practitioners) from Idaho, Wyoming, and Montana, hungry to learn and have fun in the process.

In order to assimilate the whole Montana EMS and trauma system development and assume a leadership role in our desolate state, it was imperative to attend trauma-related meetings in person; the whole teleconference concept being utilized had its inherent time and travel benefits but did not allow for face-to-face discussion. This was extremely important and beneficial for my face and name recognition; however, it did involve long hours traveling hundreds of miles to Billings, Helena, Great Falls, and Missoula where the larger hospitals were. It allowed me the opportunity to meet and speak with the players at the state level.

During the process of certification, there was a remarkable transition in the hospital and staff. The eager and extremely knowledgeable Livingston Fire Department staff was just completing their first paramedic classes and started offering full-time paramedic ambulance service to our area. I provided what assistance I could to integrate quality improvement programs, chart reviews, standardized radio communications, trauma triage criteria, etc. They were a very dedicated, talented, ambitious bunch of men and women.

Some nurses who once felt anxious and intimidated when we received major trauma now eagerly responded in full PPE (personal protective equipment), now trained and prepared to accept the new challenge with enthusiasm and much less trepidation. Our doctors felt more comfortable with hands-on ATLS. When prehospital EMS alerted us of an incoming trauma patient meeting activation criteria at 0300, our surgeon, nurse anesthetist, and orthopedic surgeon would quickly respond. With some exception, most major trauma patients were treated and stabilized, initiating necessary emergent lifesaving procedures, while arranging for expedient helicopter transport to Billings or Idaho Falls, Idaho (burn patients).

Patient outcomes improved dramatically; those who survived their serious injuries likely would not have lived with identical injuries two years prior. One such case reflects the benefit of preparation, training, and dedication.

A large gathering of hospital staff, friends, and family had gathered at our friend John's home on East River Road just a few miles south of town for a starry hot August Saturday night party on the river. East River Road runs north-south along the east side of the Yellowstone River, with Highway 89 tracing the same twists and turns of the Yellowstone on the west side in the breathtaking Paradise Valley. Highway 89 is one of only five access roads to YNP and the only one with year-round access into the park, so it was usually bustling with locals and distracted tourists at all hours.

The Rolling Stones were pounding out the jams with their 1969 hit "You Can't Always Get What You Want" on John's stereo, unsuccessful, however, in overpowering the growing gloom of multiple approaching sirens from the north. Most of those in attendance at the party had been drinking alcohol and were committed to stay put. Dear friend and personal physician Doug Wadle was sitting next to me, and we listened intently to the event unfolding from the portable radio scanner on my belt. We would sit this one out on the sidelines. It was time for the acid test.

Livingston Fire and Highway Patrol responded initially to the report of a two-vehicle accident on Highway 89 with injuries. Twenty-eight-year-old Bart Johnson had just left his home just off Wineglass Road for a moonlight ride in his Harley and had driven only a short distance on 89 before he was unceremoniously introduced to the front bumper of distracted ditsy driver Delores Daily. Montana does not have a mandatory motorcycle helmet law, but Bart, and others of my ilk, defied the un-law and wore our brain buckets religiously anyway. Such outlaws!

Bart had sustained a crushing AKA (above-the-knee amputation) of his left leg and a global distribution of road rash from bouncing like a flat rock skipping across a pond on the still hot asphalt. His helmet had protected the most vital and hard-to-repair organ, and as a result, he was fully conscious and reportedly calmer than most of the first responders attending to him. LFD contacted the ER at LMH immediately to alert them to an impending trauma alert. Bart was packaged in the usual fashion in full C-spine precautions with large-bore IVs, oxygen, and trauma dressings to his stump, while others gathered his leg and requisitioned ice from the Igloo coolers of stopped tourists in traffic from the highway shutdown and placed his severed leg atop the ice in a plastic trash bag for transport. Meanwhile, LMH had already spoken to the ER physician at DBC, and their Med Flight helicopter departed Billings to rendezvous in Livingston long before Mr. Johnson ever arrived.

Despite the best efforts of EMS, it was difficult to completely stop the hemorrhage from his mangled left leg. Johns-Hopkins alumna Dr. Michelle Donaldson (our excellent and sole orthopedic surgeon) and a locum tenens surgeon cared for Mr. Johnson along with the assembled properly attired (full PPE) trauma team with LFD assisting. Dr. Donaldson deftly ligated the arterial bleeders, while other nurses gave IV morphine, tetanus shot, IV antibiotics, and the standard "put a tube in every hole" Foley catheter and NG tube.

Med Flight landed minutes later, assumed Bart's care, and commenced to do a "swoop and scoop" hot load for the nearly hour-long flight to Billings and their awaiting surgical team. Did I forget to mention that alcohol was a determining factor in this crash?

Bart Johnson lost his leg, but not his life. The DBC staff later called LHC to compliment the excellent emergent treatment performed on his severed left leg. Every component of the continuum of care for the trauma patient was performed with expediency and professionalism. The odds of him surviving his injuries just a few short years ago were dramatically improved with the implementation of the state's trauma plan.

After a lengthy detailed on-site review, a few months later I humbly but proudly embraced the Montana Department of Health and Human Services framed plaque that proudly hangs in the main hospital hallway to this day. Livingston Health Care became the *first level IV trauma center* (aka community trauma hospital) in the state of Montana on December 14, 2006. Promises made, promises kept—in less than two years.

In addition to a loving relationship, there are three other substantial attributes that require special consideration and are essential for continued happiness: job, home, and location. Living in Modesto, we had the greatest jobs ever and a beautiful home but were surrounded by an ever-growing metropolis in the flatlands. In Livingston, we lived in frontier land in the lush Paradise Valley on the Yellowstone River in the Rocky Mountains. Our beautiful home was completely remodeled and expanded by four thousand square feet, with unobstructed views of snowcapped ten-thousand-foot mountain peaks and ample privacy. My job satisfaction scored a ten out of ten.

The aphorism *happy wife, happy life*, although not a scientific principle, still holds tremendous value in our household. Karen was not challenged working in our small two-bed ICU, and she quickly became disillusioned working at Bozeman Hospital's ICU. She even tried commuting to Billings to work at Deaconess Billings Clinic ICU, a two-hour drive in *good* weather. Her greatest trepidation was losing her advanced critical care skills that she acquired working at Memorial Hospital.

Sensing Karen's growing discontent with her career was conflicting for me, and her anguish compelled me to consider another relocation strategy where she could grow and flourish in her career. After meditating on this poser for several weeks, I presented my suggestion to Karen for her input. Our three children were still furthering their educations and career pursuits and had not yet married or settled down yet. Karen's mom and dad both had recently turned seventy, and both were in good health and were surrounded by countless Meylor relatives centered in and around Milwaukee, Wisconsin. Family is the most powerful trump card, and my proposal to resettle near her parents around the Milwaukee area, her childhood stomping grounds, met with astounding approval, cries of contentment, and repeated romantic rapture.

Focus shifted quickly again to DIY and HDTV networks for Karen to preoccupy her from the stress of staging our home, packing, and moving again over the next several months. Hundreds of homes were searched on the internet as well as exploring hospital and nursing job opportunities in the Milwaukee area. No longer would we be skiing 4,340 vertical feet of powder at Big Sky; treating mangled victims of grizzly bear attacks; white water rafting the Yellowstone River; caring for naive tourists gored and trampled by "that cute little two-thousand-pound bison"; countless remarkable motorcycle trips; and large herds of pronghorn antelope, mule deer, elk, and bald eagles cruising our property.

After we both made the decision to move again, we gave our two weeks' notice contingent upon the sale of our home. Marsha and others at work cast a spell upon us to prevent the sale of our home; it worked for over six months. Their obvious joy for our long-term happiness was superseded by their desire for us to stay. Our sale price was reasonable, but we were not under time constraints and were able to hold out for the full listed price. Just when we were feeling like no one would buy our home, a lady from work inquired about our home one hot summer day. A week later, she made an offer we could not refuse.

CHAPTER 13

Nightmare on Elm Street

*The optimist proclaims that we live in the best of all
possible worlds; and the pessimist fears this is true.*

—James Branch Cabell

Summer 2007

The move from Montana to Wisconsin was another culture shock,
despite the hospital research we did prior to moving there. We left
Montana with a wad of cash, high hopes, and our traveling circus.
Karen followed me in her 2000 Ford Mustang while I drove our
2003 Ford F-350 Super Cab FX4 turbo diesel, pulling our thirty-seven-foot Forest River Fifth Wheel Toy Trailer with our two Harleys
inside. We had packed clothes, expensive pictures and art, guns 'n'
ammo, antique crystal, stocked freezer, all my tools, and our malamute Casi. United Van Lines would follow later with a fully loaded
fifty-two-foot moving trailer when we bought our next home.

The two-day trip across mid-America was uneventful until we
were about sixty miles from our destination city, Milwaukee. My
diesel-guzzling Ford, which averaged about 8 mpg pulling the fif-
teen-thousand-pound fully loaded trailer, was beckoning for another
supersize big gulp.

"Hey, honey, turn your music down, I've got an update!" I
chirped into my portable hand-held radio. We always traveled with

our nine-channel radios so we could stay in touch for gas, potty breaks, and playful banter.

"What do you want, for God's sake?!" Karen retorted playfully, rock music resonating in the background.

"I'm taking the next exit on the right about half a mile ahead. Thought I could make it all the way, but the truck's teetering on empty, and my bladder is teetering on incontinence, it's so full. There's a gas and food icon on the exit sign, and I don't know what's up ahead." I slowed to a stop at the I-94 exit and, seeing no signs of a gas station, turned right heading south onto a two-lane county road bordered on both sides by chest-high corn fields and lush green hill-sides sprinkled with contented grazing bovines. The road meandered for two more miles before we came upon a small village in the middle of rolling-hilled cattle farms. A solo BP station was flanked by a small bodega and car repair shop.

To enter the small station, I had to swing wide to turn right off south Main on to Elm Street for about thirty feet before turning hard right again into the station's north/south-facing pumps. In tight spots with such a humongous personal vehicle, hasty decisions could get one into a parking nightmare if contingencies were not antici-pated and planned for. I had already plotted my exit after fueling, but for now, my rig was parked on an angle, temporarily blocking four pumps in two rows, not to mention the ass end of the toy trailer pro-truding and blocking the eastbound and westbound egress on Elm Street.

Now, I could probably fit the population of this rural town in the back of our trailer, and it was a stormy Sunday afternoon after church, so not much activity was going on. A blocked road for a few minutes would not be a big deal, and besides, I had to pee sooooo bad. As soon as I parked, I jumped out of the cab, located the green-handled diesel pump handle, inserted my ATM card, and pressed "pump fuel." I confirmed flow, and then I raced to the head to relieve myself while Karen fueled her Mustang next to me.

Five minutes later, I returned to my pump, and it had already shut off after reaching full at thirty-five gallons. I looked more closely and then looked over at Karen. She can read me like a Diana Gabaldan novel, so my look described the "Doom on Ronnie" expression on my face.

"What have you done now?!" she asked incredulously.

"WTF! In Montana and all the western states, only diesel pumps have green handles. I just filled our diesel truck with unleaded gasoline!"

"O-h m-y g-o-d!" she half shrieked, half laughed.

"Yep, Ronbo did it again. Time to call AAA." I dared not even start the engine for fear of freezing the motor. After the ceremonious and time-consuming telephone exchange with AAA, a big rig truck out of Milwaukee was en route with a one and a half to two hours ETA.

Realizing I had surreptitiously violated one of my own Rules of Reality Nursing, I felt doomed and embarrassed. Rule number 16, "Never make a critical decision with a full bladder," echoed through my mind. Then my inner consciousness argued this was not a clinical setting, and the argument continued unabated in my head while I contemplated our next strategy.

The *Elm Street Incident*, as it came to be called, took on a new life as the story unfolded. To make matters worse, it suddenly began to pour heavy rain like a monsoon in Viet Nam for the next hour. I notified the local LEOs to advise them of the road blockage, bought Slurpees for the inquisitive huddled masses gathering under open umbrellas in their Sunday best, and apologized repeatedly to the station manager for essentially shutting down half their gas pumps and Elm Street for several hours. This was hold-the-presses-front-page-news for the local weekly rotogravure gazette.

The AAA-contracted truck arrived in a timely fashion. Now he had to maneuver his massive truck in front of mine, facing the building to the north. Then he lifted the front end of my truck and backed his truck and our fifty-two-foot-long truck and trailer combo back onto Elm Street. From SNAFU to back-in-business in fifteen minutes' time!

The last hour of our drive from Montana was sad, to have gone without incident for nearly eight hundred miles, only to cruise into Milwaukee in tow with my perceived tail between my legs. Good

News and Bad News: fortunately, there was a Ford dealership just two miles from Karen's parents' home; unfortunately, it was Sunday and they were closed.

Next day, the gas was drained from our tanks and filled with diesel fuel. Now it was time to find jobs and buy a home. Karen took a job with a traveling nurse company and began working in various hospitals in the ICU while I took care of business and looked for homes. We looked at over thirty homes within a thirty-mile radius of Milwaukee and finally chose the last home we looked at in West Bend, thirty miles north of Milwaukee.

Our new home was a Cream City white brick two-story farmhouse built in 1890 that was totally upgraded and added on about ten years prior. So now, it was a 3,200-square-foot custom home on almost five acres, complete with the original two-story red barn and the most beautiful copper vented kitchen island. It had five bedrooms, a great room, decks, office, downstairs den and workout area, and full basement in the old house. We added a custom wine cellar, infrared sauna, and hot tub. Our plan was to live in Wisconsin on a trial basis for maybe five years, then move back home to Cali. We had the perfect home in the perfect location.

While awaiting escrow to close, we opted to live with my in-laws' home in Milwaukee and stored our travel trailer. We both found full-time jobs with no difficulty; Karen applied for an ICU position, and I accompanied her to her interview only one day after her application was filed. They did not have any ER positions full-time, so I didn't apply. The nurse recruiter asked me to apply anyway. The next day, we both had full-time jobs in ICU and ER respectively. We moved in to our new home on October 1, 2007. Little did we know that would be the snowiest year in recorded history for the local area.

It was not unusual to get up at 0300 to plow snow for two hours before usual waking time, just to clear the three-hundred-foot-long driveway and parking area. Several days during those first winters, it was not unusual to get from nine to fifteen inches of snow during the night. It was eighteen miles to St. Mary's Ozaukee, so the winter's challenges superseded those we experienced in the Rockies of Montana.

Karen worked at St. Mary's Oz ICU until we left Wisconsin. I was sorely disappointed with the (lack of) management, process and ER layout, disorganized chaos, and varied shifts that threw my hepatitis symptoms out of whack. There was not a week that I worked the same shift, and I needed some continuity in my life schedule that the nurse scheduler could not accommodate. Their claim to be a level III trauma center was not upheld; I always hoped our trauma patients would get transferred to the level I trauma center, Froedtert Hospital in Milwaukee, before they died in our ER. It was frightening working there.

St. Joseph's Hospital in West Bend was only four miles from our home, and I wanted to live and work in the same town. Six months after moving to West Bend, I got hired in the ER at St. Joe's, a small and relatively new hospital with a fourteen-bed ER and six-bed ICU adjacent to it. St. Joseph's also held state certification as a level III trauma center.

I settled in nicely at St. Joe's, but it was easy not only because of my years of experience but also because the staff there were all so wonderful. The infinity ER doctors were all top notch, and most of the nursing staff and ER techs were all young, talented, and experienced.

My services were graciously offered as educator to my ER supervisor and to the education department. My supervisor stated the staff were all nurses after all and did not need further training or experience. Their education department, the worst of any hospital I had worked in over thirty years, totally ignored my offer, despite an obvious need expressed by hospital staff. In Montana, I ran the education department, among other duties, and taught basic life support (BLS, or CPR), advanced cardiac life support (ACLS), pediatric advanced life support (PALS), neonatal resuscitation program (NRP), and all the incident command system (ICS) courses on HAZMAT, decontamination, disaster preparedness, etc. As a member of the American Heart Association's (AHA) Regional Training Center Faculty at Deaconess Billings Clinic, one of only four level II trauma centers in all of Montana, I managed my own training facility in Livingston and instructed my own students to become instructors in the above courses. Empowering others to teach gave them newfound confidence and pride. For the first time ever, Livingston Memorial Hospital had an education department that made a profit. My hospital also sponsored my efforts to hold annual "trauma symposiums" to educate others, which brought knowledge-thirsty professionals from Montana, Wyoming, and Idaho. It was sad and disappointing to comprehend St. Joseph's attitude toward educating their staff, and for no additional cost. Hell, I'd proven you can save money and even make money by teaching staff and outsiders.

Instead, I focused my efforts on mentoring and helping my fellow coworkers. My experience in ER and trauma proved invaluable, and the staff would seek me out when they had questions or became overwhelmed with patient care. Whenever a critical patient entered the ER, I would be there to lead or assist, and slowly I saw the improvement, the increased self-confidence, and improved patient outcomes over the months.

Trauma, unfortunately, was still the weakest link for this reputedly certified level III trauma center. Strike One: Our trauma program manager, a full-time nursing position, moved to Colorado soon after I hired on, and no one stepped up to take that position for almost four years. Yes, I considered the position several times, but major problems existed that would not be fixed without administrative support and the authority to effect those changes. Neither existed! Strike Two: Our "director" of trauma services was a prima donna surgeon who whined constantly and never wanted to be bothered with a trauma systems plan, let alone be bothered with a real dying trauma patient in the ER. Strike Three: *No* quality assurance or quality improvement program existed, a major component of any trauma program. A well-meaning but totally nonmedical secretary mismanaged the statewide trauma registry. No oversight, no critique, no review, no accountability. Completely unacceptable! Conspicuously absent were necessary trauma-related policies and procedures, a two-tiered trauma response criteria, and probably more than anything, consistent and effective leadership.

Hospital management was tumultuous and tentative when I began work on another saint's day, St. Patrick's, on March 17, 2008. My first manager, Greig Swiffer, was a good leader but a not-so-good manager, so one day during one of my shifts, Grieg was given five minutes to clean out his desk before being escorted off property by security. For the next few years, there was no real ER manager. A midlevel administrator filled in overseeing several departments. One of our own great ER nurses and my preceptor when I began there, Jeni Finger, subbed for several months but only managing the daily operations. Jeni was admired and respected and led from the front; she just didn't want to be full-time manager, and I don't blame her for her sage decision. Finally in 2010, a real ER/ICU manager was hired: intellectual, compassionate, professional, amicable, and classy in every aspect. She took over as manager, and an assistant ER supervisor was hired by her several months later.

Things just might be looking up. Little did any of us know how the politics of medicine would mutate over the next several months.

CHAPTER 14

Eve of Destruction

Pity? It was pity that stayed his hand. Pity and mercy; not to strike without need. Many who live deserve death. And many who die deserve life. Can you give it to them? Then do not be eager to deal out death in judgment. For even the wise cannot see all ends.

—Gandalf to Frodo, *LOTR*

Further polarizing America beyond the political arena was the fierce competitiveness of hospitals, the corporate mergers, micromanagement by JCAHO and the feds, shrinking profit margins, and the do-more-with-less corporate mentality that entraps us all. Wait until the Affordable Care Act is implemented!

My new manager—no, my new leader—Catherine Giampetroni, held a promise for improvement. She supported, comforted, listened, and acted on critical issues. There was, however, uncertainty in the air as physicians' groups sided with private HMOs and PPOs, and major hospitals were rumored to be in negotiations for a corporate merger that would affect where literally tens of thousands of "clients" would receive future health care coverage. Layoffs exceeded attrition during the corporate restructuring. No one's job seemed safe or secure.

The announcement was revealed that St. Joseph's Community Hospital entered into a merger with Froedtert and the Medical College of Wisconsin, and Community Memorial Hospital in Menomonee Falls along with the West Bend Clinics in 2008. Synergy Health had lost its community spirit, and local control was a thing of the past. Full implementation of the merger did not occur until June of 2011. This was the date Froedtert Health reemerged like the Phoenix with its new corporate logo and promise of everything bigger and better, faster and more cost-effective.

Meanwhile, trauma care still really sucked, and I was most vocal in expressing my feelings, finally reaching the receptive ears of Ms. Giampetroni. The trauma program manager (TPM) position, dormant and unfilled for over two years, was again revived, and she encouraged me to apply if for no other reason so that I could toot my horn during the interview and let others know how experienced I really was. During the interview I did just that but declined the position due to "scheduling conflicts." I pledged full support to the incoming TPM, and as a favor to Catherine, I prepared a needs assessment for our ER, a critical analysis of the necessary steps it should take to obtain or retain trauma center designation. She asked me to make the presentation to the St. Joseph's Trauma Committee Meeting *scheduled* monthly and *scheduled* for the following week on Wednesday, December 8, 2010. But there was another defining moment that was to take place within hours of our meeting together that would push me beyond the limits of conscious self-control. It was Friday afternoon, and my weekend was just about to begin.

Saturday, December 4, 2010, West Bend, Wisconsin

My day began earlier than usual due to the previous night's snowfall, so I rose early at 4:00 a.m., bound myself in long underwear, insulated Cabela's overall bibs, balaclava and goggles, wool scarf and hat, two pairs of mittens, wool socks and Sorel boots, all topped with my full-length oilskin duster coat, and blew the newly fallen snow into ever higher piles alongside the driveway with my snow blower. Fortunately, I had a forty-eight-inch snowblower attachment for my John Deere tractor that made the job much easier. I awoke Karen at 0500, and we showered and shared a light breakfast together before leaving for work, she earlier than me due to distance.

It was overcast gray and colder than a nun in a biker bar at 0645 when I drove to work. I had settled into the weekend position quite well. There were the few elite nurses who signed a contract with the hospital to work fifty of fifty-two weekends in exchange for special compensation. We contracted for twenty-four hours per weekend and were paid for thirty-six hours, ergo, a .9 FTE position. Work forty-eight hours in a pay period and get paid for seventy-two hours worked. Most nurses preferred *not* to work weekends, so the staffing was consistent and we soon became a tight-knit group that worked well together, knew each other's strengths and weaknesses, and anticipated each other's needs. It was still fun going to work, even when we knew we were short-staffed and understaffed and most likely going to get our asses kicked both Saturday and Sunday.

Shift change began at 0700, and we took report quickly to relieve the fatigued and bleary-eyed night shift crew. I did a cursory check to see if anyone called in sick for the day and checked the doctor's call schedule. That can make or break a work shift depending who is on call. Our ER doc was new, but one of our growing favorites, Dr. Robert "Rob" Riependorf, a quiet, unassuming, analytical new graduate and welcome addition to the infinity physicians group. The trauma surgeon was Dr. John Hamberline, a competent but outspoken and politically incorrect doctor and the only one I would ever trust to probe my abdomen with a scalpel. My trusted friend and charge nurse extraordinaire, Jackie Kaufman, was tasked with being charge nurse, triage nurse, and incident commander in disasters. We always greeted with a smile and a hug, as did the ER techs. Today was no exception, and when Missy came around the corner, she got a modified good-morning hug tailored to accompany her protuberant, gravid abdomen. The team was set, this was it; two RNs, one ER tech, one doctor, and fourteen patient beds. Our challenge for the day was "to let no one suffer unnecessarily, and no one dies on our shift." If we got a pee break and a lunch break, the shift would be considered a great success. Unfortunately, that is a credo that doesn't occur very often.

Part of the disappointment my wife Karen and I shared was the antiquated EMS system in Wisconsin as compared to California, and yes, even Montana! They were still twenty years behind Cali. Almost all the rural area fire and EMS were staffed by volunteers, but the city of West Bend Fire Department had the only paramedics in the county except for one small private ambulance company. The volunteers were a great bunch of well-meaning farmers functioning within a sluggish and outdated system. Emergency communications between prehospital personnel and the hospital were sporadic, inconsistent without a formal call-in format, and sometimes the med-net radio would be circumvented completely when they decided to call on their cell phones. Further complicating the issue, the radio transmissions were monitored and answered by the hospital greeter or other clerical employee up front in the ER waiting room, so oftentimes the doctor and nurses were not aware of incoming critical patients.

Thirty years prior, California had specially trained mobile intensive care nurses working in ERs receiving paramedic radio transmissions and EKG telemetry, relaying orders to them from the base hospital to be carried out. And there was always a dedicated full-time triage nurse!

This was not progressive communications, and today this sloppy lack of procedure would prove to be most detrimental. A *Sentinel* event!

Emergency departments can be very intimidating to patients and visitors. The overwhelming myriad of alarms constantly going off can be very distracting. There are IV pump alarms, cardiac arrhythmia alarms, EMS and radio dispatch noise, patient alarms, bathroom alarms, battery alarms, ambulance alarms, vital sign alarms, door alarms, alarm alarms. This particular day the alarms were in full swing by 1000, all the beds full, patient room alarms going off, while Jackie and I ran from room to room trying to keep up, sharing the occasional and well-needed smile and high-five in the Pyxis med room before running off in different directions.

While at the nurse's station, we heard a predispatch alert for a snowmobile accident just south of town on the radio scanner. It would be at least fifteen minutes before we would have to deal with that problem, and there were immediate needs to be addressed with our sick patients. IVs, EKGs, labs, x-rays, CT scans, and medications were needed for the majority of our patients, as well as entering the orders in the computer and documenting history, assessment, vitals, treatment, response, and reassessment in the EPIC Electronic Medical Record (EMR).

Dr. Rob, so named because his last name was so hard to remember when he started, was doing well keeping up, but things were getting dicey and the admissions were piling up. Patient admissions were always tedious and time consuming, but every effort was made to keep patient flow moving in the ER; but patients couldn't move if housekeeping had not yet cleaned the room or if there were no staff to care for the patient, if it occurred before/during/after shift change, during breaktime for the med-surg nurse, not available for patient report and handoff, whatever. There were always obstructions and bottlenecks to the process and an overly commensurate number of committees and ad-hoc subcommittees formed to devise new streamlined procedures to minimize admission times. Amazing to me is the fact that the same problems that existed thirty years ago are still in existence today. But I ramble. We kept our ears open for the EMS call on the med net radio in the background that never existed.

It must have been just before 1100, because I rounded the corner by the Pyxis med room and caught a glimpse of movement out of my right peripheral vision in trauma room 3 just inside the double sliding ambulance doors leading out to the heated indoor ambulance parking area. It was Tony, our 1100–2300 overlap nurse in the room with a single EMT, transferring a sleeping child from the ambulance cot to the ER gurney. The child seemed at peace, asleep, with nary a scratch on his perfect six-year-old snow-white skin. *Where did he come from?* I asked myself. We had not heard a word regarding the snowmobile crash. After my five-second-across-the-room patient assessment, none of that mattered anymore.

My mind and body went into that instinctive automatic overdrive mode that all great ER nurses possess. When the patient's skin is whiter than the white cotton sheet covering him, you are way behind in the assessment-plan-implementation-evaluation-reassessment algorithm if you have done nothing yet! It was obvious from thirty feet away that the young, lifeless obtunded body on the ER bed was either in profound uncompensated shock or dead. I ran into the room, rattling off WTFs right and left to Tony and the EMT while simultaneously ripping the phone off the fanny pack around my waist.

Tony and the EMT began CPR while I yelled as loud as I could from the most remote room in the department to all who might hear, "Code trauma, Code PALS, ER trauma room 3!"

After punching in the code number on my phone, the operator came on the line after half a ring. A strange, raspy, eerie voice interrupted a split second earlier, the oldies station KWTF puttin' out the jams. It was 1965 and Barry McGuire is trumpeting his antiwar classic "Eve of Destruction." Although released over fifty years ago, the song has become a classic with more contemporary "Axis of Evil" baddies. Ironically, a few months later, another Barry, Sergeant Barry Sadler, medic with the Green Berets, released "Ballad of the Green Berets," which I also adored and emulated immensely at the time.

The eastern world, it is explodin'
Violence flarin' bullets loadin'
You're old enough to kill,
But not to votin'
You don't believe in war,
But what's that gun you're totin'?
And even the Jordan River
Has bodies floatin'.

But you tell me
Over and over again my friend
Ah, you don't believe we're on the eve
Of destruction!

"Code PALS, Code trauma in the ER, trauma room 3 NOW!" I screamed, both angry and apprehensive, having been caught with our collective drawers around our ankles for a pediatric traumatic cardiac arrest. "Why the hell didn't you call us and give us a heads-up!?" I felt like yelling at the EMT but deferred that conversation for later when this shitstorm was all over.

Dr. Rob arrived in seconds, as did Jackie and Missy. Missy stayed to help me, and Jackie now had the remaining thirteen-plus patients in the department all to herself, to add to her multiple duties. All my other patients would just have to wait for the cavalry to arrive, but likely too late. Brendan, my unexpected six-year-old patient, was all that mattered in the whole world to me right now.

Ah, I loved Dr. Rob, and he did an excellent job for his *first ever* pediatric trauma code of his short medical career. I am never more abrupt or dangerous as when another life is in peril, and that is when that hidden, unforeseen force takes over in me and I cut right to the chase. A-B-C-D-E-F-G-H, just follow the alphabetic mnemonic of trauma, remember what you were taught, don't vary much from the recipe! Dr. Rob took the airway with RT and intubated Brendan on the first attempt, while other staff from the floor performed good CPR. I performed the clinical checks and confirmed ET tube placement with my stethoscope, and the ETCO2 monitor further confirmed placement.

Meanwhile, Tony had gone next door and came back with the intraosseous drill. *B-z-z-z-t-t,* and an intraosseous infusion was established after drilling a hole in his proximal anterior tibial tuberosity bone in his lower leg and attached to blood Y-tubing with warm 0.9% normal saline infusing wide-open on a pressure infusion pump.

As help quickly arrived, duties were assigned. The ICU nurse had a PDA for downloading all activity as it unfolded, every procedure, every med given, everything. RNs from the floor changed off every two to three compression cycles, pumping on Brendan's sternum one-hundred-plus times per minute. Pharmacy was available to provide IV medicine assistance and was busy preparing epinephrine doses according to the Broselow tape color-coding chart that I quickly placed next to Brendan off the pediatric crash cart. ACLS and PALS are both invaluable aids for drug administration, but I knew this patient needed blood, and he needed it thirty minutes ago!!

"Hey, Rob," I called from the foot of the bed.

"Yeah, Ron," he retorted, lost in a myriad quilt of emotions, decisions, and orders.

"We need blood! Can I order up some blood?" One look at Brendan and I knew he had already bled out!

"Yeah, yeah, whatever you think. Just do what you think we need."

I intuitively interpreted his response to indicate that was my carte blanche to do what needed to be done with no credit limit. He had enough on his mind being the HMFIC (not a medical term, but a slangy Marine term meaning *head motherfucker in charge!*).

I punched in the four-digit code for blood bank. "Blood bank," the lab tech replied.

"Hey, Sandy, Ron in the ER. I need four units of O-neg delivered to the ER for a pediatric trauma code, and I need them now, no questions asked. Have someone deliver them STAT to trauma room 3. If they aren't here in two minutes, I will hunt you down!" and then abruptly hung up. In a *real* trauma center, uncrossmatched O-neg blood would arrive via blood bank tech within minutes of any trauma activation in a cooled Styrofoam container with the paperwork as part of the trauma activation, but this was West Bend, Wisconsin, for dog's sake.

CPR continued while another RN started a second peripheral IV line that was also primed with blood Y-tubing for blood administration. No blood could be obtained for sample, so for now we would have no lab results. A beating heart was preferable. Epinephrine 0.2 mg, or 2 mL of 1:10,000 solution was given IV every three minutes with CPR and pulse checks. Finally the blood arrived from blood bank; it seemed like hours, but in reality, a breathless lab tech sprinted the hallways and stairs in record time and showed up outside trauma 3 in less than two minutes.

"Ron here!" I shouted over the din in the overcrowded hallway outside. "I'll take the blood!"

"I need a doctor to sign for it first," the young lab tech retorted.

I spun around and saw my doctor, Dr. Rob, leading his troops in battle to save young Brendan's life twenty feet away. He was right where he should be.

"No problem, here you go," I said as I scripted my best physician forgery in typical illegible fashion, grabbed the cold bags of packed RBCs, and dashed back in the fray.

Two units of blood now infusing simultaneously, one on pressure bag and warmer, the other bag of RBCs squeezed under the firm pressure of the hands of yours truly, I found myself for the first time skeptically hopeful.

Dr. Rob noticed my deer-in-the-headlight stare and gave me that "What?" expression.

"Remind me to tell you later," was all I could say. I know I broke some archaic rule, but like I said, when a life is on the line, I am more of the philosophic persuasion of asking for forgiveness rather than permission. Rob would later "countersign" the Blood Release Form, *as if* anyone could read the initial signature. I have always acted in the best interest of my patient and as a result have never been reprimanded or ever had a written patient complaint filed against me to my knowledge in over thirty years. This is not to say that I have not pissed off a lot of hospital administrators during my tenure; that I am proud to say is one of my strong suits. Choose your battles wisely.

Despite our most intense and invasive interventions, we were not making any headway in resuscitating Brendan. Did I forget to mention all the other distractions in the room? Oh, fuck yeah, parents, family, friends, EMS, sheriffs! Brendan's mom was never separated from his side during the whole ordeal. God bless her! She never left his left side, kneeling down to see Brendan at eye level, never letting go of him for even a second and always talking to him. "Brendan, Mommy and Daddy are here. Don't you give up. You come back to us, don't give up! We love you, please live!" Brendan's dad was pacing frantically like a caged carnivore, although not causing disruptive behavior necessitating security's intervention (that's a laugh!). He was in total denial and disbelief, screaming and lamenting his grief, banging his head and slugging the walls while running from the room, down the hall, and in and out of the ambulance parking area.

Across the hallway in another treatment room was their best friend, neighbor, and driver of the snowmobile that had crashed with Brendan on it, who had minor injuries and was transported by a second ambulance, I later discovered. Friends, family, people wailing and flailing, curious gawkers from other rooms, fire, EMS, law enforcement, and media had swarmed the hallways, making for one of those chaotic ER scenes "*as seen on TV!*"

Focus on the ABCs. Trust your sixth sense. Don't lose the edge. Follow the recipe. Failure is not an option. Improvise, adapt, and overcome. Never leave your dead and wounded behind. Never leave your wingman. Never give up. Unfortunately, there was no progress despite nearly faultless treatment.

In nearly four decades of working in ERs, I have personally witnessed only *two* people who have walked out of the hospital neurologically intact after suffering cardiac arrest secondary to blunt trauma, and to this day I have no explanation why they survived and others did not. Both of them had emergent thoracotomies. One was a young male police officer wearing a Kevlar vest shot point-blank in the sternum by a perp with a 12-gauge shotgun during a botched robbery attempt back in the mid-eighties and only minutes from our doorstep. The second was a young male motor vehicle crash victim that literally exsanguinated (bled out) en route to the hospital in our helicopter. Our trauma surgeon, Dr. Tony Tam, performed an open thoracotomy, initiated open heart massage, defibrillated the heart with internal defibrillation paddles, clamped the descending aorta, then stabilized and transported him to the OR with my hands inside his chest, squeezing the blood in his heart with gloved hands until the leaky organ(s) could be repaired surgically.

"Ron, let's do a thoracotomy," Dr. Rob stated.

"A what?" I repeated, in a somewhat lower voice. Despite all the clamor and extraneous noises in the trauma room, I had a feeling where this was headed, and I got a sick feeling in my gut.

"A thoracotomy."

"Uh, that is likely not possible here, since we don't have a thoracotomy tray," I half-whispered. When I performed my Trauma Center Needs Assessment survey, this was a BIG RED FLAG, to *not* have a surgical open thoracotomy (chest) tray, but despite my recommendations, the issue fell on deaf corporate ears. Reportedly only one person, a long-time St. Joe's nurse who was our nursing supervisor on duty today, knew of the possible whereabouts, possibly hidden under other unused trays in the OR on the bottom shelf in some corner. If no one asks for it, who needs it, right? Well, I just had a new, talented pragmatic graduate doctor from medical school and four years of ER residency ask me for one, only to deny him and our patient the opportunity because we did not have one, at least not in the ER where one should always be, *if* one claims to be a trauma center. Ironically, and sadly, I was probably the only ER nurse who worked at St. Joseph's Hospital who had the experience and knowledge with performing thoracotomies and internal defibrillation.

"You're kidding!" Dr. Rob said incredulously.

"You're kidding!" Dr. Rob inculcated.

"I wish I were. We can MacGyver something together if you're insistent. You grab a scalpel and I'll have to be your rib spreaders. Not ideal, but…" my voice trailed off.

"All right, team," Dr. Rob spoke to the resuscitation team as a whole. "We've intubated Brendan and done great CPR. We've given him warm fluids and almost four units of blood. Multiple doses of epi have been given IV with continued asystole [flat line] on the heart monitor. We still have no detectable pulses. Pupils remain fixed and dilated, GCS remains 3. Can anyone think of anything we may have missed? Anything else we could try?"

"No, no, no, you can't stop!" cried Brendan's mom.

"We're not giving up, Mrs. Dobby." I assured her. "The doc is just soliciting input from staff, is all." All I had time to do was place my right hand on her left shoulder for affirmation and reassurance as she knelt unwaveringly next to the cold stainless steel gurney holding her pale, lifeless child's hand. My mind was still in hyperdrive.

"Psst! Hey, Rob. We can needle his chest. We don't have a chest x-ray yet [should have!], he's pulseless, and we've got nothing to lose. We have no idea what's goin' on in his chest, but likely there's blood somewhere in there."

"Yeah, yeah, that sounds like a great idea. Let's do it. Do you have the equipment to do it?"

"No problemo. I'll be ba-a-a-ck," I intoned in my worst Schwarzenegger impression. Sometimes you just gotta throw in some movie trivia humor to lighten up the moment.

Now, Dr. Rob was doing an exemplary job of managing his first pediatric trauma code, but are some of you asking yourselves, "Where the fuck is the trauma surgeon?" I certainly was. It would have been a tremendous benefit to have an extra set of experienced hands, eyes, and ears of an experienced surgeon to help manage an overwhelming situation. In their defense, St. Joseph's Hospital did page the surgeon on call and the other trauma team members per hospital protocol. What was out of their control was the phone system that provided service on the surgeon's right hip pager/phone. Surgeons are obligated to arrive within twenty minutes of notification for major trauma patients 80 percent of the time or answer and be accountable for their noncompliance as part of level III trauma center designation.

Later reported as a phone system failure, our beloved trauma surgeon was likely noshing with family on a snowy Saturday afternoon and totally oblivious to the horror taking place in the ER. But, alas, all is not lost. Someone reported seeing Dr. Khaled Mario, the director of trauma services, in the hospital doing weekend rounds on his patients.

Dr. Rob was distressed when he was notified that the trauma surgeon was not available or unable to be reached. Since I had yet to see a "trauma surgeon" show up at *any* trauma during my tenure at St. Joseph's and, since I had an already acerbic angst toward them and what they failed to represent, I passed it off with a shrug. I had already seen too many others die here due to apathy, selfish narcissism, and self-absorption.

My blood's so mad feels like coagulatin'
I'm sitting here just contemplatin'
I can't twist the truth, it knows no regulation.
Handful of senators don't pass legislation
And marches alone can't bring integration
When human respect is disintegratin'
This whole crazy world is just too frustratin'

When Dr. Mario was finally reached by phone, he reportedly became agitated and defensive. He was quoted as saying he had the weekend off and could not be bothered, even after he was apprised of the critical pediatric trauma patient, inability to reach the on-call surgeon, and our knowledge he was physically in the hospital. He hung up on the caller and left Dr. Rob wearing the albatross around his neck.

After I heard what Dr. Mario said, he ceased to exist to me. The intensity of my anger and subdued rage at this moment triggered my dark side to secretly hasten his long-awaited visit with the seventy-seven virgins. My peers had seen Angry Ron. No one had seen Raging Ron—yet!

"Here you go, Dr. Rob," I stated after returning from pillaging the *locked* needle drawer across the room. "For this, all you need is an alcohol prep, strong arm, and a big needle."

This was a truism I remembered from reading Samuel Shem's classic satire of hospital internship, *House of God*, back in 1976 right after reading J. R. R. Tolkien's *The Hobbit* and *Lord of the Rings (LOTR)* trilogy hiking the backcountry in Yosemite. I still suggest this satiric yet poignant book, as well as the book you are reading, as required reading before investing years of your young lives in the medical profession. The *House of God* was a primer back in the '70s. I typed (yes, on a Royal Typewriter) the "Laws," then reduced them in size on an enormous office printer and had the sheet laminated. It was a little frayed around the laminated corners but otherwise intact and readable when I retrieved it from my fanny pack (lovingly referred to as my "man pouch" by nearly all my female coworkers) late on the night of October 2, 2011. I had carried it faithfully in my man pouch every day for all my years in medicine. Reading it takes a more close-up look with my glasses on to read the print that seems to have shrunk and blurred over thirty-five years. Must have gone through the wash? HOG Law 6: "There is no body cavity that cannot be reached with a #14 needle and a good strong arm."

I handed Rob some Betadine and alcohol preps and a 16-gauge × 1.5-inch IV catheter. He was on Brendan's right side or left side of the gurney, me on the left. Brendan's mom was kneeling so close to me I think our hearts were beating synchronously. CPR was still ongoing, with RT interspersing ventilations during chest compressions. His pale, white chest bounced rhythmically above the white sheet, and his spirit hovered above the bed, smiling down on all of us.

There was some hesitation, at least in my space-time continuum, so I just acted. Prep the site. Locate the left midclavicular line (MCL), and then palpate the ribs. Find the third rib and then insert the needle perpendicular to the chest wall just lateral to the MCL, penetrating the second rib space while gliding the needle over the superior aspect of the rib to avoid blood vessel damage. Advance needle until a "pop" is felt as the pleural cavity is accessed. Advance the catheter over the needle, secure with tape, and place one-way valve if time allows. It's a serious invasive procedure I had performed hundreds of times over my career, yet I was not "certified" to perform it at St. Joe's. But this one held special significance, and I really did not consider asking permission or forgiveness. A moment frozen in time, never to thaw, always remembered.

Quicker than Emeril could say "Bam!" bilateral needle thoracostomies were performed. Blood came out of the needle on the right, so Dr. Rob asked for a chest tube tray. I probably overstepped myself again in this medical arena, but hopefully any statute of limitations attached to this medical snafu will have expired before publication. I've performed them as paramedic and flight nurse, as well as chest tubes. I was probably more proficient at chest tube insertion than some ER docs I worked with over the years.

A tension pneumothorax causes rapid hemodynamic decompensation and left untreated you *will* die. Add medical intervention like positive-pressure ventilation to chest trauma with often higher than normal physiologic tidal volumes and rates, add iatrogenesis to the equation, and things can go south quickly. The astute clinician will notice increased dyspnea, chest pain, tachypnea, hypotension, tachycardia, altered level of consciousness, hypoxemia, decreased or absent breath sounds over the affected side, hyperresonance on the affected side, and tracheal deviation toward the unaffected side of the neck. The ability to recognize and intervene before all those symptoms manifest is key to survival and improved patient outcome. You don't want to diagnose a tension pneumo with a chest x-ray!

The thora*costomy* tray (totally different from a thora*cotomy* tray) was opened utilizing aseptic technique. The insertion procedure went smoothly as expected, until Mr. Murphy unexpectedly showed up. Like most medical equipment, they come in smaller sizes to accommodate the pediatric population. Thora-Klex chest drainage systems were no exception, and they come in pediatric sizes or larger sizes with smaller pediatric adaptors. We only stocked the one-size-fits-all adult Thora-Klex with no pediatric adaptors; surely nothing sterile in our supply that would taper to adapt from suction tube to the chest tube.

Fortunately, Nurse MacGyver was working today, and Mr. Murphy was escorted out of the room. A smaller nontapered sterile adapter was pilfered from a Salem-Sump NG tube set, and with the expertise of MacGyver, several hemostats, safety pins, and nonporous tape, a sterile airtight connection was achieved. Blood flowed from the chest tube into the drainage container on the floor while donor's blood hanging above him flowed into his peripheral and intraosseous lines as fast as it could be pumped in.

CPR continued, IV epi was given every four to five minutes, and as more family entered the resuscitation room, it became strangely quiet and voices became hushed as one, partly for respect and consideration of patient and family, partly to acknowledge that the inevitable had finally arrived.

"I think it's time we called this," Dr. Rob mumbled.

"I agree."

Dr. Rob looked around the room, making eye contact with each person and acknowledging their somber nods of approval. Everything possible had been attempted to save this young boy, but this child had already been reclaimed by his Creator for an early release of human suffering.

"All right, I'm calling it. Stop CPR, turn everything off. Time of death 1210." Dr Rob humbly spoke, his voice choked with emotion. The proverbial pin could have dropped, and even Mr. Hearing Impaired, yours truly, could have heard it reverberate off the walls.

Dr. Riependorf and I both turned our attention to the parents and family of the deceased, Brendan A. Dobby, and offered our sincerest condolences. Brendan's mom, her heart smitten with grief, suddenly became withdrawn and quiet, while Mr. Dobby became very vocal. Cries and screams could be heard echoing off the walls throughout the department.

This event was far from over. I had to speak with EMS and law enforcement, then call the coroner, the organ donor network, and clergy and speak again with the family to discuss release of the body and funeral arrangements instead of how much the UW Badgers would win by in football today. Then the monumental task of re-creating the whole (non) resuscitation in minute detail in the patient's EMR (electronic medical record). But first, I needed to speak to Dad.

We met in the chilly ambulance garage, the lingering smells of diesel and oil permeating the cloud of death, Mr. Dobby amped out, still ranting in shock and disbelief. Brendan was "daddy's boy," and it showed. Despite experiencing death a thousand times before, this death struck a deadly blow to my psyche. To this point, I had performed with the highest professionalism, but here's two dads suffering a life-altering experience with the strongest emotions in the human playbook. It came easily for both of us.

"Hey, Mr. Dobby, I'm Ron. Brendan's nurse. I'm so sorry... for...your...loss," I said as the tears just flowed like a river during a warm spring thaw. Our eyes met, I opened my arms, and we met in a man embrace that lasted minutes as we just cried silently, holding each other tightly. We both channeled our chi, and a sense of calm overcame Mr. Dobby after several minutes. No more screaming, yelling, bashing. I'm sure guilt and remorse had overwhelmed his soul. We sat and talked for several minutes, me letting him speak about the good times with Brendan. I answered tons of medical questions as honestly and as truthfully as I could, and my answers gave him some solace.

In the meantime, Mrs. Dobby was seated in a chair just outside the trauma room when she suddenly threw herself to the floor and began wailing and screaming inconsolably. Another staff member took over her charge along with her other children. I finally met up with my charge nurse, Jackie, and Sue, the nursing supervisor. The department was utter chaos, and the prospect of taking care of another patient today was the farthest thing from my mind right now. I still had hours of work processing the still-warm remains of young Brendan, who was quickly assuming room temperature.

Despite the psycho-trauma of a child's unnecessary death, I was angrier than a mosquito in a mannequin factory over the total systems breakdown, from EMS not giving us a radio call, no thoracotomy tray, inadequate pediatric resuscitation equipment, no trauma surgeon response. Everything went as well as it could have given the circumstances; however, Brendan's death was testimony to a hospital misrepresenting itself as a level III trauma center. Accountability and responsibility are assets I list on my résumé. I expect my employer to hold those attributes as well.

I was sitting at the nurses' station staring at the EPIC charting software when I felt yet another unexpected emotional crash that overwhelmed me. A wildfire was burning out of control with no expected time of containment. I totally broke down in full view of my peers, patients, visitors. I explained to Jackie and Sue, as well as Dr. Rob, I was done for the day. There was no way in hell that I could go into another patient room and function to my expected abilities. My emotions were way out of control, and I really needed to chill. Sue quickly went to work calling our short list of off-duty ER nurses to cover my shift, as well as another ER tech. I learned later that my excellent ER tech Missy had experienced her own breaking point and couldn't continue her shift. She was eight months pregnant and had two children at home near Brendan's age. Her unborn child had felt the seism.

> *The poundin' of the drums,*
> *The pride and disgrace*
> *You can bury you dead,*
> *But don't leave a trace*
> *Hate your next door neighbor,*
> *But don't forget to say grace*
> *And, tell me over and over and*
> *Over and over again my friend*
> *Ah, you don't believe*

Later that day, I had the opportunity to speak with Dr. Riependorf. I learned only then that this was his *first* pediatric trauma code, despite years of residency in pediatric ERs. I told him about my document forgery to procure blood products. We hugged (yes, real men *do* hug!), shared some laughs, shared more tears, and parted ways after speaking with a few lady social workers who guaranteed us there would be a CISD posthaste. The nursing supervisor got a sympathetic nurse to come in to cover my shift that allowed me to follow through with the paper trail. The coroner was a friend and local volunteer fire/EMS who assured me he would give me a quick COD (cause of death). Content with that, I could not wait to get home.

After hours of contemplation alone, Karen got home from her ICU shift at St. Mary's Oz (Ozaukee) and immediately knew something was not right. Funny how a woman who shares her bed for over twenty years with a man can sense these nebulous feelings. While she changed out of her scrubs and put things away, I lit some Shoyeido Evening Zen incense, started a fire in the fireplace, and decanted a bottle of 2002 Sonoma County Cabernet.

We cozied up underneath our red fox faux fur blanket, then raised our glasses to each other, and I could see the sparkle in her blue eyes from the roaring fire.

"A toast?" Karen asked, quizzically.

"Yes, a toast," I responded hesitantly. I know it makes her crazy when I drag things out when I'm normally more decisive.

"To?"

"To us. To us moving back home to California. To us, to be with our children again. To us, to be back with our old friends. To us, to work in a real hospital that's cutting edge again. To us, to not have to plow any more snow. I think it's past time."

"Wow, sure I'm ready. Let's do it!" she replied confidently. God, I love this woman!

We talked on for hours about what had transpired earlier and discussed moving till the wee hours. The market was flat and not many people buy in December, but it was time to begin. That night I slept little; the strong images of the day were too frightening to invite sleep.

First thing Monday morning, December 6, 2010, I met with my manager Catherine and we had a long talk about the Saturday SNAFU. I gave my verbal two weeks' notice to sever my employment contingent upon selling my home. Someone, I was told, was working on the issues I had documented in the Post Trauma Critique Form. Remember, no radio call, no thoracotomy tray, no internal defibrillator paddles, inadequate pediatric chest tube accessories, failure of the surgeon notification system. I agreed to her request to attend the trauma committee meeting as planned on Wednesday. I explained I would be brutally honest and not pull any punches in my evaluation. Saturday only reinforced those strong feelings.

Karen was already taking down wall hangings and had brought home boxes from work to begin the packing process. Excitement filled the Martin household, but terror and anger filled the mind of the master of the house. I didn't know if I could carry the weight of another unnecessary death on my watch, ever. The fuse was growing dangerously shorter.

Wednesday, December 8, 2010, 0800 hours

The meeting took place in the swank Board of Directors room with long faux wood table with high-back leather swivel chairs. The usual Robert's Rules of Order prevailed. Minutes were read and approved, then on to old business. When new business began, Dr. Mario unexpectedly went off on a rant that would have made Dennis Miller chuckle. Since he didn't exist to me since his Saturday refusal to help out, I tuned out most of what he said and instead tuned in to KWTF…

> *Don't you understand what I'm tryin' to say?*
> *Can't you feel the fears*
> *I'm feelin' today?*
> *If the button is pushed,*
> *There's no runnin' away*
> *There'll be no one to save,*
> *With the world in a grave.*

At the end of his tirade, he even had the audacity to bad-mouth hospital staff for bothering him on his weekend off. He was sick and tired of being bothered by young, dying trauma patients, even though I cannot recall him ever showing up for a major trauma patient. Shortly after his rant, he tendered his resignation as director of trauma services. There were no objections to his decision; he was whiny and obstructionist, not to mention being a total asshole and a black mark on the human race. Good riddance.

Below is the Trauma Center Needs Assessment I presented to the emergency committee that day. Nine general areas of concern were identified as severely deficient. Item 3, "Restructuring of Trauma Activation Criteria," should have been a simple trauma policy with clear, concise anatomic and physiologic criteria identified. The policy was given to nurse Marcella Martin, the director of clinical services, where it had remained, lost and unapproved for over two years. When pressed for it at the meeting, she went to her office and returned, stating she didn't know where the policy was. Marcella was the anti-Ron, Bizarro Ron, the total antithesis of everything I represented. She was meddling, indecisive, monochromatic, pretentious, insincere, and a micromanager with no experience or credentials for the job.

Froedtert Health St. Joseph's Hospital
Level III Trauma Center Designation
Needs Assessment

1. Administration
   A. SJH Board of Director
      Letter of Commitment
      Financial support
      Transfer agreements

2. Physicians & Staff
   A. Surgeons—Clinical support
   B. ED physicians and staff

Conceptual support
Education (ATLS, TNCC, continuing education)
Job descriptions: Trauma Medical Director & Trauma
Program Manager

3. Restructuring of Trauma Activation Criteria
   A. Level 1 Activation
      Surgeon presence mandatory
   B. Level 2 Activation

4. Trauma Policy Implementation
   A. Multiple policies necessary

5. Equipment Needs
   A. Surgical airway
   B. Thoracotomy
   C. Internal defibrillation paddles
   D. Pediatrics

6. Performance Improvement & Patient Safety
   A. Peer Review
   B. Multi-Disciplinary Trauma Review

7. Education, Outreach & Prevention
   A. ATLS, TNCC
   B. Community involvement
   C. Disaster management
   D. Staff education & continuing education

8. Trauma Registry & Reimbursement
   A. State Trauma Registry
   B. National Trauma Data Bank
   C. UB-92 Trauma Billing reimbursement

9. EMS Pre-hospital Trauma Care
   A. Education

B. Call in format standardization
C. Disaster management

10. References
A. Resources for Optimal Care of the Injured Patient 2006: American College of Surgeons, Committee on Trauma (ACS-COT)
B. Advanced Trauma Life Support: American College of Surgeons, Committee on Trauma (ACS-COT)

I was so familiar with the ins and outs of trauma center designation that I could quote chapter and verse from the above references. I had gone through several trauma site surveys in the past and knew the critical issues all too well. As far as I was concerned, St. Joseph's trauma program was in total shambles. No trauma medical director, no trauma program manager, no CQI, no education, no training, surgeons who don't want to be bothered, no policies, no peer review. In short, major changes were needed. Major bottom line to take to the board of directors meeting: patients are dying unnecessarily!

When the meeting adjourned, I did not wait around to shake the outgoing director's hand. Everyone at the meeting knew what had transpired the past weekend. I just slipped out quietly to attend my second critical incident stress debriefing (CISD). Talking promotes healing, and I had some gaping wounds; you just couldn't see the bleeding from the outside.

Ah, you don't believe, we're on the Eve of Destruction!

CHAPTER 15

Go West, Young Man

*Washington is not a nice place to live in. The
rent is high, the food is bad, the dust is
disgusting and the morals are deplorable. Go West, young
man, go West and grow up with the country.*

—Horace Greeley, July 13, 1865

Summer 2011

It didn't take long for Karen to get in the spirit of moving. She has always been adventurous and loves to drive and travel. We began packing up nonessentials and storing them in our ample barn. The excitement of moving back to California kept us going through the winter months. Selling a home is stressful. We were great real estate "stagers" who took pride in our home, so it was always in show condition in case our realtor called with a prospective buyer while we were both at work.

Over the next year, we would lower the selling price of our home by over $50,000. The market was bleak, and we couldn't afford to take a loss, so patience prevailed over profit. The sale of our home was also complicated by our already planned three-week European vacation in August. That was going to happen, and the sale of our home would have to work around this engagement.

Karen's side of the family has dozens of relatives scattered over southern Germany, and most of them have come to America to visit. We were long overdue to see their country, so for the last five years we had slowly planned a European vacation as a twentieth wedding anniversary gift to ourselves. Every aspect of the trip was planned out, every step first-class. It would be worth the wait.

Summer came and went, and despite over thirty prospective buyers and two offers, our home had not sold. For the next month, nothing mattered but our extended vacation. With a house sitter and doggie hotel arranged for Casi, our malamute, we were picked up in a limousine and dropped off at the O'Hare international terminal. The next twelve hours flying in an aluminum human transport tube would be the only hardship we would encounter for the next three weeks. We drove over 2,500 miles all over Germany, Switzerland, Austria, Italy, and the Czech Republic in a luxury BMW hardtop convertible and stayed in five-star hotels when not staying with relatives. This was a once-in-a-lifetime luxury trip, and we had the greatest time of our lives.

It was fall when we returned to West Bend, and our realtor agreement was about to expire. Karen and I discussed taking a break and not listing the house until the next spring but decided to push on and keep it on the market since we were still getting lookers. We were almost half packed, and our barn was stacked high with rows of boxes and furniture. We felt displaced in our own home, not having a lot of our usual comfort items (hot tub, espresso machine, massage table). If only our home would sell, we could move back to California to be united with our family and friends and Karen and I could get nursing jobs in *real* hospitals again. We were both getting anxious to move, constantly looking at homes in California on the internet. I had already secured a realtor, a dear friend of over thirty years, to help us purchase our home out west. Just like in past moves, during the listing and sale of our homes, Karen became obsessed with DIY and HGTV on the tele when not watching the Food Channel. It's her way of coping and keeping her dreams alive, and I loved it.

Karen was happy in her ICU job, I was frustrated and looking forward to working in a real ER in California, and we both anxiously awaited change and challenge in a new hospital out west. Rainbows and unicorns. Hopes and dreams.

But dark angry clouds were gathering on the horizon, and Thor's thunderous rumblings intensified. An unexpected yet distinctly familiar storm was about to rain down with all of Mother Nature's fury, and I was in the eye of the storm. It would be a life-altering event.

CHAPTER 16

The Day the Earth Stood Still

*True courage is not about knowing when to
take a life…but when to spare one.*

—Gandalf the Grey

Froedtert Health, St. Joseph's Hospital, October 2, 2011

I have always been an advocate for hospital staff safety as priority one, but it wasn't until the attempt on my life with the shotgun-toting junkie that I donned cape and cowl to become a nurse crusader for staff safety. I was quick to point out real and perceived hazards to my supervisors, but I had already sustained over sixteen concussions in my lifetime to this point, and banging my head against the wall with an unresponsive administration was not in my best neurological interests.

Fortunately for me, nearly all our ER staff (nurse, techs, PAs, doctors) felt the same, and most of them were even *more* vocal than me in expressing their angst about lack of hospital security measures. Maybe my advanced experience had given me the strategic edge in tact. The warning signs were overt; the alarm had been sounded by ER staff. Only four days prior to the storm, my coworker Stefani, an excellent EMT and ER tech attending nursing school while working full-time, had sent an urgent email to our manager Catherine Giampetroni stating, "Someone is going to get hurt in this ER if something is not done now." That was September 29, 2011—that calm, still moment during a Midwest storm just before the tornado strikes. I was not made aware of Stefani's admonition until weeks later.

"Ladies and gentlemen, the story you are about to hear is true. Only the names have been changed to protect the innocent, and the dead...

"This is the city. West Bend, Wisconsin. I work here. I'm a nurse. It was early Sunday morning, October 2. It was colder than a witch's tit in a brass bra. I was assigned to the day watch in the ER division. My job was to ease suffering and let no one die on my shift. My partner Nurse Jackie is here. My supervisor is Louise. It was a typical weekend shift: short staffed, no overlap nurse during the busy afternoon time, and everyone tired from working extra shifts to make up for our huge pay cut from last June. My name's Martin. I carry a stethoscope."

With that lousy Sgt. Joe Friday personification behind us, Sunday was just another typical aforementioned day in the ER at West Bend. The love, camaraderie, and respect for my fellow staff members and their loyalty to get out of bed and drive to work in blinding snow, knowing what hardships lay ahead each workday, were responsible for me getting through a lot of shifts, even though I was twice as old as most of them and routinely gobbled Advil like Skittles to survive twelve-hour marathons, most with no breaks or lunch.

The day got busier as the hours passed, much like the lunch break most employees are afforded also came and went. Shoulder dislocation in room 8 requiring 1:1 nursing care during a conscious sedation procedure, chest pains, exacerbations of COPD, lacerations, and a seemingly nonstop flow of patients in the waiting room.

Since we had *no* formal triage, every time a patient came to the ER for care, the charge nurse, my partner Nurse Jackie, had to leave the department to go out and perform triage and assign an emergency severity index (ESI) number rating from 1 to 5—1 being emergent and 5 meaning we'll get to you but it's going to be awhile. The ESI scale is a five-level tool that is used in emergency departments to rate the severity and urgency in which patients are seen and treated. A cardiac arrest (ESI 1) or cardiac chest pain (ESI 2) always supersedes illnesses that can wait, like a sore throat or "I want a pregnancy test" (ESI 5). We don't care that you have no ID, no address, no insurance, no teeth, track marks, and someone broke into your home and only stole your bottle of 100 oxycodone tablets for your chronic pain from a car accident twenty years ago, and now, on Sunday, you need your prescription refilled. R-i-g-h-t! When there are only two and sometimes *three* nurses for the whole department, including the charge nurse, things can go south literally in a heartbeat. A lethal arrhythmia loomed not far away.

Much to the chagrin of administration, infection control freaks, and "the Joint Commission," nurses occasionally nosh at the nurses' station while simultaneously computer charting, talking to the ER doctor, and taking a critical troponin 1 lab value of 2.4 mg/mL from the lab tech while concurrently visually scanning and listening to the EKG monitor screens for cardiac arrhythmias for the whole department.

When we don't get our lunch break, we get hypoglycemic and crabby. A handful of M&Ms can sustain an ER nurse for thirty minutes and help mitigate an imminent estrogen or androgenic storm. Today was no exception. I was the M&M pusher, and all my coworkers were my willing return clients. With no hope for even a short break, let alone a real thirty-minute lunch break, it was a simple matter of supply and demand. The M&Ms, audaciously displayed in a yellow (unused) emesis basin, disappeared quicker than a female intern's virtue at a William Jefferson Clinton Cigar Club meeting.

While I was eating at the nurses' station doing the above tasks, I overheard the EMS med net radio in the background while quasi-ignoring the repetitive and irritating *clang-clang-clang* of the ambulance alarm indicating another ambulance had just arrived.

"St. Joseph's Hospital, this is Jackson Fire, Unit 12. We are en route to your facility with a fifty-two-year-old male patient accompanied by Jackson Police. Patient was found passed out on a sidewalk and has strong odor of alcohol on his breath. Vital signs are stable, but the patient is very uncooperative. He was placed in handcuffs by PD and is being transported to your hospital for evaluation."

All the rooms were full. The waiting room was backed up for hours. Jackie looked over in my direction and gave me one of *those* looks. We had worked together for so long that words were often unnecessary to convey one's thoughts. Her beautiful blue eyes batted at me, and I knew her exact thoughts.

"Oh, Ron, can I give this one to you?" she asked in her most demure voice. What could I do? Say no? Due to a lot of factors, some being age, experience, size, and being of the male persuasion, I was oftentimes assigned patients who were drunk, obnoxious, aggressive, crazy, or on death's door. I truly did not mind, because I was protective of *all* my staff, 95 percent female, whenever there were unruly patients. Often I would close the room's glass doors and curtains and have a serious one-on-one talk with the disruptive or aggressive patient after they had inappropriately touched or uttered sexually suggestive comments to my female coworkers. Behavior patterns changed dramatically after our hands-off discussions. Warren Beatty once said, "Always thank your nurse. Sometimes they're the only one between you and a hearse." I can speak their language and make my point crystal clear.

"*Si, no problema, senora.* Help me get room 5 out of here, and the bed will still be warm when this joker arrives." I could hardly wait. Due to budgetary restraints, a totally inept system for dealing with mental health and alcohol/drug-related patients, and the burden of the hospital to determine whether the patient is impaired due to his favorite inebriant *or* from getting drunk and then falling and striking his head causing a subdural hematoma, the average time from door to transfer to an appropriate facility took from four to five hours on average.

That knowledge essentially quashes the "Meet 'em, greet 'em, treat 'em, and street 'em" ethos of the ER. Some are truly metabolically or psychologically ill, but most are just an expensive five-hour endeavor in babysitting incontinent, obnoxious, stinky, snarky human parasites. It does get old though, seeing the same "GOMERs" (get outa my ER) who frequent the ER like a revolving door. Off to drug or alcohol rehab, only to return in a week or two totally shit-faced with a blood alcohol concentration (BAC) of between 0.35 to 0.60 mg/100 mL. In the US, most states cite a BAC of >0.08 to be legally intoxicated. Do the math; four to eight times the legal minimum, and still conscious! For a young or neophyte drinker, a BAC that high can be fatal.

I glanced up at the clock: 1625 hours, nine and a half hours into my shift and no breaks or lunch except for a handful of M&Ms, coffee, and 800 mg of Advil. Making it through the last three hours was going to be a challenge.

Republic of South Viet Nam, Summer of '69

Unbeknownst to me at the time, twelve thousand miles away on a six-hundred-acre farm in upstate New York in the town of Bethel in the Catskill Mountains, one of the most extraordinary musical events of the century was about to take place. Max Yasgur had provided his farm land for a three-day concert celebration that would bankrupt the sponsors but change the world. Think small yellow bird, friend of Snoopy and Charlie Brown. Yeah, Woodstock! My future wife PJ, whom I would meet two years later, was attending Woodstock while I was counting the days before I came home.

I was on the night duty crew, so I hadn't gotten much sleep before I set out to visit some of my Vietnamese friends in a small village about ten klicks south of Da Nang not far off Highway 1. My comrades all had other plans, so I decided to head out on my own. Stupid is as stupid does! Checklist: sunglasses, camera and film, gum and candy treats for the kids, M16 with two magazines. No flak jacket; it's too fucking hot already.

It was always an exciting challenge when visiting an American-friendly (at least during daylight) 'ville, or village, as everyone was warm and friendly, and I just loved the little children. If we did not win them over, they could grow up to hate and kill Americans. Today was no different. I visited with Lindas and her family, shared a meal of rice and "catch o' the day," and washed it down with a warm Tiger beer. The children all loved to be photographed, and it was an even greater thrill to give them their pictures and see their eyes light up with joy at a later visit.

The sun had moved far to the west and it was time to pay my respects and make it back to Highway 1 and hitch a ride back to base in Da Nang. Dark clouds were gathering as I departed, and the wind became so calm and still I could feel my heart beating in my chest. The temperature was at over 100°F, and the humidity was stifling, probably 90 percent or more, so my camos clung to my body like a second skin. Sweat rolled down my forehead into my eyes, stinging them continuously; the sweat ran down my arms in small rivulets before taking the huge plunge, landing harmlessly on my boots or the ground. When the wind calmed, it was like a signal flare went off nearby alerting all female *Anopheles* that a warm-blooded creature with six liters of prime O+ blood was in the area. Mosquitoes swarmed my body, and they were so thick I had to breathe through the nose or with clenched teeth, lest I swallowed some of the swarm.

I continued walking quietly through the jungle following a narrow, worn dirt trail surrounded on both sides with dense green growth. The stillness was unsettling to me. It reminded me of my days as a kid growing up in Kansas. My brother and I were latchkey kids because both our mom and dad worked long hours each day and didn't get home until late afternoon or evening, so my brother Rich and I had to fend for ourselves. We would often sit on the picnic table in the backyard my dad had made and gaze at the dark ominous clouds above, looking for funnel clouds while air raid sirens wailed in the distance alerting all in hearing distance of a tornado warning.

As my mind wandered about returning home, a special guest DJ on KWTF radio howled in my mind's eye. It was Wolfman Jack himself spinning the platters tonight. The impenetrably ambiguous refrain of "Blowin' in the Wind" rang out with acoustic guitar and harmonica as Bob Dylan's words resonated in my brain.

> *How many roads must a man walk down*
> *Before you call him a man?*
> *How many seas must a white dove sail*
> *Before she sleeps in the sand?*
> *Yes, how many times must the cannon balls fly*
> *Before they're forever banned?*
> *The answer my friend, is blowin' in the wind*
> *The answer is blowin' in the wind.*

It was but a few steps further along this windless lonely dirt trail before my life would inexorably change forever and the earth stood still.

At 1630, the beyond-obnoxious ambulance alarm wailed, signaling the arrival of Jackson Fire & Rescue. My patient was delivered to the still-warm gurney in room 5, vacated only minutes before by my previous and now discharged patient. I patiently listened to the medic's verbal report and then listened as Jackson police officer Jenkins gave his account. He stated that the patient was not officially under arrest, so we asked him to remove the handcuffs from his wrists that were secured behind his back so we could better evaluate and treat him.

James A. Carvelli was a fifty-two-year-old male with a long history of alcohol abuse and dependency. Once he was entered in the hospital database, I accessed his EMR (electronic medical records) and looked at past visits; this was not his first visit to the country club in the last six months for similar hijinks. JAC had unkempt hair, unshaven face, large bloodshot eyes larger than Marty Feldman's or Adam Schiff's, ruddy and puffy face, despicable oral care, and filthy clothes over his sallow, skanky skin that covered his lean malnourished body. He could have stood in as a stunt double for the pitiful but loathsome Gollum Smeagol in *Lord of the Rings*.

He arrived cussing like a sailor, calling me names I've heard a thousand times over. My partner Stefani and I worked quickly and quietly, placing soft wrist restraints instead of the handcuffs and securing them to each side frame on the gurney. Then we placed him in a gown over his birthday suit since we removed his smelly clothes so we could more effectively evaluate and treat him. Noninvasive BP, heart monitor, and pulse oximeter were placed and set to repeat every fifteen minutes. Next, Stefani started an IV in his left distal forearm and drew a "rainbow" set of blood tubes that would cover most any test ordered by the doctor later. Then a twelve-lead EKG was done. Simultaneous with all this, I performed a thorough physical exam by looking, listening, and palpating his body, then documenting my findings in the computer-based EPIC medical record.

Two other major evaluation tools still needed to be performed on the patient and documented. Every patient placed in *any* type of restraining device requires a physician's order with specific time periods, reasons for restraint, and parameters requiring meticulous documentation every fifteen minutes they are restrained.

The primary evaluation tool for assessing the level of impairment and treatment for withdrawal from alcohol is the CIWA-ar Scale (Clinical Institute Withdrawal Assessment, alcohol revised). It measures ten categories that are associated with alcohol withdrawal with each category measured on a scale of 0–7 except for Orientation, which measures 0–4. All subcategories are added to arrive at a final score from 0 to 67. The higher the score, the more likely the patient is to suffer significant withdrawal. It is not precise, as some categories are easily measurable, while others rely upon the patient's subjective responses, but it remains a fairly accurate and useful assessment tool. A threshold of <8–10 usually indicates minimal symptoms no longer requiring pharmacologic intervention. The protocol is discontinued once the patient has three consecutive CIWA scores <8.

> ➤ Nausea/vomiting
> ➤ Anxiety
> ➤ Paroxysmal sweats
> ➤ Tactile disturbances (itching, bugs crawling on skin, etc.)
> ➤ Visual disturbances
> ➤ Tremors
> ➤ Agitation
> ➤ Orientation
> ➤ Auditory disturbances
> ➤ Headache

JAC's first CIWA score was very high, I believe 27.

Do not think for a second that JAC lay patiently while each of these tasks were performed. He obstinately fought and pulled against anything we tried to do, which took much more time, effort, and inner strength.

"Fuck you, you motherfucker! I'm goin' to kill you!" he yelled to me.

"No thanks, I have a headache, *and* good taste," I retorted. "There are other sick people in the department, and I would appreciate it if you would keep your voice down and not use profanity." Yeah, right.

"Fuck you, you bitch!" he yelled at Stefani.

"That's not a nice thing to call a lady. Please don't say that again," Stefani replied.

"Fuck you, bitch, and you too!" he screamed, looking at me with wild red Schiff-ty eyes.

"Okay, you ready, Stef?" I asked.

"Officer?"

Both of them answered yes in unison. Urine specimen collection for urinalysis and toxicology screen was the final test to perform before we could wrap him in warm blankets and wait for the doctor and mental health to do their parts. It would surely pose another challenge. The sooner one gets it done and gets the results, the quicker we could transfer his sorry ass out of here.

"Then, let's git 'er done," I said in my best Larry the Cable Guy impersonation.

The police officer and I each took a leg and held them while Stef performed a quick in-and-out urine cath. Just as we were finishing, the officer let go of his right leg before I was ready and was promptly rewarded with a couple of swift kicks to the chest with the police officer witnessing the event from two feet away.

My feminine side overruled my impulsivity. "Listen, mister, you are not under arrest *yet!* Don't ever do that again or your ass is going to jail tonight. You understand!"

"Fuck you, you motherfucker! Leave me alone!" was all he could muster. Why bother? I thought to myself. One should know it's a frivolous waste of time to try and rationalize with a shit-faced drunk. Linda, a social worker for Washington County, had already arrived, but unfortunately, Mr. Carvelli was too intoxicated to be questioned. Stefani and I finally left the room with JAC covered in warm blankets under the watchful eyes of Linda and Officer Jenkins. CIWA score in hand, I sought out my ER doc or PA (physician's assistant) to get an order for restraints, a "banana bag," and an open-ended order of IV Ativan, a long-acting benzodiazepine to help ameliorate his symptoms based on his CIWA score, also giving me some breathing room to see my other six patients.

The PA, Beth Stone, wrote orders for labs, x-rays, head CT scan, IV fluids, and Ativan IV p.r.n. (as needed). The "banana bag" is a liter bag of isotonic 0.9% normal saline with multivitamins (MVI), thiamine (B_1), magnesium sulfate ($MgSO_4$), and folic acid. The MVI is dark malodorous yellow and turns the IV fluid yellow; ergo, "banana bag." I could give 0.5–1.0 mg of Ativan every fifteen to thirty minutes based upon his CIWA score until he scored <8. IV hydration and benzos should help him through this crisis or till 1900, whichever comes first.

The Ativan actually helped for a short period. JAC dozed/slept while we waited for lab results. Officer Jenkins had been tied up with Mr. Carvelli for over two hours now, and since he was asleep, he asked if he could go back to Jackson.

"Sure, go catch some bad guys. I think we have things under control here. Thanks for your help. See ya later," I replied. If ever in my life I could have eaten my words and said the opposite, this would have been the moment. It was almost 1815, just forty-five minutes left before shift change, hot tub, warm beautiful naked body snuggling next to mine, and an icy margarita.

Unfortunately for me, my life was about to take another dark turn.

The narrow trail I had occasionally traveled over the past year seemed eerily different today. Call it sixth sense, instinct, gut feeling, something just wasn't right. The trail meandered slightly to the right, taking me on a northeast heading toward Highway 1. The mosquitoes had taken several blood samples from numerous locations, so now I itched on top of the profuse sweating, causing further discomfort. The clouds were angry and dark, and daylight was waning.

Up ahead about ten feet I noticed the trail intersecting at an acute angle. In a few steps I came to the intersection and was surprised to see two children, a boy and a girl in typical black pajamas and ubiquitous conical woven bamboo hats. They couldn't have been more than twelve or thirteen years old. Because of the intersecting angles of the trail junction, they were facing slightly away from my position. Under normal circumstances, we would have just smiled, nodded, said hello, and continued on our separate ways.

Except this inescapably dark day, both children were not smiling and carried Russian Kalashnikov AK-47s!

The Ativan only worked for a while. Soon JAC was screaming and cursing again. During our short absence from the room, he had managed to urinate all over himself and the bed, concentrated foul-smelling urine trickling down all over the floor. His gown was soaked in urine, and he had managed to wriggle the gurney sheet into a ball along with his wet blankets. Attempts to clean and wash him were met by him clenching the linens in his hands and refusing to let go. He refused and again greeted us with the now familiar phrase, "Fuck you, you motherfucker! Leave me alone! I want to go home!" We certainly had other much sicker patients that required our care, so we let him ferment for a while in his foul-smelling urine. One of us literally had to check on him every few minutes to ensure he didn't get out of his restraints or pull out his IV. The time was 1830, T minus thirty minutes until my shift would theoretically end. I was hungry and had a full bladder; and the sugar boost from the M&Ms was long gone.

A full three hundred seconds had elapsed before the social worker Linda in JAC's room came out of the room and yelled for me to come into his room right away. She said there was blood everywhere.

Stefani and I rushed into the room to find that he had managed to pull and tug his wrist restraint until it finally pulled the plastic IV cannula in JAC's left distal forearm out. Sticky IV fluid and blood now ran all over the floor, and blood soaked the gurney, side rails, and most of his naked body.

We looked at each other with that knowing look, laughed at the folly of it all, and grabbed towels, four-by-fours, tape, and gloves. Stefani's smile was contagious, and she made me laugh a lot when I should have been screaming. She will make a great nurse someday.

"Okay, let's get the bleeding site covered and dressed, then we'll clean him up. We're going to have to release his left wrist restraint in order to dress his IV site and stop the bleeding. I'll hold his left arm while you slap a dressing on his arm."

So by now, nearly everything in a five-foot radius of JAC was splattered with blood, sticky IV fluids, all with a heavy undercoating of skanky stagnant urine. Everything was wet and sticky.

"Leave me alone! Fuck you, motherfucker, I'm going to kill you!" he intoned over and over.

I was temporarily distracted again by Wolfman Jack's platter selection from Dylan's 1963 album, *Freewheelin' Bob Dylan*, back when one could actually understand Bob's lyrics.

> *Yes, how many years can a mountain exist*
> *Before it's washed to the sea?*
> *Yes, how many years can some people exist*
> *Before they're allowed to be free?*
> *Yes, how many times can a man turn his head*
> *Pretending he just doesn't see?*
> *The answer my friend, is blowin' in the wind*
> *The answer is blowin' in the wind.*

Once his left wrist restraint was removed, his demeanor changed and his anger escalated exponentially. Stefani tried to cover his bleeding site, but he flailed his arm so wildly it became difficult to even keep it still, and tape sticks better to nitrile gloves than it does to wet bloody skin, so a usually simple procedure would take more than two people to complete. His left arm got loose, and he swung at both of us with his fist, blood flying in all directions from his IV site, then quickly went to work trying to release his right wrist restraint.

At this point, I instructed Stefani to grab his left hand and I would go over to the other side of the gurney to secure the right and hold him down from the right side. Things were spiraling out of control. Our main focus besides our personal safety was to prevent him from getting free and climbing or falling out of bed. Both siderails were still up at this time.

Stefani regained control of his left arm after getting struck with a fist to her shoulder. He twisted to his right while simultaneously trying to sit up and climb over the right side of the bed. I tried to hold him down, but he was slippery as an eel, and it was all I could do given the situation just to keep him on the bed. We were both engaged with all four hands so we had no way to call for help.

Then suddenly, Mr. Carvelli caught me totally by surprise. I was amazed at how he became like a wild animal and possessed astonishing strength. He had become Gollum at the base of Mount Doom in the desolate land of Mordor, fighting, swinging, kicking, biting, pinching, spitting. He swung his hips up and right. Both legs free, they became battering rams. Stefani grappled to gain control of his left leg.

The right leg still free found its target. Leaning over the side rails of the gurney had left my torso and head exposed. Still trying to keep him from climbing out of bed and making matters worse, I did my best to hold him down.

Thump, thump, thump! His coiled right leg landed several direct blows to my sternum, left ribs, and right side of my head as I turned away from his head kick. My head jerked back just as everything in the room turned intensely crimson red and reason was supplanted by madness and rage.

I glanced down at his exposed neck and remembered from my Marine Corps training how to crush a man's trachea with one well-placed punch just as things started getting dark, thinking, "I'm going to KILL HIM! I'm going to kill my fucking drunk, skanky, abusive asshole patient!"

I will never forget my Marine Corps basic training, because I have employed it numerous times and it has been responsible for saving my life many times over during my lifetime. Today would be no exception.

The two Vietnamese children stopped in their tracks when they saw me and stood motionless like two wooden statues. By sheer good fortune, my tactical position was favorable since I was facing forward toward them, and they were facing slightly away from me in a westerly direction at my eleven o'clock with the barrels of their rifles facing north.

Their dark wide eyes locked on mine, and mine fixed on theirs, unblinking. Even though my eyes burned from the sweat running down my face, and it was late afternoon with dark storm clouds overhead, there never was such clarity of vision and of all the senses.

The hair at the nape of my neck tingled and stood at rigid attention. My pupils were dilated, eyes wide and hypervigilant. My chest tightened, my breath deepened, and my heart rate accelerated and felt like it was going to explode out of my chest like an alien parasite. My abdominal organs shut down as blood was shunted from the gut to the brain, heart, and lungs. My mouth was so dry my inner cheeks stuck to my gums and teeth. I could smell the soil beneath me, the pungent aroma of the abundant foliage, and my own bromhidrosis (BO), caused by bacteria breaking down sweat into acids. My auditory sense detected the heart pounding in my chest and acknowledged the surreal silence of our surroundings; no wind, no birdsong, nothing. I sensed each and every one of the thousands of arrector pili muscles that contracted simultaneously on each hair follicle causing my body hairs to stand on end, making my skin look like saturated dripping goose flesh.

The sympathetic branch of my autonomic nervous system was in serious hyperdrive and had accomplished all those complex bodily functions in a nanosecond. Oohrah for hormones! My mind flashed back to my bike crash at age three, first day of kindergarten, first kiss in grade school, camping in Yosemite, Matterhorn Mountain at Disneyland, high school graduation, my only grand slam homer, my friends and family at home thirteen thousand miles away. My psyche peppered me with a myriad of rapid-fire thoughts all at once. *Is this really happening? Am I going to die? Are these two brother and sister? Where is their mom, and what are they doing carrying rifles of my supposed enemy? Are they VC, and if so, are there more VC heading my way? Do they want to kill me? How can I possibly get out of this? And where did all the fucking mosquitoes go?*

This moment would define me and likely haunt me for the rest of my life. The plethora of feelings, emotions, and major bodily functions under involuntary autonomic nervous system control and fueled by the endogenous catecholamines epinephrine and norepinephrine prepared my body for the "flight or fight" response that all primordial animals possess to help prevent them from becoming the catch of the day and tomorrow's leftovers for the hyenas and vultures.

In my short nineteen-year tenure on planet Earth, there were few days that I could recall that were major life-changing events. This day would definitely change the course of my life forever—assuming I made it out of this mess alive!

Klaatu Barada Nikto!

Those three words uttered by the dying humanoid alien Klaatu (portrayed by Michael Rennie) to Helen Benson (Patricia Neal) were to be delivered to Gort, the giant indestructible metal alloy robot in the event of his death to prevent the destruction of Earth in the classic 1951 sci-fi movie *The Day the Earth Stood Still.* Gort yielded to Klaatu's delivered message and delayed Earth's destruction and later brought Klaatu back to life aboard his flying saucer.

His journey to Earth was to warn world leaders about the careless use of nuclear weapons causing a disruption affecting the entire solar system. After he was unceremoniously denied an audience at the United Nations, Klaatu devised a scheme that would get the whole world's attention. At precisely twelve o'clock noon, a worldwide power outage caused a major planetary disruption for precisely thirty minutes. The Earth stood still!

It seemed to me that Klaatu had rendered a warning to the world and to me on this fateful day. It was twelve o'clock noon somewhere on Earth. The Earth stood still for what seemed like thirty minutes but in real time was closer to three seconds.

In boot camp at MCRD San Diego, we trained and qualified with the M-14 rifle, a 7.62 mm × 51 mm NATO (.308 Winchester) rifle. It weighed nearly eleven pounds with magazine and ammo, stood just over forty-four inches tall, had a muzzle velocity of 2,850 fps, and a maximum effective range of 460 meters. My unit was assigned M-14s initially, but the M16 had been in use in Viet Nam since around 1963 and the M-14 was being replaced by the next generation assault rifle, the M16.

Manufactured by Colt, the M16 utilized 5.56 mm × 45 mm NATO ammunition in a twenty-round clip (later modified to accommodate a thirty-round banana magazine). Its loaded weight was three pounds lighter than its predecessor, nearly five inches shorter, and much improved muzzle velocity (3,250 fps) and maximum effective range of 550 meters. Both "theoretically" could fire between seven hundred and eight hundred rounds per minute, but considerably less in a sustained fire situation. In full auto, firing off twenty rounds of ammo could take about as long for one to say "Holy shit!"

We were given no formal training on the rifle, and we were left to practice with them shooting cat-sized rats on our visits to the garbage dump, I guess. We were also not advised of its predisposition to jam when the round in the chamber failed to extract from the right ejector port. Maybe the data had not been collected, collated, examined, interpreted, and disseminated back to the troops by 1968. Mine had never jammed during test firing, so the aphorism coined by Thomas Gray (1716–1771), a British poet, historian, and scholar educated at Eton College, seemed suitable to the situation: "Where ignorance is bliss, 'tis folly to be wise." Only in this case, better to be alive and foolish than ignorant and dead!

The young trio of hesitant combatants continued looking into each other's souls through deep, dark, penetrating orbs for thirty minutes in Klaatu time, frozen in the fourth dimension, unable to move or speak. Almost imperceptibly I noticed an insidious narrowing of the boy's eyes and a twitch in his right arm (the one that extended to his index finger that was attached to the trigger of the AK). No one as yet had blinked, and the young girl just to his left and to my right two meters ahead at eleven o'clock remained frozen.

It was high noon on October 26, 1881, in Tombstone, Arizona, at the O. K. Corral. The moment of truth. Decision time. Live or die. Kill or be killed. What's it going to be, Wyatt?

It must have been 12:30 somewhere Klaatu time, because maybe three seconds had elapsed since our chance meeting at the trail crossing. The boy moved first, pivoting on his right foot, turning in my direction. As I iterated earlier, I had full tactical advantage. He and the girl had to turn their muzzles nearly 180 degrees to their right to point them toward me, whereas I had the barrel of my M16 pointed at them spot on. I had the selector switch located on the left just above the trigger guard set to full automatic when I left base, mainly because anyone who has been shot at or shoots at someone else is scared shitless, and full auto paints a wider kill zone, slightly increasing your odds of hitting someone.

Before either of them had moved ninety degrees right, I instinctively sent my brain an emergent message directing the motor neurons to transmit an urgent message to my right index finger, enabling it to flex at the proximal interphalangeal joint and remain so until directed otherwise.

Now instead of stop-action, as the world began moving again, everything occurred in slow motion. Five feet away from its target, the roar of my rifle interrupted the quiet stillness of the afternoon with startling, lethal, mechanical clarity. The first several rounds struck the boy, and then the girl, their bodies jerking in spastic disunity, skin and flesh ripped from their bodies, blood spraying everywhere. Their faces became bloody, grotesque, misshapen death masks.

Somehow in my mind's eye, the Wolfman Jack on KWTF interrupted my thoughts...

> *Yes, how many times must a man look up*
> *Before he can see the sky?*
> *Yes, how many ears must one man have*
> *Before he can hear people cry?*
> *Yes, how many deaths*
> *Will it take till he knows*
> *That too many people have died?*
> *The answer my friend is blowin' in the wind*
> *The answer is blowin' in the wind.*

Not five seconds had now elapsed since first contact, and just like that it was over. The smell of gunpowder, blood, and death now invaded the senses. Upon checking my weapon, it was found to have a spent brass casing in the breech; the ejected magazine still had five rounds in it. Damn, a jam in the Nam, Sam! Fifteen rounds were fired before an extraction failure had occurred, but I gave it little thought at the time. Clear the weapon and move on. Hmmm. I was one of the fortunate soldiers who did not have the misfortune of sustained battle on a regular basis to further test the extraction failure percentage.

I forced myself to take a breath; it had been thirty Klaatu minutes since I last drew breath. Training, instinct, and the will to survive had spared my life yet claimed two children. Gort's intervention could not change their sealed fates. I no longer felt the multiple red indurated *Anopheles*'s blood bank withdrawal sites. I no longer noticed the wetness of my skin and sweat-soaked fatigues. I no longer *felt*. What should I feel? I asked myself. Horror? Isolation? Remorse? Exhilaration? Resentment? Confusion? Empathy? Conflict? Emptiness? Guilt? Anxiety? Panic? Terror? Shame? What had just happened? Was it murder? Were these children really enemies of my country? Who really *was* the enemy? Was it child-slaughter? Was I a baby killer? Was it self-defense? Two enemy KIAs? What the hell are we fighting for? Don't ask me, I don't give a damn! My body was in that sympathetic autonomic "fight or flight" mode; I ended the fight, and now it was time for flight.

All I knew for sure was that there would be two less bowls of rice at their parents' dinner circle tonight. Two of God's children had just stood before me seconds ago; living, breathing human beings who would never again play in the mine fields, never have mutant children from Agent Orange, or live to see their children and grandchildren grow up.

Still fearful of others nearby who now would know my relative position by the distinctive sound of the M16, I hastily raced down the trail, leaving the children, possibly from the same village I had just left, lying where they fell dead. With twenty-five rounds left, I was not prepared for even a brief encounter. Mr. Murphy must have been following me that day; to make matters worse, those angry black clouds decided to drop their payload of stored dihydrogen monoxide in a deluge of rain that was so heavy it was hard to see far ahead. I only stopped running once to briefly throw up before making it "safely" to Highway 1 without taking one in the back of the head.

I quickly caught a ride north in an empty northbound Army canvas-covered (thankfully!) deuce-and-a half that dropped me off right at the east entry gate into Da Nang Air Base. Fortunately, the torrential rain had rinsed most of my bloodstained body and uniform, but later I discovered dried blood in the recesses of my face and neck.

Thus ended my days of Vietnamization and traveling to the outlying villes to make friends with the locals. The emotional toll that disastrous event had taken on me was immeasurable. My experience in no way could be compared to the physical and emotional trauma experienced by the grunts that were faced with enemy confrontation on a regular basis. Thanks to a caring sergeant major stateside, I was (unjustly, in my unsolicited opinion) exempted from that nightmare because of my intellect and worked on computers instead of participating in "search and destroy" missions. No way in hell did I feel the expected high of taking another life that I was so convinced of while sitting in my warm, secure home in Kansas. Quite the opposite.

I became isolated, depressed, withdrawn, and antisocial for a long time. Nightmares and graphic flashback reenactments haunted me in the shadows of sleepless nights. I was an emotionally fucked up nineteen-year-old who had tremendous difficulty dealing with my deep wounds on my own, and psychological counseling and postwar readjustment were not high priorities for the hundreds of thousands of returning veterans. Most younger Americans looked upon returning vets with disdain and hostility, no one wanted to hear our story, and even more importantly, we were not willing to talk about it; forty or fifty years later maybe, but not then.

It was not until thirty-five years later in 2004 that I first spoke about that infamous day with a social worker assigned to my disability claim working for the VA who was a combat medic with the Navy during Viet Nam and determined I had PTSD, which the US government, of course, *denied.*

There is not a day that goes by that I do not see the ghostly images of those children's faces, and the nightmares will continue to

invade my dreams. The last image etched on their retinas was a confused, conflicted teenaged bumpkin from Kansas and bright flashes
of heated gases and brass shredding their young bodies.

That day had even more profound meaning in other aspects of
my life as well. My desire to take another life had vanished. I realized
that I could make more of an impact in other people's lives by helping and healing than I could by taking another life. The horror I felt
toward taking two children's lives profoundly influenced me in my
decision to pursue nursing as a lifelong career. Those two children
were my inspiration to strive to be the best at what I did, to help others and give those fortunate few a second chance on life. Many other
horrible experiences occurred during my tour, but none affected me
with such intensity and mental anguish.

The other outcome of that iniquitous date in history pertains
to a more deleterious aspect of my life. Thirty years later, it was discovered that I had a chronic virulent strain of the hepatitis C virus
(HCV). During my investigation of the illness, my blood contact very
likely occurred during that brief bloodbath, slitting a man's throat, or
from the multiple air-propelled vaccination shots given during boot
camp. The government conceded infection from air propelled vac-
cinations was biologically plausible but reported no *proven* cases of
HCV. That practice has since been discontinued, and HCV infections
among soldiers have decreased dramatically since the Vietnam era.

Just a month or so after rotating back to the US in late 1969,
I was rejected as a blood donor candidate three times because my
liver function screening tests (ALT, SGOT) were very high, but they
were normal before leaving the US. I had done intense research on
HCV and was initially more knowledgeable than my treating family
physician. I also discovered that there could be more than 3.5 million
people in the US who have HCV, and as many as 75 percent of those
infected are totally unaware. An inordinate amount of those infected
are veterans, and Viet Nam era veterans comprise over 62.7 percent
of all veterans infected. One in ten military veterans has HCV; the
number jumps to over one in five for Viet Nam vets.

There was no reliable testing for hepatitis C until the early nine-
ties, and only in 2001 was there a specific test that was able to detect

99.9 percent of positive results, so most infected veterans like myself were chronic carriers for over two decades before even being diagnosed. The chemotherapy treatment in 2000 consisted of oral ribavirin and alpha interferon injections every other day for a year that I self-administered in my abdomen or let nursing students practice giving injections. The side effects of the drugs nearly killed me, yet I have coexisted with the disease for nearly fifty years and have learned to accept the devastating side effects over the years. Same response from the VA when I filed for disability for hepatitis C: *denied!* I felt abandoned and betrayed by my own government over a measly $125 a month.

The totally unexpected rage welling up within me had exceeded all the combined anger spanning the last forty years. I was once again placing myself, and my friend, in physical danger trying to protect a drunken, inconsiderate, and abusive patient. My head was reeling from the blows of his kicks. Just as I began to be consumed by blinding uncontrolled red rage and planned to strike back to protect myself, another ER tech, Kris Janes, walked by the room and heard a commotion, so she poked her head in the room and was aghast at what she saw.

"We need help now. Call a code green!" I yelled to her.

Kris ran out of the room with hospital phone in hand to call the operator to announce a code green, but more importantly, she shouted it out to the entire ER staff from the main hallway. Within seconds, there were ten staff members swarming over our exposed Gollum. Each of his extremities were seized by two staff members while Stefani's husband, Big Tom, RN, took JAC's head, deftly turned it ninety degrees to the left, and put him in a headlock while another placed the opaque netted spit mask over his head. I still had a very firm grasp on his right wrist and shoulder, and I admit to severely twisting his arm beyond the normal range of motion until it became still.

Heading up the rear of the procession was PA Stone. She sidled up next to me and gave me the most incredulous look. "Ooh, what are you doing to him, Ron? You're hurting his aaaarm!" she accusingly whined.

The smell of burnt wire permeated my aura as the motherboard in my brain had a giant meltdown. Blind rage filled every fiber of my being. My inner self was saying, "Fuck you, bitch. Do you even have a remote clue as to what just transpired here?" But instead, I found a crumpled piece of paper on the floor that was an as yet unused coupon for "One Random Act of Kindness," so I did the noble thing; I spun on my right foot and strode out of the room without speaking a word, throwing the symbolic coupon in the trash can on my way out. I sat down at the nurses' station, picked up the phone, and dialed the Washington County Sheriff's Department. I would never work with PA Beth Stone again. *B-i-o-t-c-h!*

"Sheriff's Department, Officer O'Neill speaking."

"Officer O'Neill, my name is Ron Martin, a nurse at St. Joe's ER. I need an officer to respond here to arrest one of my patients and I would like to press charges against him for assault."

"Did he assault you, Mr. Martin?"

"Yes, sir, he did, and one of my coworkers too. There were three witnesses including a Jackson police officer and social worker. This was my *third* serious assault at St. Joseph's involving arrests and charges being filed, all three attributed to alcohol."

"We'll send a unit over right away to meet with you and take any statements."

"Thanks, goodbye." I felt like a missile on the launching pad that had ignited its engines for takeoff, but some lackey forgot to untether the security chains. My chest hurt and my head throbbed. I made it to 1900! I gave report to Melissa, then finished up charting in Mr. Carvelli's EMR.

Now came even more documentation. The nursing supervisor Louise was notified. A hospital incident report form had to be completed and mailed to Employee Health. When the sheriff arrived, I gave him an oral statement then spent the next hour filling out a victim's statement. It kept me focused, and it allowed me to have minimal people contact.

An eerie presence appeared to add more insult to injury. The director of clinical services, Marcella Martin (no relation), my polar opposite, my Bizarro Martin, my antithesis, somehow materialized directly behind me much like Almira Gulch (aka Wicked Witch of the West) appeared in Oz after a house from Kansas fell on her sister, except no red smoke emanated around her. I would not doubt she flew on a broom to work.

"Ron, are you okay?"

The lackey who forgot to release the tether chains from the gantry structure must have atoned his sins, because I sprung out of the chair with thrust to spare.

"No, goddamn it! I am *not* okay!" I declared as I slammed both fists into the desktop while my afterburners kicked in and I flew out of my chair with surprising quickness.

"O-kay," Bizarro Martin meekly squeaked as she wandered off to perform some other nonessential task. At least she was away from me and out of my face. I was in no mood to talk to her. A familiar faint aroma wafted from her direction as she left. Now, what was the name of that perfume? Hmmm…Repulsion? Oohrah, nailed it.

It was past 2130 when I had finished filling out reports and documentation, and playing with the staple remover and paper clips, while eating my dinner at the nurses' station in obvious defiance of the sacred JCAHO scrolls. I almost welcomed some supervisor, albeit remote on a late Sunday night, to challenge me so I could bite her head off like *T. rex* in Jurassic Park and swallow it whole. I was really pissed off!

The oncoming night shift ER doc and trusted party friend, Mary Lewis, asked me if I wanted to be seen through the ER as a patient for my injuries.

"Thanks for offering, but I was supposed to be off work two and a half hours ago, and I just want to go home and go to bed. I have a class back here at 7:30 tomorrow morning. If I still feel this way in the morning, I'll go to Employee Health. They should have my incident report in their inbox by then."

So, fourteen and a half hours later, I arrived back home, happy that I had heeded the Grey Wizard Gandalf and chosen to spare a life, not take one. Karen had beat me home after working her twelve-hour shift at St. Mary's Ozaukee ICU and had a glass of cabernet decanting next to "Archie's chair." She has seen me too many times come home from a horrible day at the office, but she sensed something was frighteningly different this time. Our wine-enhanced debriefing went on as I ranted like Kanye West after losing best rap album to "a Drake" at the Grammy's. I was tired, frustrated, hungry, angry, incredulous, and I felt betrayed, abandoned, and powerless. I had a mandatory EKG class at 0730 the next morning, but we turned in well after midnight after watching Aaron Rodgers run for two touchdowns and pass for three more in the Packers rout of the Denver Broncos prerecorded on DVR.

Sleep did not come. My night was spent fighting the racing thoughts, flashbacks, and dark thoughts that attacked my brain faster than a knife fight in a phone booth. The pain in my head and chest continued to preoccupy my consciousness. Morning could not come soon enough. I still had a lot to get off my chest since last night, and I fully expected to speak with my supervisors directly after my mandatory meeting and a stopover at Employee Health to get checked out from my injuries.

Karen and I had only been back from our wonderful vacation to Europe three weeks prior. Each day we were there, I kept a detailed daily journal to chronicle the trip and for identifying and viewing photos later. Something in my head stuck during the crazy all-night mind trip I'd just experienced; the voice in my head said, "Start an ass-ault journal!" If this case turned out to be a felony case, I wanted to document, document, document—just like any good nurse. It evolved into a much more comprehensive piece in the healing process, as it gave me focus and a ready place to vent my intense feelings with no fear of judgment or reprisal. A log was kept on whom I spoke to on what date about what subject at what time. It proved invaluable as time passed.

I didn't have any answers yet. They were blowin' in the wind…

CHAPTER 17

End of Days

*Forgiveness is not always easy. At times it feels more
painful than the wound we suffered to forgive those who
inflicted it. Yet, there is no peace without forgiveness.*

—Marianne Williamson

*Froedtert Health, St. Joseph's Hospital, October 3, 2011,
0700 hours*

The next morning, October 3, I arrived early for my scheduled class,
only to discover that it had been canceled the prior Friday, but the
education department failed to notify me that not enough had signed
up and they canceled the class. I discovered this tidbit Monday at 0735
from someone in the education department I found walking the halls.
It was all I could do to maintain my professional decorum. I was barely
holding it together as it was, and this was another kick in the teeth.

As I rounded the hallway corner, I ran smack into my two bosses,
the aforementioned Ms. Catherine Giampetroni and the newly hired
ER manager, nurse-child, Lenore Limbs. At first glance, Catherine
knew something was seriously wrong by the forlorn, haggard look
on my face.

"My god, what happened to you, Ron?" Catherine inquired.

"Something horrible happened last night in the ER, and I was
coming to see you both to discuss it, but I need to stop by Employee

Health first and get checked out. Can I meet up with you in an hour or so?"

"I have an admin meeting at nine, but Lenore will be free to talk," she replied.

"Good. I've got a lot to say. See you in an hour or so."

Catherine was genuinely concerned by my appearance and gave me a big, warm hug. I think Catherine knew the basic premise of what had happened, the inevitable, and it had happened to the best, most well-trained nurse in the hospital. Dread filled her dark eyes.

Froedtert Hospital, St. Joseph's Hospital Employee Health, 0800 hours

Angelina Stefanovich, RN, nurse practitioner, was St. Joe's employee health nurse and workers' compensation nurse for the hospital, and she was wonderful, caring, compassionate, and a great listener. After consulting my previously filed incident report, she performed a thorough physical exam and medical history, then ordered a chest x-ray and left rib detail. Further, my blood pressure was extremely high, and she felt I was not cleared to return to work until I was evaluated by a doctor at West Bend Clinic (WBC) for my BP. My x-rays were negative for any fractures, but what it did not show was my broken heart!

After visiting Employee Health to open my *work-related* claim, I went straight to Lenore's office located in the bowels of the ER and closed the door. We had an intense one-hour discussion with most of the manic dialogue coming from me, which is unusual for my casual laconic laidback demeanor. Lenore was a new hire and younger than my grown children—well-meaning and kind, but inexperienced and naive.

Just as I walked out of Lenore's office, there was the ubiquitous Catherine standing before me and our eyes met. My eyes got misty, prompting another hug. We spoke briefly about the Day the Earth Stood Still, part two. She gave me another reassuring hug and whispered to me that I should see someone from EAP (Employee Assistance Program). She asked me if I would like to talk to the director of human resources, Doby Lowenbrau, thinking it would be beneficial to inform others about the southern direction the hospital was headed. I gladly agreed.

In the locked office of Ms. Lowenbrau, I prefaced my conversation by stating that what I had to say would be totally candid and would probably not be looked upon favorably by some of my superiors. I expressed my hope that what I divulged would not cause me to lose my job, but even if it did, I needed to express my concerns that were collectively shared by everyone in my department and most of the rest of the hospital.

Two hours were spent discussing understaffing with resultant low morale and staff burnout, unsafe work environment, no staff response to code census, code trauma snafus, no backup resources when we were overrun, lack of required trauma resuscitation equipment, trauma center certification issues, the Bizarro director of clinical services, and lack of administrative support. She assured me she would take these issues to the executive committee, composed of upper management including the CEO and CFO that coincidentally was meeting later that afternoon.

Still plagued by a splitting headache, I left the hospital and drove the four miles back home, took a Vicoprofen, lay on the couch, and watched our Milwaukee Brewers beat the Arizona Diamondbacks 9–4 in game 2 of the National League Division Series. Karen fixed a nice dinner, and I finally fell into a fitful sleep on the couch.

CHAPTER 18

Betrayal!

*Those who don't know the value of loyalty can
never appreciate the cost of betrayal.*

—Anon

Home, October 4, 2011, 1000 hours

The morning sun shone in through the eastern and southern windows of our 1890s farmhouse. It was a sunny, warm, beautiful day for working outside in the garden. Karen had gotten little sleep the night before, so she decided to sleep in. It was past harvest time, and we had put up more than one hundred quarts of canned veggies and frozen even more. We were blessed with the bounty God had provided. As a native Kansan, I have always had a fondness for the Kansas state flower, the sunflower. One of my God-given gifts was my green thumb; I routinely grew sunflowers eight to ten feet tall with flowers sixteen inches in diameter. This year was a record setter. The flowers were hanging in the barn, drying upside down, winter food for the local birds stupid enough to stick around Wisconsin in the winter.

But the sunflowers posed a problem; their stalks were two inches in diameter and their root systems were broad and tenacious. They surrounded my entire fifty-by-sixty-foot garden. I decided to pull every one of them out by the roots, load them in the back of my pickup, and haul them to the county refuse disposal site where the processed green waste was ground into free mulch. I drove my truck behind the barn near the garden and left the doors open with the stereo blaring '60s rock and roll while I worked.

The bed of my F-150 was overflowing with giant stalks, yet many more loomed in the once-thriving and now dormant vegetable garden. My headache had gotten increasingly worse, and a runaway freight train now rumbled in my head. Purple stars permeated the golden unicorns, and the cosmos twisted into a sparkling celestial pretzel. Lynyrd Skynyrd was playing "Free Bird" on the radio, then suddenly the bright sun overhead turned black as a sack of assholes, the world spun like a child's toy top, and the ground rose up to meet my face with a suddenness that sent me tumbling down the rabbit hole on my Mis-Adventure in Underland.

Everything ceased to exist until a beautiful elven face surrounded by a bright halo of bright light spoke as she looked down at me lying supine on the ground.

"Are...you...all right...Ron?" an angelic voice spoke. Karen leaned closer, the bright midday sun directly behind her head.

"What...who...are...?" I responded, dazed and confused.

It was 1230 when Karen decided to wander down to the garden to check on me and surprisingly found me diaphoretic and barely conscious lying on the ground not far from the truck that was still running. She stated it took great effort to get me loaded in the truck and drive me to the house where she somehow got me up the steps into the living room where I once again collapsed on the floor. She brought me food and water along with four Advil for my headache. After an hour with no relief in my pain, I could take the pain no longer and I asked her to drive me to the ER. Over the past fifteen years, with the exception of stitches in my head (duh!), every time I have gone to the ER, I have been admitted. So it is a rare thing for me to *want* to go the ER as a patient. As opposed to Karen who has never been a hospital patient since giving birth to Katy over thirty-seven years ago!

Around 1500, I arrived delirious and hypertensive back in my own ER. My blood pressure was 214/130, and the pain in my head was unrelenting. The usual "syncope workup" was ordered with EKG, comprehensive metabolic panel, CK and troponin, and head

CT scan. Hydromorphone (Dilaudid) finally mitigated my headache to a tolerable level. My BP had lowered somewhat from earlier, but I was still hypertensive. I was admitted to the telemetry unit with postconcussive syndrome and syncope, rule out seizure or cardiac dysrhythmia. All I remembered was that I required a nurse escort to get up to pee in the middle of the night. The following morning after repeat cardiac enzymes, I was discharged home.

The following day I had a 1000 follow-up reevaluation by Angelina Stefanovich at Employee Health. She deemed me physically and mentally unfit to return to work and called West Bend Clinic to schedule an immediate appointment to see the doctor for my high blood pressure, insisting I drive directly there to be evaluated by my doctor. Before October 2, my blood pressure had been normal, ~135/80. I was taking *no* prescription drugs except the occasional Vicoprofen for the painful exacerbations of my hepatitis C. My life's goal was to go to my grave taking no routine pharmaceuticals.

Dr. Robert (Bob) Gibson was no stranger to the ER, and he and I shared some intense moments recently in the ER when one of his young thirty-year-old female patients came in by ambulance one morning when he was in-house rounding his patients. Misdiagnosed by prehospital staff as a narcotic overdose and unresponsive to the antagonist Narcan, she arrived "fish breathing" and I immediately called a code. She was immediately bagged with BVM and intubated, but her condition rapidly deteriorated, going into cardiac arrest. Because she was a frequent ER visitor and well-known to me and the staff, we pumped her full of steroids and IV Solu-Medrol in addition to dopamine and Levophed after defibrillating her heart several times. The end result of an acute adrenal crisis almost claimed this young mother of three children. She finally saw an endocrinologist, got her steroids adjusted, and lived happily ever after…

So, we shared a common unbreakable bond similar to that shared by soldiers in combat, a sense of closeness and brotherhood that cannot be explained by mere words. He listened, he heard, he understood all my pain, anger, resentment. He also agreed that I was unfit to return to work and prescribed lisinopril 5 mg daily for my BP.

Later that afternoon, I met with Kerry Lampwick, social worker with Employee Assistance Program (EAP), a free service provided to all employees to provide early, temporary mental health counseling, family issues, etc. Maximum of five visits allowed I might add. I rambled on for my hour that seemed like five minutes, laying the groundwork for what had occurred over the last several days. She was very supportive and a good listener but seemed sadder than me and Eeyore combined. More than anything, I felt she wanted to go outside and puff on a cancer stick. She seemed unhappy and troubled and had smoked too many cigarettes for too many years. Nurses know just by looking, believe me. She listened quietly but offered no feedback at all!

My headache returned at 2100, refractory to repeated Vicoprofen (hydrocodone [Vicodin] 7.5 mg and ibuprofen 600 mg). I spent another fitful night sleeping on the couch so I wouldn't keep Karen awake in bed with my tossing, turning, and moaning.

At 0800 I was startled suddenly by a phone call from Angie, the employee health nurse. She also sensed something was not right. My BP was 210/120; she insisted I come see her and get checked out again. My lisinopril dose was increased to 10 mg daily.

Meanwhile, back at the ranch...Our ER went on ambulance diversion for several days due to dangerously low staffing levels. There were times when our ER was staffed by only one, yes, one ER nurse, after the department was short two nurses plus an extra night sick call. My heart pined for my coworkers, but it was not my problem. It was time to take care of me for a change.

Now ten days since my assault, Jules Sampler, RN, St. Joseph's workers' compensation nurse liaison, contacted me at home and was unable to answer most of my questions. Koran, the representative for Sentry Insurance, our workers' compensation carrier, stated she had received no paperwork from Jules Sampler. I sensed frustration welling up inside me. The individuals who should be most informed about my Worker's Comp claim seemed to be the most uninformed. Only a week had elapsed and things were getting hinky. My anger and stress levels were still beyond the red zone, and the hypertension and headaches were becoming as common as a high-paid hooker at a DNC political convention.

The following day I went to the sheriff's department and obtained copies of the case file and witness statements. I also discovered Carvelli went to Fond du Lac for alcohol detox, spent three days incarcerated, and was released. Koran called to advise that Sentry Insurance had declared my case "compensable" and checks should be forthcoming. I made another doctor visit to Dr. Gibson. He prescribed Ativan 0.5 mg every four hours and added clonidine 0.1 mg every hour to keep my BP < 160/90.

Two days later, on October 13, I discovered that my very supportive supervisor, Catherine G. was given five minutes to clear out her desk and was escorted off hospital property. Fired. No notice, no explanation other than "You don't fit here anymore," and out the door! I believe she was fired for supporting me and her department, and not fitting the preferred managerial mold of obsequious sycophant. A few weeks after losing her job, she was diagnosed with cancer. I could imagine the staff in employee benefits sniggering behind their desks. I had another follow-up visit with Karry Lampwick at EAP, more headaches, and my first normal BP reading in eleven days.

Over the next several days, I became even more agitated and frustrated when I was given more misinformation and misdirection from Ms. Sampler and Michelle from the Benefits Customer Service Center regarding my rights and benefits under workers' compensation (WC). None of my WC checks had arrived, and the hospital miscalculated my compensation based on the previous fifty-two weeks worked, which ended up paying me over $400 less than I should have received. I was told by Ms. Sampler that I had not worked enough hours to qualify (total bullshit) for FMLA (Family Medical Leave Act), so I only qualified for two weeks of FMLA leave. Ergo, since I had already missed two weeks' work, my position in the ER was forfeit and it could be given away.

That was another proverbial straw that broke the camel's back. The pent-up emotions of the past few weeks finally manifested itself in a monsoon of tears and uncontrollable sobbing that lasted five hours. The untimely news came just as I pulled up for a hair appointment with Charlotte at Creative Cuts. Charlotte cut my hair in silence without questioning my grief and didn't charge me or accept a tip afterward. Earlier that day I made first contact with my soon-to-be attorney, Monika Hartl, RN, BSN, JD. Her office passed my phone message to her, and she called me from *Italy*, where she was ending her vacation, and we made an appointment for the *next* day! Oohrah!

Sleep evaded me again that night, and I was having another intractable headache and a BP of 180/112 despite taking clonidine hourly. The pain was so severe I asked Karen to take me back to the ER, but she called Dr. Gibson's office and got an appointment to see him at 1040. Karen's assertive ICU nurse came out during the doctor's visit, and she insisted the meds I was taking weren't effective. He agreed, and I was switched to propranolol 40 mg twice daily and hydralazine (Lopressor) 10 mg every hour for BP > 160/90. He added Ativan 1 mg every four hours p.r.n. and oxycodone 10 mg every four hours for my headaches. The oxycodone unfortunately continued at increasingly higher doses and frequency for *six* years! That will require greater explanation in a later chapter. If this didn't work, he suggested admitting me to get my BP controlled.

Ninety minutes later Karen and I sat across from Attorney Monika Hartl and spent two hours consulting with her before signing documents to retain her as my attorney. She talked formulas and financial compensation and life-long salary replacement for lost wages, but I was more interested in justice. I'd take the money if we ever saw any. Monika was supportive and was a fast talker; luckily, Karen was there to interpret later, because my mind was preoccupied with pain, fear of having a stroke, flashbacks, and dark intrusive thoughts.

She felt reasonably certain I had a strong case, but it would take a while to arrive at a settlement. Until such time, I was a POW (prisoner of Wisconsin) and could not leave the state. It was almost winter, and our home was still on the market during one of the slowest times of the year for home sales, and this was a depressed seller's market. One day at a time, I thought. Just get through it. Persevere. Never give up. Improvise, adapt, and overcome. And, *never* fuck with a US Marine!

We spent over two and a half hours with Attorney Hartl, only to return to our parking space to find a $22 ticket for being thirty minutes late on a two-hour meter. At least my eighteen-hour headache had temporarily surrendered to oxycodone.

Five days later on October 25, Dr. Gibson increased my propranolol to 80 mg twice daily and added Micardis 80 mg daily along with hydrochlorothiazide (HCTZ) 12.5 mg daily. He also extended my time off work for two more weeks. It was twenty-three days since my injury, and still no check from workers' compensation; Koran said it was "in the mail" when I spoke with her. Because my psychological symptoms were getting worse instead of better after nearly a month, my doctor referred me to see a psychologist, Dr. Kelly Smerz.

Dr. Smerz has taken workers' compensation patients in the past, and treaded cautiously. She even wrote a letter to our comp carrier, Sentry Insurance, requesting permission to treat me prior to our first visit. She was approved by Sentry, so we had our first meeting on Tuesday, November 1. On the way home from our meeting, I had a minor meltdown; a lot of old and fresh wounds were opened. More locked doors would be breached and monsters freed from their dark sanctuaries before this would be over. It was decided we should meet once a week.

Meanwhile, vivid flashbacks of the assault infected my mind, and when sleep did come, which came more infrequently, my sleep was interrupted by graphic nightmares. The fatigue, the lack of sleep, the nightmares, and the nearly continuous headaches were wearing me down. My personality had changed. Human contact became repulsive; I couldn't stand to touch or be touched. I also felt like Austin Powers after Fat Bastard stole his *mojo*. My isolation became more intense. Since I had retained an attorney, I was given a gag order to not speak to anyone regarding my case. It could only be presumed that my ER friends were advised to sever contact with me as well, because my phone didn't ring much.

My headache had held sway over me for thirty-three hours at 0900 on November 3 when I contacted the district attorney's office to inquire about Carvelli's case.

"What do you mean? We mailed you a letter on October 6 with all the information. Didn't you receive it?" the receptionist asked.

"No, I have received no correspondence from your office."

I scheduled a meeting to meet with Mr. Peter Cannon, prosecuting attorney at 1100. In the meantime, I called Stefani and asked if she received a letter from the DA since she also filed charges.

She stated she got her letter two or three weeks ago. I drove to the hospital and went to the mailroom and asked around. No one knew anything. I checked with Dorothy, who was the ER mail guru, and she gave me the Sgt. Schultz "I know nothing" response. When we filed our statements for the sheriff, we were instructed to enter the hospital's address as our home address, so the perp could not easily locate us; really, all he had to do was look up our names in the phone directory—duh! In the ER nurses' lounge, each employee had a mail slot and I had a small mostly empty locker that I never locked. This is where we received hospital mail, memos, etc. When I visited Employee Health, each time for my checkups, I checked my mail slot before going home, and no such letter ever made it to my mail slot.

At 1100 I was promptly ushered into DA Cannon's office. He informed me that since I had not contacted their office, he was going to file two misdemeanor charges and accept a plea and probation, no jail time. I pleaded with him for felony charges and lots of jail time. He agreed to postpone the case, asked me to get Dr. Gibson to write a letter explaining my physical and psychological complications, and assured me I would be able to testify before the judge before sentencing.

More feelings of anger, betrayal, and abandonment surged in my blood. Had the hospital "lost" my letter from the DA in order to avoid a trial and bad press from the media? My headache was exacerbated by my conspiracy theory, real or imagined, my BP was up, and the pain meds were not working. Two hours later I was in the ER again. A follow-up head CT scan was negative for subdural hematoma, and several IV doses of Dilaudid once again masked the pain in my head where I could care for it at home. Finally at 1800, my headache went away after forty-two hours. When I lay down in bed, I was stricken with night terrors again and couldn't sleep. Another night spent staring at the ceiling from the sofa.

Two whole days passed without a headache before the dragon returned with its bare-toothed, flaming fury. At least four potential buyers looked at our home that day, and our realtor thought one of them was going to place an offer. My BP was 210/120 despite hourly 10 mg hydralazine × 4. Yet another trip to Dr. Gibson's office, and more pharmaceutical changes. Increase propranolol to 160 mg daily, increase Micardis to 80 mg daily, and increase HCTZ to 25 mg daily.

The Marine Corps celebrated its 136th birthday on November 10. We celebrated by selling our home! The interested couple from two days ago put in a generous offer and quickly accepted our counteroffer. Oohrah! Ten months on the market, and it sells just before Christmas. Who woulda thunk, huh? Let the serious packing begin!

The following day, Veteran's Day, I was scheduled to meet with Dr. Wojohowitz for an independent medical exam (IME), a meet-and-greet with Sentry Insurance's sponsored spin doctor. We met in his small office, which faced south and looked out over the huge busy parking lot through large floor-to-ceiling windows. I sat on a table in the classic open-back hospital gown watching spectators outside spectating inside while Dr. Wojo performed a most cursory exam. I performed more thorough physical exams on my ER patients that he did on me. Total time spent together was about fifteen minutes, and whatever decision this doctor came to would be binding for Sentry, overriding the findings of my private internal medicine physician and psychologist. And, he was not medically qualified to render medical decisions pertaining to my mental health.

Two weeks of intense furniture packing passed and still no checks from workers' compensation. I placed a call to Attorney Hartl and sent her an email. Later that day, I received a letter from Sentry Insurance denying my claim *entirely*. Mystery solved! Ergo, I had no insurance coverage, no worker's compensation benefits, and no money at all, thanks to my discompassionate employer, Froedtert-St. Joseph's Hospital.

Now a major conundrum arose. We likely would have to vacate our home before Christmas. I could not leave Wisconsin until the court case settled. So we had no place to live, no home, all our household belongings were to be placed in a long-term storage warehouse (our Harley motorcycles included!) at $1,300 per month, and our income had taken a spiraling $72,000 annual pay cut, which equates to around $125,000 in California if I ever worked as an RN there; my wife still does.

Mom and Dad to the rescue. Karen's parents Patrick and Rosie Meylor graciously opened their home to us and Casi, our eighty-pound Alaskan malamute. They live in a beautiful large home on historic Wisconsin Avenue just five miles west of downtown Milwaukee. On December 1, we moved into their spare bedroom on the main floor at one end of the house, offering relative privacy. They slept upstairs, and the basement was a music room, workout room, and rec room with pool table. Casi was eleven years old, and never lived near the city or around zooming cars and buses. She was a mountain dog who always had room to roam and was comfortable walking next to a horse or American bison (buffalo for y'all city slickers) but had no common sense in urban situations. Left off the leash, she would take off running, oblivious to city dangers. So, at least four to six times a day she would have to be walked on sidewalks around the city blocks to pee and poop. It really made me wonder sometimes who was the master of this relationship. Casi made me get up at all hours, follow her snuffling nose for blocks, then pick up her shit in a plastic bag and carry it back home for disposal. You the reader can decide.

Probably not on any son-in-law's bucket list of things to do before he dies, the decision to live with the in-laws in my sixties was actually an easy decision, because I loved them both and called them mom and dad also, and told them that in my heart they were my parents, as both my mom and dad had died years before. They were wonderful and gracious and made a difficult transition pleasurable. Dad is a vocal conservative who listens to AM talk radio and watches Fox News and *The O'Reilly Factor* and Sean Hannity with undying loyalty. If Karen and I were secular progressive liberals, we wouldn't have lasted there any longer than a Lindsay Lohan stopover at the Betty Ford Rehab Center. Fortunately, we were already O'Reilly fans, and we all agreed there had not been a worse, more corrupt usurper of the US Constitution than B. Hussein Obama since Tricky Dick Nixon.

We joined the Wisconsin Athletic Club (WAC) just one mile from home and ironically conspicuous in the shadows just across the street from Froedtert Hospital and the Medical College of Wisconsin, the level I trauma center. The WAC was a full-activity center with every known workout amenity. They had excellent yoga instructors, and they met at times that were convenient for both of us. Our mornings were spent from 0800 until around noon each day working out, practicing yoga, and soaking in their co-ed hot tub. On or about 1900 each night, Mom and Dad would bid us good night and retire upstairs to watch TV in bed, giving us total private access to the main floor. They awoke before us and ate their breakfast before we rose.

The one communal time was evening dinner. Mom cooked on days that Karen worked, and Karen agreed to cook on her days off. The guys were the real winners here. We were not allowed to pay them for living in their home, so we splurged on lavish dinners prepared by my lovely gourmet cook wife, and exposed Mom and Dad to great cheese, hearty breads, and organically cooked meals. Salsa and horseradish were still frequent table condiments. We even had desserts with relative frequency, a heretofore no-no in both households. We continued to drink great cabernets and merlots while Mom and Dad maintained their perversely misunderstood loyalty to the four-liter red box wines. A good time was had by all, and looking back, view those days spent together with fond memories and great times together.

Some things did not change. Like my uncontrolled blood pressure, almost continuous headaches, and my PTSD. Weekly sessions with Dr. Smerz continued with regularity, but progress was slow. Dr. Smerz wholeheartedly agreed that the incident of October 2 caused me to experience post-traumatic stress disorder.

Furthermore, this horrible event triggered the release of repressed memories that had remained conveniently locked away in the brain vault for years. Now my memories of the horrors of war returned with a fiercer intensity. Nightmares and graphically vivid reenactments of the thousands of patients whose tragic gory deaths I witnessed visited me nightly. I was so sleep deprived that I desired sleep but was also paradoxically apprehensive, because the demons still ruled the night.

More often than not, I spent more nights "sleeping" on the sofa, which equated to staring at the ceiling all night, in the living room because my erratic behavior prevented Karen from sleeping. The only caveat was that the sofa was right below Mom and Dad's bedroom upstairs, and many nights I would awaken them or the whole household screaming out during many of my nightmares. Many nights I lay wide awake counting the number of ambulances racing to Froedtert during the night or counting the number of times the snowplows passed the house.

On November 11, Dr. Smerz advised me that Sentry Insurance, who had previously approved Dr. Smerz, had now refused to pay any of her medical bills and totally denied my claim as "not work-related." After two sessions and only ten days, Sentry denied the claim in its entirety, not from November 1 our first meeting, but from *October 2, the day of the assault.* So essentially, Sentry Insurance, Froedtert-St. Joseph's Hospital workers' compensation carrier, denied the whole existence of my claim and I was personally responsible for all my incurred medical bills! She casually dismissed it with a wave of her hand and said it was just part of the game that had to be played, and assured me not to worry. She even advised me that she would defer payment for her services until the case had settled; she knew I had a slam-dunk case.

The number of pharmaceuticals continued to grow as psych medicines were introduced to treat my PTSD. Unfortunately, so did the deleterious side effects. Sertraline (Zoloft) 100 mg daily, an antidepressant selective serotonin reuptake inhibitor (SSRI); and the benzodiazepine clonazepam (Klonopin) 0.5 mg daily; both had been proven clinically effective in treating PTSD. Zolpidem (Ambien) 10 mg nightly was prescribed for my sleep disorder. With the addition of these three medicines, it increased the list of drugs I was taking now to *nine!* Add propranolol, Cozaar, HCTZ, amlodipine, hydralazine, and oxycodone. Pharmaceuticals do not cure disease; they mask symptoms and create more problems with their multiple side effects. I could have secured a walk-on starring role in the *Walking Dead* without an audition, because I looked and felt like a zombie; no acting necessary, just pure raw, sluggish, starry-eyed zombie. Synthetic medicines have never been gracefully accepted by my body.

Taking greater than three prescription medicines has been shown to increase adverse drug reactions (ADR) and drug-to-drug interactions (DDI) exponentially, and with the addition of each new drug, the odds increase. The most common ADRs are gastrointestinal upset (99%), headache (96%), postural hypotension (95%), and vertigo (94%). All of them were nearly daily occurrences, plus xerostomia (serious cotton mouth!), confusion, loss of fine motor coordination, impaired concentration, increased fatigue, blurred vision, urinary frequency, and syncope!

Ironically, most of the side effects worked reliably well; however, the intended purpose of most of the drugs was ineffective. The five antihypertensives were not adequately controlling my blood pressure. The Ambien didn't help me sleep; a placebo would have been just as effective. The oxycodone masked and diminished my pain but rarely made it go away completely; maybe I could have taken more, but I carefully monitored how many I took each day and didn't usually exceed my daily limit. That's a road I did not choose to go down if it could be avoided. The PTSD/antidepressants only exacerbated my feelings of despair and distress.

Each time I met with Dr. Smerz and we discussed returning to work, she noticed my anxiety level spike upward. Besides my continued fear of experiencing a stroke, my greatest obstacle was returning to the clinical environment. I expressed to her that I could not go back under any circumstances. That uncrossable, intangible line between preserving life and destroying life was violated and had become indistinct since I consciously wanted to kill Carvelli. Trust was a big issue in this case. Could I ever trust a patient again to not strike out at me? More significant and much more frightening was how I would respond to a threat, real or perceived. I was terrified that I would now act instinctively without regard for the consequences of my actions. Retribution would be swift, deliberate, and unrestrained. Human touch, one of the most valuable tools in the Bat Utility Belt of all nurses, was lost from my utility belt and instead replaced with anthropophobia and mistrust. Another unrelated benign phobia I have is hippopotomonstrosesquippedaliophobia. Yes, it is a real word.

A later excerpt from yours truly during testimony at my third hearing on April 22, 2013, expressed my concerns that I

> *might reactionarily strike out and cause great harm to one of my patients…If I were touched inappropriately, anything could set me off but basically, yeah, just being hit, struck by a patient be it in an altercation from drugs, a head injured patient from a bicycle accident or a person with Alzheimer's Disease that is confused…I can't guarantee with certainty I won't hurt them. I would pretty much say that would be my first response. Somebody hits me; I'm going to strike back. Kind of like teasing a cornered rattlesnake. You are eventually going to get bit. Yes, my skills and training are—will be with me the rest of my life. But can I go back into the clinical setting and take care of patients: I would have to say my answer would be,* **absolutely not**.

Despite the continuity of my symptoms, it was approaching four months since the assault, and Dr. Smerz was tasked with imposing permanent restrictions for my eventual return to work. We discussed each bullet point in detail, and I suggested one final addition. When we finished discussing each item and finally agreed and settled on all items, a wave of relief flowed over me, bathing me in renewed hope. She had determined that certain psychological traits were permanent and that it was her opinion that I had come to an end of healing, meaning I would not get any better but could get worse. She confided to me that when she guaranteed me I would never be forced to return to patient care ever again, a profound calmness washed over me.

As much as I loved and enjoyed nursing for over thirty years, in my heart I knew unequivocally that the night on October 2 would be my Waterloo. Now it was official and signed by a licensed psychologist. She gave me a Return to Work letter to present to my employer, allowing me to return to work with restrictions effective February 15, 2012, about five weeks away. That night I slept like a puppy dog.

After over ten weeks, our home finally closed escrow on Inauguration Day, January 20. A huge snowstorm struck southeast Wisconsin and eight inches of snow fell in a few hours. We drove thirty-five miles north to the title company to sign papers and collect our money. The drive back to Milwaukee during rush hour traffic in a blinding snowstorm took over two hours, but we had a wad of cash for our last big move "back home" in California.

Snow was again falling heavily on January 25, 2012. The big day in West Bend Municipal Court was scheduled for 1315. I arrived early and met with Ali from the DA's office, who notified me that James Carvelli (JAC) was back in jail for probation violations and public drunkenness. He was twenty-fifth on the trial docket for the day, but since I showed up to testify, she had it moved to the top of the pile. His defense attorney, a public defender, was disgusting to look at. He was young, morbidly obese, wore a dark-blue suit whose shoulders were littered with excess dandruff, and poorly fitted, which accentuated his fat folds. His hair was unkempt, his skin unctuous, ruddy, and creepy. He was totally unprepared for the case as he had only learned twenty minutes prior that JAC spent the night in jail for alcohol intoxication *again.*

When JAC was finally ushered into the courtroom, he got the Martin Death Stare from me. When the judge discovered the public defender was unaware of his client's whereabouts only twenty minutes ago, the judge gave the fat man a strong admonishing glare and not-so-friendly dressing down for being an idiot. After the scolding, the judge rescheduled a new trial date of February 15, 2012, at 0800, ironically the day I was scheduled to return to work, with restrictions.

As the days came and went, I was still plagued by uncontrolled hypertension, the debilitating headaches, chronic body pain and fatigue from my hep C, and the omnipresent nightmares and flashbacks from past and present psychotrauma. I continued to see my psychologist and Dr. Gibson but also tried acupuncture and massage and continued my spiritual yoga practice. I was still an unwilling

POW stuck in Wisconsin until all this went away. We still enjoyed our special time with our parents, ate excellently prepared gourmet meals, and spent hours each week searching the internet sites for homes in California in and around the town of Oakhurst where our combined families' three children all attended Yosemite High School and grew up. It was "our hometown" more than all the towns and states in which we have lived.

On two separate occasions, we thought we had found the right home. It was a buyer's market as home values had plummeted and interest rates were extremely low. I flew out twice to meet with realtors to look at the homes we had only seen pictures of on the internet, and as a photographer, I know all the tricks of the trade like cropping; wide-angle lens shots; how to not show any deleterious signs of wood rot, erosion, and mold; and not show the house next door only twenty feet away. These two visits included some quality time with two of our kids, but the homes did not come close to matching our expectations or needs. You don't really know squat unless you see firsthand what and where the homes really are. They turned out to be disappointing cross-country flights salvaged only by a three-day visit with a few of the kids.

February 15, 2012

Today was showdown day at my hospital. The previous day I was contacted by Human Resources and asked to meet with several administrative types about my job status. The tribunal consisted of the polite director of human resources (HR); the emergency department manager, my "new" direct boss since Catherine had been fired a week after standing up for me and her staff; the totally inept micromanager director of nursing and clinical services; and the vacuous nurse representative from the hospital's worker's compensation department.

When I walked into the conference room, the ladies were all seated. I asked where the praetorian guards were as I laughingly envisioned two gilded Roman guards with chest-high shields, belts clad with razor-sharp swords, Mithril hauberk tunics, topped off with a long spear standing at attention on each side of the table. That was my overt way of criticizing the hospital for not having real hospital security.

The previous night I was awake all night with a horrible headache and out-of-control hypertension, so I really looked like Hillary Clinton on November 9, 2016, at 0337 EDT when she found out she lost the election to Donald J. Trump, a job for which she felt "entitled." You get the message, I felt and looked like shit.

HR began and did almost all the talking. She wanted to discuss the "harsh" restrictions imposed upon me by my doctor and psychologist and began very s-l-o-w-l-y reading each one to me and asked if these were in fact correct and if they were my ideas or those of my doctors. I iterated that the restrictions were the strict instructions from them with the exception of item 5, which I suggested to them as they would not have been aware unless you worked in a hospital.

To Whom It May Concern:

Below is a list of permanent work restrictions for Mr. Martin:

1. No work or contact in the emergency room/ department.
2. No patient contact or patient care.
3. Can only work day shift hours.
4. Work hours limited to 4 hours per day, 12 hours per week.
5. Cannot respond to any hospital "Code" involving patients, visitors, etc.
6. Because of chronic headaches, computer work should be limited with frequent breaks allowed.
7. No work in areas that involve high demands, fast pace, time pressures, or critical decision making.

I facetiously complimented HR for her great reading skills and confirmed that the permanent work restrictions read-back was indeed correct. My attorney informed me weeks before the meeting that it was the responsibility of the hospital to find me a job with my "restrictions and disabilities," not me. About three days before the meeting, I received a job offer working in interventional medicine in radiology caring for both inpatients and outpatients (like crazy ER patients). HR asked if I would accept the position and I explicitly refused as it violated nearly every restriction listed above. I informed them it was their responsibility to find me a compatible position in the organization.

HR informed me that it was my responsibility to log on to the Froedtert job website and search for jobs just like a prospective job-seeking new employee, resubmit my résumé they already had on file for five years, and they would inform me if I qualified. As an ER nurse, chief flight nurse, trauma case manager, education manager and instructor in BCLS, PALS, ACLS, PALS, EMT and paramedic instructor, mentor to new nurses and paramedic preceptor, trauma program manager, and excellent policy writer spanning four decades, it seemed the administration could surely find me a position meeting my restrictions. Nevertheless, I did apply, at the direction of my attorney, for two non-nursing positions. One I didn't "qualify" for and the other Froedtert-St. Joseph's never got back to me.

Each one of my permanent work restrictions had merit and were resolutely explained and defended with calm, eloquent elegance by my psychologist during her four-hour testimony during my court hearing, including cross-examination by the snide, eye-rolling, debasing Adam Henry (AH is a LEO radio acronym for "ass hole") hospital-appointed suit, Snidely Whiplash. She also stated in her report that I had reached the "end of healing," which essentially meant my condition would never improve but it could get worse. Certainly, it was not worth me killing or maiming a patient to test the theory. I agreed.

Some excerpts from my psychologist stated,

> *On October 2, 2011, the patient arrived in the ER by ambulance. He was physically combative and verbally aggressive. Patient was placed in restraints so that he would not pull out his IV. However, several hours after admission, the patient managed to pull out the IV, was bleeding "everywhere" are [sic] urinated on the bed. Patient's left arm restraint was released to address the bleeding. While Mr. Martin and a care tech attempted to physically restrain the patient while they addressed the bleeding, the patient began kicking. He kicked Mr. Martin several times in the head and chest. He also threatened Mr. Martin stating "I'm going to kill you (Mother Fucker)."*
>
> *...It is my professional opinion that this incident was a direct cause of Mr. Martin developing an anxiety reaction in the form of posttraumatic stress disorder (PTSD) and secondary depression. Mr. Martin has had a very distinguished professional career in critical care nursing, including his role as the chief flight nurse in a Flight for Life program in California. But for the incident of October 2, 2011, I believe Mr. Martin would still be working in his role as an ER nurse and would not be experiencing the symptomatology for which I have been treating him.*
>
> *My diagnosis of PTSD is based on Mr. Martin's presentation of the following symptoms: 1) Mr. Martin experienced the incident at work as a direct threat to his physical well-being. He also began to fear for his life when the patient indicated wanting to kill him. He experienced an intense fear reaction. 2) Re-experiencing symptoms: Mr. Martin reported a ruminative preoccupation with the event, with recollections being intrusive, bothersome, and unresponsive to his efforts to distract himself or con-*

trol the thoughts. He reported nightmares about the incident, intense anxiety in reaction to the thought or returning to work, and physiological reactivity in the form of hypertension. 3) Avoidance symptoms: Thoughts of returning to work triggered anxiety, panic, and difficulty coping. Patient also manifested symptoms of depression and attendant features of anhedonia. 4) Hyperarousal: Sleep disturbance, concentration difficulties, and anger issues have been prominent since I began treating this patient.

Mr. Martin is unable to return to work in any type of inpatient, hospital setting. The cumulative effect of occupational stress, combined with the 10/02/11 incident, has compromised Mr. Martin's ability to tolerate stressful, face-paced [sic] work environments where critical patient care decisions must be made under time pressure.

My attorney also scheduled an independent vocational evaluation by a certified private vocational rehabilitation specialist from the state of Wisconsin, Department of Workforce Development. His conclusions supported the imposed restrictions and placed me in an odd-lot employment situation, meaning that I had total loss of earning capacity for workers' compensation purposes.

Then of course, the hospital sent me to see their company-paid obsequious sycophant psychologist for a comparative psychiatric evaluation. He was actually very personable, but he emoted more than the villain in a melodrama in my opinion. He complimented me way too much, praised my "exemplary" professional nursing career, called me a living war hero, and oozed so much sugarcoating I felt like I needed to take a shot of insulin (I'm *not* a diabetic!). We only talked for maybe an hour, versus weekly visits with my own psychologist over a period of nearly eighteen sessions; then he gave me a battery of three psychological evaluation questionnaires containing over 450 total questions. An MPS, a TSI-2, and one more I do not recall. I'm sure he and especially Froedtert-St. Joseph's were hoping these tests would discredit my case.

Well, ESAD (eat shit and die), ye nonbelievers and agents of lies and betrayal. The tests confirmed exactly what my doctors had been telling my employer for months: the patient has a serious case of work-related PTSD and secondary depression, anxiety disorder, sleep disorder, chronic headaches, and hypertension. It made me feel like Mad Bum, Madison Bumgarner, after setting several World Series pitching records during the SF Giants World's Series in 2014. No time for gloating, but at least four independent medical professionals now agreed and it proved I was not malingering or making up symptoms. My physiological responses were overt and statistically measurable (BP, no sleep, weight loss, anxiety, headaches, and syncope).

Time passed and the winter was record-setting for snow in Milwaukee for the third straight year. I was forced to retain my POW status until the case settled. Routine turned to boredom, boredom supplemented my depression, and the depression urged me forward to finish this unholy nightmare a winner. We continued searching for homes in our hometown on the internet, but the choices that met our criteria were scarcer than a Vespa scooter at the annual Sturgis, South Dakota Motorcycle Rally.

Did you forget about my court date for my testimony, restitution, and sentencing trial date with Mr. Carvelli on February 15? It was postponed again until March 5 due to the evils of Satan's spirit, *alcohol.* So sayeth the church lady, and she scares me! I met early with Ali at the DA's office and met with the DA, Peter Cannon. I felt high because I awoke feeling rested, refreshed, no headache, and no HCV blahs. When I testified, I went on a rant that even Dennis Miller would have been proud and impressed, holding nothing back including the threats and foul language he used on October 2, 2011. It felt really good to say "Fuck you, motherfucker" out loud in a crowded courtroom!

Carvelli pleaded no contest and showed no remorse for ending my nursing career. The judge was going to sentence him to three months and six months probation, but after my testimony, he increased the sentence to fifteen months in the Washington County Jail and two years probation and was ordered to pay yours truly over $10,000 in restitution to cover my mounting medical bills. If I would have held my breath waiting for one penny in restitution from Carvelli, I would be bluer than Papa Smurf! Once again, since my injury of October 2 was "work-related" according to my employer, Froedtert St. Joseph's Hospital, they refused to pay my medical bills. My workers' compensation insurance carrier, Sentry Insurance, refused to pay benefits, stating my claim was "non-work-related," refused my claim retroactively from the moment of injury, and also refused to pay my mounting hospital and doctor bills and did not pay workers' compensation benefits to me. So the onus was upon me to pay the bills until this nightmare ended.

Just to exemplify the shortcomings, overcrowding, and lying running rampant in our criminal justice system, Carvelli spent less than three months of his fifteen months in jail. He was released "early" on June 6. Another roach released early to crawl around in society unchecked, no jail time, no rehab, no justice, and no cash for me, not that I had high expectations. I felt angry and betrayed once again by the court bargaining at the expense of the innocent victim. BOHICA (bend over here it comes again!), Ron, and don't expect any KY jelly this time. It reminded me of Sam Montalvo, the shotgun-wielding psychotic meth addict who tried to kill me in the ER eighteen years prior. His felonies were pleaded down to misdemeanors and he walked out of the courtroom a free man, no jail time except time served awaiting his speedy trial. The LEOs do their job, the attorneys prosecute, and the judges give little or lenient sentences to felons.

My trust in the criminal justice system has greatly diminished. B. Hussein Obama is emptying our prisons and released five dangerous terrorists from Gitmo for an American deserter and traitor, Bowe Bergdahl, who was dishonorably discharged but received no prison time from the military JAG.

Spring and summer slowly passed, and I continued to suffer from sleep deprivation, headaches, uncontrolled hypertension (still!), and my nightmares; and the dark still ruled the night. Each day we felt nearer to closure and the final testimony phase coming soon. We did normal summer stuff: barbeques, visiting friends and relatives, going to Brewer's games, and hanging out on Lake Michigan. On August 13 I finally received the long-awaited letter from the Department of Workforce Development with a hearing date set for October 8, 2012. My attorney said after this hearing, we could make plans to move to California. We could not wait to see our kids and not spend another winter in Wisconsin.

CHAPTER 19

Lookin' Up

Things do not change, people do.

—Henry David Thoreau

Melting snow, now brown slush, was the harbinger of spring in Milwaukee, the snow and ice thaw bringing forth hope of an early settlement to my case. In early April of 2012, Karen and I saw "the home" in Coarsegold, just seven miles south of Oakhurst. We decided to gamble again and hopped the red-eye to Fresno on April 16, then partied most the night with our son Eric and his girlfriend Heather. We got up way too early, but it had just snowed and the air was cold, fresh, and crisp, garnished with the smell of woodstoves and pine trees.

We looked at every home Mary Pence from Century 21 had to show in a twenty-mile radius from Oakhurst, even homes way above our mortgage comfort zone. It really was a no-brainer. The first home we viewed was the home we had been drooling over for two weeks, and no other home came even close. We spent several hours closely inspecting for mold, rot, infestation (OMG, yes), and plumbing (many leaks) and walking the perimeter of the vastly overgrown seventeen-acre forest surrounding the home.

The home was actually a complete horse ranch with fenced irrigated paddocks; metal no-climb fence; lighted riding arena; trails, long since overgrown; lighted corral; and a barn with 1,800 square feet of storage, tack room, and three air-conditioned enclosed stables.

The home was a 2,800-square-foot two-story with a spiral staircase leading upstairs to a bedroom/office that afforded views both north and south. The main floor had three full bathrooms, three bedrooms, a huge steeple-shaped twenty-eight-foot-tall great room that sported an inefficient noncompliant woodstove, and nearly floor-to-ceiling single-pane large windows facing north and south looking on high mountain peaks surrounding us. The master bedroom was nearly four hundred square feet with not one, but two large walk-in closets; the other bedrooms only had one large walk-in closet each. The en suite was big with two separate sink areas and a four-by-eight-foot sunken tile shower/bath with three separate showerheads on three different walls and a skylight above the shower. Shower for six, anyone? Got grapes? An attached two-car garage faced east with about one thousand feet of asphalt driveway with two circle drives and a remote-controlled gated entry to the property.

We loathed the carpeting, paint scheme, '70s kitchen appliances, inefficient windows, and fake wood flooring (poorly laid Pergo) with lots of "Waldos" in the great room. The entry tile and woodstove tile hearth were both ugly poorly done white marble, lots of "honey-do" repairs, none of which I could not fix/repair.

This was to be my new full-time job, to care for the animals; maintain and repair the ranch, home, and barn; and clear the property while cutting down hundreds of dead oak trees that had died from seven straight years of drought. I have a lifetime supply of *free* firewood, much cheaper than propane. These downed oak trees, of course, created huge brush piles that had to be cut, dragged, and stacked in huge piles, then burned during the winter months when allowed to burn by the San Joaquin Air Pollution Control District Hazard Fuel Reduction Program that one had to call each day to see if it was a "burn day." The good news was that the house was priced at nearly 50 percent of its sales price six years prior; the bad news was that there was already an offer placed on the home.

We spoke with our realtor Mary, a friend of nearly forty years, and she stated the one offer was a sight unseen low-ball offer from LA that the owner refused outright. On April 19, 2012, we submitted an offer and the following day on Karen's birthday ("420") it was graciously accepted. Did I mention that this was a "short sale," the ultimate oxymoron, and the last step taken before complete foreclosure proceedings began? Since I remained a Wisconsin POW, we could be patient until the sale completed and then move our belongings to California; the mortgage with property tax and insurance combined was cheaper with our down payment than the fees being charged for monthly storage of our possessions stored in a cold Wisconsin warehouse.

We flew back to Milwaukee with a renewed sense of purpose. Luckily, I had the forethought to not pack in storage our previous tax returns, income statements, and other important papers. We faxed documents back and forth across the country for months. Our broker/loan agent was our oldest son, Eric, who lives in Oakhurst and works for Pence Supreme Lending (now Granite West Funding, LLC), locally managed and owned by Drew Pence and his brother Jesse, sons of our realtor Mary Pence, and Eric's boss and BFF since childhood. It was quite the family affair, with all parties coming out ahead financially; everyone got their commissions.

Finally, the fog was lifting, and just like Archie Bunker's neighbors, the Jeffersons, things were indeed looking up.

CHAPTER 20

Movin' On Up

Trust takes years to build, seconds to destroy, and years to repair.

The remainder of 2012 passed slower than Congress passing bipartisan legislation. Tension, angst, frustration, and despair continued to manifest itself in unthinkable ways, as my adverse daily symptoms and drug side effects continued to exacerbate. The hearing date for October 8 was drawing ever nearer. A new ray of hope? We continued our established routines, went to Brewer's games, traveled to Door County, visited family, and marked off a big red *X* on the calendar each day before breakfast as *the* day grew closer.

When D-day finally arrived, I awoke with fever, chills, along with the expected headache, muscle and joint pain, and a BP of 206/116 (thank dog I kept a detailed daily journal during these years). Snidely Whiplash, the hospital-appointed arrogant, presumptuous, eye-rolling suit spent the whole day questioning my psychologist Dr. Smerz while I sat quietly fuming in my chair. The day passed painfully slow and there was not enough time for me to testify, so the judge ordered a continuance, date to be announced later.

Karen took me after the hearing to Eddie Martini's, a very expensive and chic restaurant, paradoxically also right across the street from Froedtert Hospital. I had not taken two sips on my drink before the big meltdown began. Uncontrollable shaking and sobbing brought many strange looks from the gathering evening crowd. My defense mechanisms had again surrendered completely, and I felt release, not embarrassment, for my behavior. It just was what it was.

Now we were faced with another long delay before the next hearing where I could speak my mind. Surrender was *not* an option!

On December 12, we traded our older Ford pickup and bought a crew cab Ford F-150 King Ranch with topper on the back for our much-anticipated move to California. It's un-American to own a ranch and not own a pickup, and I've owned one most of my adult life. During the transaction with the purchase of our new vehicle, we received a wonderful phone call from our realtor, Mary Pence. Our escrow had officially closed that morning, and we were now proud owners of a seventeen-acre horse ranch in Coarsegold, California, we named Martin's Flying Monkey Ranch. We bought a new truck and a new house all in the same day. Oohrah! It was truly a time to celebrate one small victory.

Despite our combined elation and euphoria, my sleep that night was interrupted with an apocalyptic nightmare of a modern-day US civil war with atrocities, mutilations, decapitations, and brutal take-no-prisoners conflict. I couldn't shake it, waking in a cold sweat, headache, and BP of 172/116! Still think PTSD is a pleasant mental illness to live with?

For the holidays, Karen and I flew to California and rented a huge chalet on Bass Lake, about five miles from Oakhurst and twenty miles from our new home. All our children and their spouses-to-be slept and partied in the chalet, and then we had the first official family Native American Indian herb smudging in our new home. We did some minor repairs, turned on the gas and electric (no heat or lights!), and walked our lush green, snow-tinged, mossy-smelling property several times, while concurrently in the planning, pragmatic part of my brain, I was plotting riding trails, tree-thinning mostly drought-dead oak trees, burning brush piles, and poison oak abatement. A local cleaning company spent one eight-hour day cleaning windows and scrubbing the house from top to bottom. A bug and bat exterminator followed with their toxic sprays and clever bat deterrents. Our house was definitely overrun by several nasty species, which had lived unchecked the last two years our home lay vacant. In a few months, I would come to realize just how true that was. We had a great visit with our kids, and they were all ecstatic we were moving back "home."

We got home on the red-eye flight New Year's Eve and arrived in Milwaukee at 0300. Waiting in our stack of mail was a letter stating the next, and hopefully last, hearing date would be Monday, February 11, 2013. More great news. I only had six more weeks to go. Ms. Hartl, my attorney, said I could be released from my POW status in Wisconsin and could move to California after the hearing.

One of my favorite pastimes during my internment was reading—books, journals, and almost any articles about PTSD, head injuries, depression, trauma to nursing staff in hospitals (and how hospitals try to discourage reporting and cover up the truth!). One day, I read an article on CTE (chronic traumatic encephalopathy) and realized I experienced many of the same symptoms.

On January 8, I spoke with Cliff Robbins, the brain study coordinator at Boston University. After a long talk, during which I briefly described my sixteen major concussions (now nineteen!), my sports and military history, it was determined I met inclusion criteria and became a candidate for brain and spinal cord study; the only caveat was that testing had to be conducted on postmortem autopsy. I kindly informed him my brain was not currently available for extracranial study but did register at Boston University's School of Medicine Center for the Study of Traumatic Encephalopathy. The day my spirit in human form assumes another energy path, my brain and spinal cord will be removed with no charge to my survivors to be studied for CTE. I even included it in my living will (durable power of attorney for health care) and am a card-carrying donor as well as organ donor. It is worthy of note and no coincidence that one of my favorite actors *at that time*, Will Smith, portrayed forensic pathologist Dr. Bennet Omalu in the movie *Concussion* that was released Christmas Day 2015 about his discovery of CTE.

I finally made a list of my known concussions, some of them related to me by eyewitnesses, and gave copies to my doctors, hospitals, and Boston University. The listings are terse but nevertheless inclusive enough to extrapolate serious chronic trauma to my head and spine. Below is that list:

Ron Martin Concussions:

1. 1952: Age 3. KC, MO. Tricycle over six-foot retaining wall onto concrete sidewalk, landing on head. Also head and leg lacerations, sutures.
2. 1957: Age 8. KC, MO. Bicycle crash on gravelly asphalt turn. LOC, multiple abrasions.
3. 1965: Age 16. KC, Kan. Baseball vs. head sliding into second base. Also facial laceration from player's knee to face. Taken out of game, sutures.
4. 1965: Age 16. KC, Kan. Football, helmet-to-helmet contact, with axial load on spine during football practice.
5. 1966: Age 17. Turner, Kan. Baseball, ran blindly into four-inch steel fence post chasing home run. LOC, taken out of game and carried off the field.
6. 1966: Age 17. KC, Kan. Football, helmet to helmet/ground. LOC, removed from game.
7. 1968: Age 19. Viet Nam. Basketball game. Jumped up, another player accidently ran into my legs, and I fell directly on my head onto asphalt. LOC, nausea, vomiting, headache.
8. 1968: Age 19. Viet Nam. Concussive blast from explosion. Blown backward about ten to fifteen feet from fifteen-foot rooftop onto hard ground below. LOC, shrapnel in left thigh.
9. 1970: Age 21. SD, CA. Hydraulic lift gate (400 lb.) fell on my head while sitting under gate working on truck. Hydraulic line burst. Ambulance to hospital. Compression of axial spine, ripped hair out by the roots. Fractures of T-4, T-5, T-6, and T-7.
10. 1971: Age 22. La Mesa, CA. Motorcycle accident on rain-slick on-ramp at 50+ mph. Not wearing helmet (no helmet law in CA 1971). Closed head injury, sprained ankle, second-degree leg muffler burns.
11. 1990: Age 41. Toele, UT. Solo rollover MVC at 65 mph. Concussion, head laceration, contusions.

12. 1998: Age 49. Modesto, CA. Tripped over family dog, head struck stationary cabinet with hyperextension of neck and unknown LOC. Lay on floor three to four hours with temporary paralysis. Karen came home from the movies with our kids and found me on the floor. Ambulance to level II trauma center. Admitted with C-5 and C-6 subluxation and permanent spinal stenosis.

13. 2003: Age 54. Livingston, MT. Weighted fence post driver slipped off top of post, full force onto top of head. LOC in pasture for unknown time.

14. 2008: Age 59. Livingston, MT. Shot rattlesnake under fifth-wheel trailer. Raised up quickly, hit head on sharp-edged angle iron. Fell to ground, head laceration, sutures.

15. 2009: Age 60. West Bend, WI. Retaining wall work, five feet below ground level. Rose up under my overhanging Ford truck bumper frame. Head vs. hard metal surface. Fell onto boulders. LOC, bruised ribs, neck and left shoulder pain/paresthesia.

16. 2011: Age 62. West Bend, WI. While working as an RN in St. Joseph's Hospital ER, assaulted by drunken patient, hit and kicked on right side of head and chest multiple times. Syncope, postconcussion syndrome, bruised sternum and ribs, blood and urine exposure. Developed chronic headaches, sleep disorder, uncontrolled hypertension (for over five years!), and PTSD (confirmed by five separate psychologists). Have not been able to work since assault on October 2, 2011.

17. *2015: Age 66. Coarsegold, CA. While raising garage door, two guide wheels on door track came off. Garage door fell on top of my head, knocking me onto cement floor and pinning me under garage door. Large head contusion, severe headache.

18. *2016: Age 67. Huntington, CA. I have been an expert downhill skier for over forty years. While skiing one early freezing morning at summit of China Peak, slipped on icy surface and slid two hundred yards face-first downhill on

bumpy ice. Skis did not release until I dragged them on the ice, then I flipped, rolled, and finally stopped. Brief LOC, severe head and severe neck pain. C-spined by ski patrol, transported to ski patrol hut, then ambulance to helipad, and helipad to level I trauma center by helicopter air ambulance. Concussion syndrome, right shoulder sprain, broken right ribs, and bilateral laminar fractures of cervical spine at C-2!

19. *2018: (May 12) Age 69. Flying Monkey Ranch, Coarsegold, CA. While trying to corral a male goat, missed flying tackle, then my left frontal lobe vs. four-by-four post in barn. Lemon-sized hematoma, abrasions to head, left shoulder. Down for twenty minutes before able to move. Three *symptomatic* hyperextension injuries to the cervical spine occurred within two weeks.

(* denotes concussions sustained after court hearing.)

These are all that I recall, or have been recounted to me by direct observers, friends, and relatives. Somehow there is a haunting absence of head injury from 1971 to 1990, the age period of high-risk male behaviors. Certainly, some likely occurred and passed forgotten, as my stubborn recklessness most assuredly continued during that twenty-year span. It does not include the subconcussive blasts potentially incurred while in Viet Nam with far too frequent mortar and rocket attacks in my 1968 and 1969 tour there.

In mid-January 2013 I flew back alone to California for a week and slept on the upstairs carpet with borrowed pillows and blankets provided by Eric and great hot potato soup from Heather. The inside garage was masked and painted (it never was painted and looked horrible). Satellite TV, phone service, and DSL were installed, trash pickup established, and the movers showed up the next day. It took two days to unload a fifty-two-foot moving van filled to the brim, and we were "downsizing" from a larger home in Wisconsin. All the boxes fit in the newly painted garage, and the onus was on me to set up the big furniture, most importantly our bed. Then a few days later I was leaving on a jet plane to Milwaukee to await the next hearing.

The hearing was scheduled to begin at 1300 and finally the judge and court reporter showed up and we began late at 1340. My BP just before leaving home was 200/124 despite my meds, and my headache was my main preoccupation. It was not as hard as I imagined, and it was not difficult to defend myself, the witnessed-by-many-incident of October 2, my character, professionalism, and terrible well-documented symptomology that was a direct result of the assault. I was examined and cross-examined by both attorneys until the judge ordered yet *another* continuance. This meant I would have to move to California and then fly back to Milwaukee sitting in coach round trip with my knees pressed on the seatback in front of me. At least we were on our way to California one way or another, which posed another conundrum.

Karen and I went window shopping at one of the nearby indoor malls to get out of the house. The weather outside was abhorrent for all but polar bears and penguins. We began discussing how we were going to drive the filled-to-the-brim pickup with an eighty-pound malamute taking up the back seat, as well as a stuffed Audi A6 from Milwaukee to Coarsegold with just the two of us. I did not feel physically capable of driving across town, let alone cross-country, and Karen had done almost all the driving since my hospital incident of October 2, 2011.

"I think we should rent a car trailer and tow the Audi behind the pickup and that way you can drive and I'll navigate," I said.

"Amazing, I was just thinking of the same thing. I don't think you should be driving cross-country the way you feel."

"I agree. With my headaches, dizziness, and uncontrolled BP, it might take us a week or more to get there. Plus, I'd be under the influence of all the pharmaceutical drugs I take."

"Then it's agreed!" Karen chimed in. She drove home in time for dinner with the parents. Dad stopped drinking alcohol for over thirty years, but in recent years, he had reacquired a predilection for inexpensive "box wine" with a spigot. That trait was not passed down to his only daughter, who has always possessed a keen nose and love of fermented grapes bottled with corks and expensive price tags.

The O'Reilly Factor was on FOX, a daily ritual in the Meylor household. To interrupt his program is a serious transgression, much like when some wives decide to vacuum the carpet in front of the TV when it's fourth and goal on the one-yard line with no timeouts and ten seconds on the clock. Yes, that really occurred in a prior lifetime.

Suddenly out of nowhere, Dad muted blathering Bill, tapped his thrice-filled glass of wine with a spoon, and said, "Okay, everybody quiet down and listen to me, 'cause this is some serious important shit." The alcohol had worked its magic, and Dad always talked much louder as if we had all suddenly gone deaf when he drank one too many glasses. We all tuned in and gave the elder sage our undivided attention.

"Your mom and I have been talking while you were out, and we came to a conclusion and there's no discussion about it."

"What are you talking about?" Karen and I simultaneously chimed in.

"Jinx, one, two, three," I jokingly interjected to Karen as I gave her a gentle love slug to her exposed arm. When I was a teenager, when two persons spoke the same thing simultaneously, whoever called jinx first got to slug the other in the arm or thigh, only we punched as hard as we could. Stupid game played with male friends only, and it toughened us up and formed a stronger nonsexual bromance bonding, I guess.

"We've been talking about your car situation when you two and Casi drive out to California, and we came to a conclusion. There's no discussion about it, and that's final!" Dad blared. "Your mom and I don't think Ron should be driving that far, so we have decided that we'll drive your Audi to California and you, Ron, and Casi can drive your truck and you'll be together. We'll leave a week later and take about a week to drive there. We want to stop along the way and take it easy driving out." Living in the same household for over a year, Mom and Dad had seen me lose my balance, pass out, experience the blinding headaches that confined me to the couch with sky-high blood pressures, and many other of my "weirding ways." We could see through the thin veneer of alcohol and recognize that Dad's words were full of sincerity, concern, and love.

"Wow!" Karen exclaimed, breaking the code of silence. "Ron and I were just discussing the same dilemma on the way home, and we thought we would rent a car trailer and tow the Audi behind us so Ron won't have to drive. Are you sure that you two are up for driving 1,500 miles and then flying home on a plane?" Mom and Dad would rather be hung by their thumbs than fly in an aluminum tube six miles above Mother Earth, so this was a huge sacrifice on their part, and they had done so much to help us already. At the time, they were eighty years old. That's what parents do for their children, don't they, no questions asked? Unconditional love.

"From the bottom of my heart, I want to thank you both for your generous offer. Your solution relieves a lot of stress on us. I just want you to consider what you've committed yourselves to, is all."

"We've thought it over for a long time, and we want to do this for you. This way we get to see your new home too!" added Mom.

Karen and I looked at each other through teary eyes of happiness and nodded to each other in agreement. What a strange twist of fate, even more eerie because all of us had been dwelling intensely on the same subject on this particular day and time.

Sharing the same thoughts simultaneously was not covered under the "Jinx, one, two, three" rules, by the way.

Moving day finally arrived on February 27. The back of the truck was filled with all the clothes not in storage, guns and ammo, and liquids not allowed by the moving company, including six cases of ten- to fifteen-year-old expensive red wines, just in case we got lost or stranded on our way. The back seat of our crew cab was stuffed with pillows, blankets, and dog-proofed with an old quilt on top of everything so Casi could have some space. Thankfully, she was a great traveler and lay down or slept most of the way. She wasn't one of those hyper dogs who have to have their head out the window with the wind blowing in her face.

Karen drove the whole way, and it's fortunate that she loves to drive—always has. Part of it is a control thing, I know, but to her credit, she is an excellent driver of both cars and one of the safest motorcycle drivers I've ridden with. Between sightseeing and navigating, I passed a good deal of time adjusting my heated leather seat in the full recline position, trying unsuccessfully to find a comfortable position or pain relief.

We left the morning of February 27 and pulled into our driveway in Coarsegold at noon on March 1, a two-and-a-half-day easy drive. As soon as we opened the metal entry gate to our seventeen acres, I opened the back door and let Casi loose to run at her new home. She had been virtually a prisoner since selling our home in West Bend and moving in with our parents. Unfamiliar with the lunacy of city living, she had to always be kept on a leash every time she went outside, and inside she lived in our bedroom. Our hearts lit up with joy, seeing her run amok, sniffing, peeing, and exploring. We had finally reached our destination after being POWs for sixteen long months. We were *home at last*!

CHAPTER 21

California Dreamin'

Nemo me impune lacessit—No one harms me with impunity!

On the first night in our new home, Karen decided to barbeque on the back patio. Our son Eric and his friend Matt Sands came over, and conversation and alcohol flowed freely as the tri-tip steak, baked potatoes, and corn on the cob simmered on our Charmglow barbeque. A pleasant time was had by all, and it felt really good to be closer to our kids again in the neighborhood where they all went to high school together, and I should never have to put the forty-eight-inch snowblower on my John Deere tractor again.

Just prior to their arrival, I opened the rear French door exiting to the back patio. The bottom portion of the threshold is raised slightly higher due to the exotic design of the doors. As I stepped out with my right leg, my left foot caught on the threshold lip and I felt my knee "pop." It hurt but I shrugged it off, since my left knee has popped since I had football-induced medial malleolus cartilage surgery when I was seventeen, though none of those hundreds of "pops" really caused distracting pain.

We slept in *our own* bed for the first time in nearly two years, and it felt really good. My body has endured more than its share of pain over the decades. In the middle of the night, I awoke with burning pain in my left knee. On closer inspection, my knee was warm, indurated, and the size of a cantaloupe. I knew right away that synovial fluid had extravasated throughout my knee area, and the swelling was putting pressure on nerves, tissue, and muscle causing the intense discomfort. The pain was intensely unpleasant.

By morning it was time to go to the Oakhurst Urgent Care. The unfortunate caveat was that Karen's health insurance expired the last day of the month of employment, February 28, so we had no insurance and decided before we left not to pay for the very expensive COBRA interim health insurance. I explained our plight to the staff and requested the doctor only remove the extra fluid causing most of my pain. No lab, no x-ray, no meds. We got a "room charge" of $1,500 and $300 in miscellaneous charges. We went to town and bought a nice knee brace and a pair of crutches. I decided to wait it out until Karen got a job and health insurance.

Of course, it did not take long for her to find a job. She was interviewed and hired at Fresno Heart and Surgical Hospital affiliated with Community Medical Center in a matter of days, working in the cardiac ICU caring for patients who have just had open heart surgery, receiving them fresh from the operating room with the surgeon, anesthesia, respiratory therapy, and a spiderweb of IV tubing, four to six chest tubes draining blood, Foley catheter to monitor the patients' urine output, endotracheal tube assisted by a pressure-controlled ventilator, fresh blood and fresh-frozen plasma (FFP) piggybacked into a central line site along with vasopressors (epinephrine, norepinephrine, neosynephrine, vasopressin, dobutamine, etc.), arterial line, nasogastric tube, and a host of hospital staff to stabilize.

It's a truly amazing job Karen does, and I am so very impressed with her skills and calm in stressful situations. She has them extubated and walking within a day of having open heart surgery! Anyway, with the job came a huge pay hike from Wisconsin wages and a great health insurance program, but we had to wait two months before it became effective, so I hobbled on crutches with daily temperatures in the one hundreds, another scorching drought-ridden summer in California.

Before my surgery, I received my final hearing date in Milwaukee on April 23, so I packed my bags and headed east solo on American Airlines walking on crutches. Of course, a blizzard decided to begin during my travel time at transferring airports (either Denver or Salt

Lake City, can't recall), which made for a more interesting trip. The small commuter jets with narrower aisles and seats closer made it a real challenge. I requested an aisle seat on the right side on all my flights and plane changes so my left leg that refused to bend enough for it to fit underneath the forward seat could be strategically placed so as to not trip flight attendants or passengers seeking to relieve themselves. Adding insult to injury, I had to change planes coming and going. The smaller jets were forced to park away from the terminal, departing the plane via portable roll-up stairs to the front of the plane for exfil, then an arduous walk on several narrow raised snowy walkways to the main concourse.

After a painful and stressful but no-fall-down-go-boom flight, I arrived safely in Milwaukee, drove directly to my lawyer's home, and discussed strategy for the next day. I could have not felt more prepared to testify and find some closure. Despite nearly two years of counseling, I still felt the sting of betrayal, had PTSD symptoms, headaches, and hypertension refractory to the barrage of meds my doctors prescribed. It was reported to me later that my testimony was awesome and flawless.

The only SNAFU that occurred during the hearing was when I tried to push myself up on the empty chair to my immediate left to stand during a break, the chair slipped on the recently waxed government floor tile and I went airborne, landing on the hard, shiny concrete floor—on my head of course. It was witnessed by both attorneys and the court reporter. When the judge reappeared and heard of the incident, he wanted to call for another continuance to which I voiced my discontent (through my attorney Monika) and told him I wanted to continue. The paramedics were called to evaluate me (and I *evaluated* them!) before he would continue the hearing, and they took my vital signs, performed a lousy cursory exam, then left when I explained to them I was okay and knew the signs to look out for more serious injury. Now my head was hurting more than before, and I could do nothing but persevere. A few months later, the unnamed ambulance company sent me a needless bill for over $500—and I didn't even want an ambulance called. It was the court's decision, not mine, but Ronnie Jim got hosed again and paid up!

We completed the hearing late in the afternoon, and Monika and Judge Martin were so concerned about my welfare they summoned security for a wheelchair and I was personally escorted to Mom and Dad's awaiting van at the curbside. We chatted along the way, and in my heart I knew then that I had won my case. The truth was exposed, the evidence was overwhelming, and the respondent, traitorous Froedtert St. Joseph's Hospital was in total denial and chaos.

Four and a half months passed by patiently waiting, and then on September 4, 2013, a final decision was received via mail in a pregnant manila envelope from the State of Wisconsin Department of Workforce Development, Workers' Compensation Division in Madison, Wisconsin. It was addressed to "Applicant, Ronald Martin vs. Respondent, St. Joseph's Community Hospital Froedtert Health, and Respondent, Sentry Casualty Company."

An excerpt from the judge's decision read, "Considering all of the evidence presented, I find that as a result of the work incident of 10/02/2011, applicant sustained physical injury, psychological injury as well as aggravation of underlying psychological conditions, including PTSD. I find the opinions of Dr. Smerz to be the more credible of the opinions submitted in this case with regard to applicant sustaining permanent partial disability....I find that applicant is entitled to worker's compensation benefits, including but not limited to temporary total disability benefits already paid, as well as apparently unpaid benefits from 02/07/12 to 03/02/12." Both respondent and insurer were given twenty-one days to settle up and pay the winning team.

After twenty-three months, the decision was *final*. The court had ruled in my favor—*we won my case*. Froedtert Hospital and Sentry Insurance were at fault and medically and financially responsible for all incurred costs since the date of injury, October 2, 2011. They also had to pay for my out-of-pocket costs and mileage that I paid for some of my medical bills, including one bill I received for evaluation and treatment the day after my injury when I went to Employee Health, which is what the law and hospital policy dictates for any *job-related injury*.

My wonderful psychologist was paid 100 percent since she so kindly deferred any payment until my case was settled, knowing her diagnosis was correct (corroborated by the hospital-appointed shrink, my private physician, and a social worker), and I had a slam-dunk case. My attorney was paid off. My personal financial settlement totaled up to less than three months' pay, and paid for with great sacrifice, pain, anxiety, POW status for fifteen months, and tremendous stress on my whole family.

The monetary settlement was less important to me than truth and justice being served and my integrity, character, and honor intact. It would have been nice to receive a settlement check for years of lost wages for fifteen years, since my nursing days are now far behind me and I know in my heart I could never return. At least I won my suit, and being the better man, I decided to forgive Froedtert for their betrayal and treatment of one of their exemplary employees.

The Froedtert organization is truly amazing, does great things and helps treat thousands of patients, and has saved countless lives. They just treat some of their employees like second-class citizens. Hopefully, they will wake up and come to the realization that the doctor sees the patient for ten minutes a day; the other twenty-three hours and fifty minutes, the nurse cares for and keeps the patient safe and alive. Employees, mostly nurses, are a hospital's greatest asset, and hospital administrations still don't get it.

Hospital violence against employees should not be hidden under a stack of bureaucratic red tape, denied, and covered up to protect their image, which eventually interprets into increased revenues in the end. It's all about the money! It should be confronted, addressed, then rectified. Once again, the critical-mass effect may intervene and stories such as mine might just wake up a sleeping congressman whose vote on a critical issue could break the tie and bring about positive change. Rant over.

Sadly and very discomforting was the brutal murder of Nurse Practitioner Carlie Beaudin on Friday, January 25, 2019, at 0100 in Froedtert's Parking Lot 1 that captured the attention of the nation on news and social media. Try to sweep that tragedy under the rug, Froedtert! Their administration refused to answer questions regarding hospital security and protocol, how often garages are patrolled, surveillance cameras, how many incidents of complaints they received, or how many incidents have occurred over the years.

Stephen Schooff, a spokesman for the hospital, commented, "We continue to work closely with law enforcement and remain vigilant about the emotional and physical safety of every person who works or studies at, is cared for by, or visits our campuses, clinics, and hospitals." Pardon me while I choke on the PC bullshit! I hope Froedtert retains Snidely Whiplash for this Charley Foxtrot fiasco. Oh, how I would love to testify at that trial!

Meanwhile, back at the ranch…

As an elder, unwilling participant of the California Summer Scorch Trials of 2013, I slowly and frustratingly became proficient in moving ladders, boxes, hoses, and tools walking with crutches in 100-degree heat every day. It was hot and slow going, but it was a lesson in patience, self-determination, and recognizing the symptoms of heat exhaustion. Improvise, adapt, overcome! Nevertheless, two months later when our health insurance became effective, I saw an orthopedic surgeon in Fresno and he ordered an MRI of my left knee. It was a month before I got to see him again and the MRI indeed revealed three tears of my left meniscus cartilage. Surgery was scheduled a few weeks later, and the procedure was uneventful.

My rehab and physical therapy took place on our Flying Monkey Ranch where I continued working mostly outdoors, using my crutches and *trying* not to overdo it. Many times Karen had reminded me that the word *moderation* was suspiciously absent from my vocabulary. Two months later I was on my hands and knees (I *almost* always wear knee pads) mixing cement and building two large man-made ponds with six-foot waterfalls, all with shovel and hand trowel, all mixed in my wheelbarrow. My knee was still swollen, and its range of motion was still limited but improving, so I assumed some very awkward positions during the whole process and got an awesome *full-body tan* (sans left knee in brace). Any co-ed naked cement work, anyone? Of course, my private doctor chastised me for my deep Cherokee tan when she saw me a few weeks into the process for an unrelated matter.

"We all gotta die from something, Doc. My instincts tell me this [skin cancer] is not the way I'm going out. Besides, when these projects are done, I'm spending the rest of the hot summer hiding out in my cool air-conditioned home." Unknown to her was the fact that I had to drive my JD tractor pulling a trailer all over our seventeen acres loading up large and sometimes huge boulders to use in my rock creations. Some I lifted and carried next to my chest, swinging my crutches forward using my squeezed armpits. Others were so heavy I had to roll them to the back of the trailer and awkwardly roll or pry them in the back. Then there was the transport, unloading, and placement and cementing in place of said boulders. "I promise to use sunblock, I usually do, but you do realize that it's been over 100 degrees for umpteen days in a row?" I replied. "I'm like the mad scientist Baron Von Martinstein, who becomes so absorbed in his work that food and sleep become nonessentials. I just added sunblock to the list of essentials." I kept my word and incidentally had my first precancerous lesion removed from my face the following year. Now it's shirt, socks, boots, hat, gloves, bandanna, and pants. Most hot days I just wore my old hospital scrubs because they are cool, lightweight, and dry on my body in minutes when they get wet.

It soon became quite apparent that running and maintaining our ranch was a full-time job, especially for the first four to five years. Our home was empty for two years and poorly maintained for years prior to that. Ridding the population of insects, scorpions, black widow spiders, bats, ground squirrels, and a nearby nest of rattlesnakes became priority one. There was a new sheriff in town, and the rules had changed. Spraying for insects on the surrounding three acres, including the barn and greenhouse, was easy and took no time at all. The more persistent pests, ground squirrels and rattlesnakes, took over a couple of years to eradicate.

Ground squirrels dug holes all over my chicken enclosure and dug dangerous tunnels that livestock could break a leg on, *and* they stripped my fruit and nut trees in one day! It's time for all of you to move on, guys and gals. In one sitting for fifteen minutes in my lawn chair in the backyard, I easily shot over a dozen squirrels on a daily basis for days, leaving the fallen dead on the battlefield for their Sciuridae neighbors and relatives to see, plus it made for easy cleanup for the vultures and ravens. I was the Ground Squirrel Darth Vader Invader.

Last year we had a banner year of apples and made apple crisps, apple pies, apple sauce, apple juice, and treated the chickens to all the nonedible apples. We have not seen a ground squirrel on our (three-acre fenced living portion) property and only two tree squirrels all summer the last three years, and our nut and fruit trees are all unmolested and heavily laden with fruit. My destructive little rodents have my other fourteen acres to party and cavort to their hearts' content. Ground squirrels are also a plentiful food source for snakes, and when the squirrel population disappeared, the rattlesnake problem resolved as well—almost.

Having lived in Oakhurst just ten miles north of Coarsegold for many years, I had never seen a single rattlesnake on any of my properties. The first summer at the Flying Monkey Ranch, I killed thirteen rattlers within thirty feet of a door access to our home. That included the one coiled up in the corner of the master bathroom sunken shower (fortunately, it was me that stepped in the shower and not Karen) and the two in the garage, one, a twelve-button who slithered between my legs while I was washing my truck. My inside weapon of choice was usually a shovel for decapitation after several cleansing breaths and a prayer. Outside, the shotgun proved more safe and effective.

Many of the rattlers I killed were small, indicating a nest nearby. One morning I entered the chicken coop and all my hens were perched, but one lay dead next to the food and water. Ironically, this "hen" was the only one of many chicks who was incorrectly sexed, day-old hatchlings I had raised from day one. Madonna, the young virgin male rooster gave his life for his personal harem of hens before he was old enough to service them. So sad! I took one step inside for a closer inspection, leaned forward, and was abruptly met with a warning tail rattle of (hopefully the mother) a huge snake coiled and ready to strike, and I was in its striking distance. Slowly walking backward, I yelled for Karen to bring me the shotgun and a few rounds. I didn't want to spook my other hens because they could jump down right on top of the rattler and create more havoc and death. The Krutch Killer of Kalifornia took dead aim, remembering the mnemonic I have never forgotten, learned on the firing range at Camp Pendleton in the Marines fifty years ago: *BRASS—breathe-relax-aim-slack-squeeze*. A nanosecond later, the head and tail of the crotalid disappeared into a thousand fragments, the body untouched. What a clean shot! No need to bury the head. When I lifted its life-less body with my nearby "chicken coop snake shovel," she stretched out to about five to six feet long sans head and tail. My knees were shaking and sweat poured from my pores, burning my eyes with the saline sweat, making it hard to see clearly. My other hens survived and barely flinched when the shotgun discharged inside the coop. My ears were ringing, but then again, they have for fifty years since Viet Nam, only exacerbated a bit by the blast. "Just another day on the ranch," I thought. The very next day I opened the door to the coop and was met by a "chicken-coop-snake-shovel" sized rattler, and I smote him/her before it had a chance to coil and strike.

One day we had just given our dogs a bath and were preparing to put them in the backyard where it's mostly grass for them to lay on and dry off. By happenstance, I walked in the backyard and noticed from about thirty feet away what appeared to be a long stick under a huge ponderosa pine surrounded by green grass. I keep a clean home-stead, and I knew there was no branch there a few hours ago. As I walked closer toward the stick, I first noticed its tail that meandered to its head five feet away. It was stretched out in the shade of freshly watered grass and therefore was not very active, so I walked no fur-ther but instead took one well-placed shot to the head with my .410 shotgun. It disintegrated, never to be found, and the carrion-fowl had a delicious dinner later that evening. The second summer, twelve more rattlesnakes fed my ravens and vultures.

This year I've seen only one, and it was on our fourteen acres of woods while I was cutting brush, so we believe we have finally erad-icated the rattlesnake nest near us. Our curious dogs still get their annual rattlesnake vaccine since they roam the property, snuffling and exploring along the way. Yes, I know there's controversy over the vaccine, but if it helps save their life after an envenomation, it's worth the twenty-eight dollars a year.

Due to the drought, well over 110,000,000 (yes, that's one hundred ten million!) ponderosa pines have died in the sad, dry sanctuary state of California. There are only a handful on our property, but it is covered with several species of oak, many of which have died as well from the ongoing drought. My other priority has been to create a safe perimeter around the house and also all around my property. We had a professional tree service remove two huge oaks that were a glaring fire hazard, covering most of the garage and parking area and hung so low my pickup scraped the hanging branches, and two in back that were ready to fall on the house, fence, and chicken coop. These trees required pros with ropes, pulleys, and tree climbers who are amazing to watch. One side branch on one of the oaks in the backyard, about sixteen inches in diameter and the inside of it hollowed out, fell during a storm, missing our house by three inches a few years ago, so we felt it best to be proactive rather than reactive with an oak tree in our laps and have this majestic tree removed. It did improve our view of the high country that was blocked by their huge leafy branches, however, an added bonus.

There are three wide gates providing access to the fourteen acres of wood and brush, plenty of space for a fire engine to enter. The riding trails and access roads I've been clearing allows access to about 90 percent of our property now and are wide enough to drive a large truck and tall enough to accommodate fire trucks, or ride two abreast on horses comfortably. Burning the oak keeps the home warm all winter, and there's nothing more fun than burning brush piles on a cold rainy winter day! Cutting firewood is hard but rewarding work and a Team Martin effort. I cut and limb the trees, and Karen loads, hauls, and stacks the wood. A hot tub soak with hot chocolate, while looking up at the Pleiades, Orion, Taurus, and Pegasus at the end of the day, really feels great for aching muscles.

On our main three acres of living space, there are over thirty-six standpipes with faucets; over a dozen are connected to drip irrigation timers, and there are four water timers and countless anti-siphon valves, many of which were leaking from freezing temperatures and no insulation on the PVC pipes when we moved in. Something is *always* breaking down on these systems, so I am constantly walking the line, checking for and repairing water leakage and broken emitters.

Managing over a mile of horse fence, horse corral, riding arena, and fenced paddocks is another never-ending task. Walking the fence line looking for critter holes dug under the fence is the worst, because that means my critters can get out as well. Once the hole is sealed with large branches, dirt, and rock, it is rarely used again. Our fence has been struck six times by out-of-control cars since we moved here. One crash took out three hundred feet of fence along Highway 41, and the CHP ruined another one hundred feet by insisting the car be towed sideways down into the creek bed and up a steep slope to the highway instead of kindly speaking with the homeowner. I could have opened one of the side gates and the tow truck could have pulled right up to the smashed car, which had amazingly ended upright on my inner road. It was now suddenly my responsibility to ensure none of my animals escaped onto Highway 41 and were safely corralled. At least the occupants were not seriously injured and their insurance was quick to settle and fix my fence, thanks to my persistence and pesky insistence.

Three of the fence crashes occurred to the front of our property. Our west paddock, about an acre in size, faces the road next to our entry gate and is a wooden fence reinforced with metal no-climb horse fence. Our non-county-maintained road takes a moderate left dog-leg turn at the corner of the paddock going steeply downhill toward Highway 41, and some of our transient disreputable neighbors a mile up the road have a propensity for getting wasted and speeding down our dirt road out of control on a regular basis. The third fence strike knocked over a long section of fence and looked strangely malicious, so law enforcement became involved. All I got was an "I'm sorry" and the deputy's card with a case number. The perp, whom one of my neighbors told me he witnessed hit my fence, was pretty obvious with all the noticeable damage and green paint transfer to the front end of his car every time he drove by our home, but he never stopped to apologize or claim responsibility. He just got a death stare from me each time I saw his car when I was down by the road. Karma will intervene when the time is right.

In the meantime, I had to replace a forty-foot section of wood and horse fence and paint it. In order to prevent future occurrences, I constructed a guardrail with six-inch-by-six-inch treated wood posts buried three feet deep and then moved several large boulders from my property with my truck, barely able to drag them in four-wheel drive, dragging the boulders behind the truck with half-inch chain and then had my neighbor place them strategically with his bigger Kubota tractor at both ends of the guardrail. If some out-of-control driver veers toward the fence now, the guardrail and rocks will really mess their car up big-time and my fence will be undamaged. They will likely be captured on video as well; there are hidden game cameras and a security system all around my property now, taping 24/7/365.

We had all new Anlin dual-pane windows installed in our home, a major undertaking. The whole inside of the home was repainted. Our floor was ugly, with poorly laid fake wood in the great room, and even uglier Berber carpet that refused to be cleaned with any machine covered the remainder of our home. We decided to redo the floor throughout the whole house including all the closets with rustic solid oak flooring and new four-inch double ogee floor molding. Only the kitchen and the bathrooms retained their tile floors. Ron the Plumber, installed three new 1.5-gallon flush ecofriendly toilets with seats that close slowly and don't slam down of the toilet ring. All the thirty-year-old corroded brass shower, bath, and kitchen plumbing fixtures were replaced with brushed nickel fixtures.

Ron the Tile Setter, now sans crutches, painstakingly removed the equally ugly tile front entry and the matching hearth tiles surrounding the inefficient, illegal, and outdated woodstove. Beautiful complimentary slate tile with detailed accents replaced the old marble, and I also added a three-foot-by-four-foot tile artist rendition mural, painted by the renowned Thomas Hill, of Upper and Lower Yosemite Falls, on the wall behind the woodstove. Mr. Hill's studio located inside the park in Wawona near the Mariposa Grove of Giant Sequoias was completed in 1884, and he was modestly profitable as Wawona's resident artist. In 2009, Hill's Studio became the Wawona Visitor Center, renovated and preserved by the Yosemite Conservatory.

The old woodstove now houses succulent plants and ivy adjacent to the driveway outdoors, and a new Lopi Liberty woodstove with brass accents and a glass-etched window to view the flames now adorns the great room, and it warms the whole house. If you put on a big oak log before retiring for the evening, the house will stay warm all night, and all one has to do in the morning is toss another log on the all-night fire. The kitchen got a facelift with contemporary awesome lighting and all new stainless steel appliances: dishwasher, side-by-side refrigerator/freezer with a bottom freezer door; convection microwave oven; large electric oven; and a five-burner heavy-duty Jenn-Air gas range. And there's a twenty-five-cubic-foot freezer in the garage for extra food storage, much of the space occupied by organic home-grown food from our garden. With electricity, we could literally live for over six months without leaving home for food. Our well water is good but had a slight iron taste, so we installed a water softener and water purification system for the whole house. That made a great difference.

The landscaping on our property was seriously lacking, sporadic, and completely overgrown, with lots of mature dead bushes, trees, and flowers. Twenty-five unwatered, nearly dead rose bushes lining our driveway that did not bloom and were in serious need of resuscitation—water, pruning, fertilizer, and love combined with my green thumb produced amazing results. Today, close to fifty roses thrive and bloom nearly all year long on timed drip irrigation with proper pruning. Many of the trees and bushes surrounding the house were so overgrown they covered walkways and blocked access to three doors to our home. Some required mega pruning before the movers arrived so they could access the house with our belongings. Today, a diversity of perennial flowers, bulbs, and flowering bushes bloom year-round. I've actually run out of places to plant flowers. I inherited the green thumb from my mom, ambition from my dad.

My mother became enamored with hummingbirds when she finally moved from Kansas to California after my dad died, and they soon became her passion. Karen and I, well, me mostly now that she works so hard and I'm retired, have carried on Mom's tradition. There are four feeders on our back patio, perfect for viewing from inside or outside that need to be filled twice or more daily because those little critters literally suck the feeders dry. It's a lot of work, so I make three gallons of hummingbird food at a time. We are frequented by robins, jays, bluebirds, ravens, turkey vultures, wild turkeys, wrens, finches, red-headed woodpeckers, quail, hawks, and the occasional eagle, all of whom seem content to share their airspace with my much larger, *mostly* docile tree-dwelling flying monkeys.

In just a few short years of living in California, we had established our Rivendell, a beautiful mountain ranch that reminds us each day that we're living in a resort home. There is a view of a pond and waterfall from every room in the house, including the bathrooms and garage. Many enjoyable times are spent in our hot tub on the deck outside our master bedroom, or just sitting outside enjoying the distant mountain views, or lying in the hammock for two and star gazing.

Now that we had a ranch, we needed animals. My love of animals almost supersedes my love of mankind. The famous author Mark Twain said, "The more I learn about people, the more I love my dog." Casi, our malamute, sadly left us from old age and the extreme heat a few years back. She was thirteen and gave us a good life together, a spirit creature with unquestioning love and devotion. I held her in my arms when she died, and I still mourn her loss. We started looking for "rescue animals," and Blue chose us first. A rambunctious two-year-old mutant Jack Russell, pit bull, border collie (?) with a left blue eye that would have made Peter O'Toole jealous. Blue was an ignored city-raised dog from Fresno who needed space, attention, a little training, and love. He is "momma's dog," very smart and totally devoted to Karen, except when it's feeding time; then and only then, I suddenly take on the lead role.

Along next came Precious (named after the One Ring), a local rescue kitten who grew up with Blue, so they are best friends; she rubs against him and they often sleep together. Blue tolerates her advances passively in the house, but when they are outside, he will chase her up a tree just to let her know the true hierarchy of the animal kingdom. When she climbs down, she will approach Blue as if nothing happened and they're best friends again. Precious is as ubiquitous as the Cheshire Cat in the classic tale *Alice in Wonderland*. Whenever we go out of the house, she seems to appear, sans toothy Cheshire smile, from out of nowhere. She speaks cat-speak whenever we are near and frequently accompanies us and the dogs on our one-mile walks around our property, climbing trees along the way like our own private security.

Soon after that a beautiful two-year-old spayed, vaccinated, and chipped chocolate Lab female chose us. Karen found an ad in her hospital's newsletter at 0300 while working at the hospital and texted the owners, in part saying, "We would Love Love Love to have a chocolate Lab!" Paradoxically, just days before I had mentioned to Karen that I would like to have a chocolate Lab as a partner for Blue, since Casi had died not long after Blue entered our lives. At 0700 I got a phone call at home from an unknown pleasant lady asking if we were the family who wanted a chocolate Lab.

Let's get one thing clear: Ron doesn't do mornings very well. My chronic sleep disorder, headaches, body pain, and occasional nightmares still continue. Most nights I awaken between 0200 and 0400 whether I retire early or late, from body pain, headache, and/or unrelenting abdominal pain; and I then transfer from bed to recliner chair so I don't disturb Karen's sleep. My body knows when the pain precedes sleep. The daily morning routine includes taking my prescription BP meds, followed, if the body concurs, with morning vitamins, all chased with a glass of milk. Then I read or do crossword puzzles to divert my attention from the pain. Positive affirmations and other alternative natural therapies seem to help, and after a few hours, I feel alive enough to function, and the pain has usually reached a tolerable level.

"Excuse me, could you repeat that again?" I asked, more than a little confused.

"You texted me at 0300 about our female lab, and your note just grabbed at my heartstrings," she replied.

After a moment of mind-sleuthing, I put two and three together and realized it had to be Karen. "Yes," I replied tentatively. "My wife works night shift at Fresno Heart, and she probably texted you. We are very interested. Karen should be home in about an hour, and I'll have her call you back."

"Oh, she likely saw it in the ad I just posted in the hospital newsletter. I work for Community Medical Center as a nurse too," she acknowledged.

"Aha. That's cool. I'm sure you will be getting a call within the hour."

At 0815 when Karen got home from her 1900–0700 shift, we had a lot to talk about, and she came clean. We called the owner back and asked her if we could drive to Fresno and check out her female, Molly. She agreed, so we loaded Blue up in the truck and arrived thirty minutes later in front of Molly's beautiful but cramped home. We decided to take Blue so the two dogs could intermingle and we could see how they got along. Blue was immediately smitten, and Molly loved to frolic with Blue, so it was meant to be. Her husband wanted to see the new home Molly was going to, so we had to wait until 1700 for Molly and his family to make it from Clovis to the Flying Monkey Ranch in Coarsegold, a thirty-minute drive. In the meantime, Karen caught some serious shuteye. When Molly's owners drove up our driveway and saw the seventeen acres where she could run and frolic with her friend Blue, they did not hesitate.

"My uncle wanted Molly for a hunting dog, and she would be locked in a cage most of the time except when the hunt was on. We want her to run and be free, and I think this is just the place."

"We agree!" Karen and I said in unison. I didn't call jinx on her this time, letting her off easy and saving me from the embarrassment of having to admit she married a crazy fool to our guests. I still sometimes play "Slug Bug" with old VWs, especially Yellow Slug Bugs. They left happy, we were happy, and the dogs were happy. Happy, happy, happy!

Molly, who earned many nicknames like Molly Brown because she's dark brown, and our son Forrest's wife Margot's brother's daughter is Maya Brown, and Karen mistakenly calls Maya Brown (the Unsinkable) Molly Brown. Got that, because I'm sure confused! Probably the most well-earned moniker was that of Molly Baggins, master thief. She has the nose of the bloodhound and will appear at the kitchen from a deep sleep at the other end of the house when the refrigerator door opens and a chunk of cheese still in its wrapper is removed. Before she was trained properly, I caught her with a two-pound salmon filet in her mouth she had snatched off the kitchen counter, preparing to chow down in the living room after turning my back for a minute. So Molly became Salmon Dog, Cheese Dog, and several other names of endearment. She fit in perfectly with our ever-growing menagerie.

Pippin, named after the famous Hobbit Peregrine Took, cousin to Frodo and one of the nine selected for the Fellowship of the Ring, was an abandoned four-week-old black kitten with white socks found next to Highway 41, malnourished and near death. She still fit in the palm of my hand. It took some special handling and love to bring her around, but her early cat-hood traumas left permanent scars, and she never became an overly friendly cat. She is very skittish around everyone but me, but not quite feral. I can still pick her up and pet her on occasion, but she likes to live under the radar and lives in the barn, our tipi, and garage rafters and hunts for her food. The perfect barn cat! Both cats have a refuge via a modified cat door into the laundry room from the garage where there's always food and milk and a warm refuge from the wet and cold winter nights.

Early in the spring of 2014 we bought eight one-day-old chicks and raised them from babies. As they got older, I gave them all diva names. In a few short months, eggs started showing up in their laying spots. Then slowly one by one, my chickens began disappearing. At the time the pen was completely fenced but open on top. One day I witnessed as a bobcat hopped the fence with a chicken in its mouth and found the feathery remains the next day. Improvise, adapt, and overcome. I covered the roof with steel horse fencing and thought I had sealed up every opportunity for predators to get in. Christmas Day 2014 and all the kids and spouses were here to celebrate family together. Just before the traditional turkey dinner was to be served, we all heard six of our dogs barking at the back fence, and they wouldn't come when called. My sixth sense told me something was not right. With .22 rifle in hand, I discovered why the dogs were going crazy.

Staring me right in the eye was a forty-pound bobcat; my two last favorite diva hens, Oprah and Lady Gaga, lay dead in their enclosure with Oprah still in the bobcat's mouth, its neck snapped and mis-shapen. Something inside me snapped too.

The bobcat took four head shots and a neck shot before he stopped moving. My whole brood of chickens decimated in one sea-son by a bobcat and a rattlesnake! I found out later that likely this same bobcat had been wreaking havoc on my neighbors' small ani-mals as well as on the Hogan's Mountain. I have not seen another one since, and my 2015 season's brood of chickens all survived and provided enough eggs for us and Eric's family. They're free-range chickens, no antibiotics, and no government control. The ladies also played an integral part in recycling and contributed to the natural home ecosystem. My girls are Lady Gaga II, Xena, Oprah II, and Lucy.

Owning and brushing seventeen acres can be a tedious, tire-some job, and I needed some help. For months I had been consider-ing buying a breeding pair or goats but knew nothing of ruminants, so I did what most millennials do: I googled it and came across a most interesting website called the Happy Hobbit, a site run out of the home in the Santa Cruz Mountains by two extremely talented, published, soon-to-be famous, beautiful, but sort of nerdy sisters Kelli and Alex Rice (aka Kili and Fili), J. R. R. Tolkien lovers. They grew up doing 4-H activities since age nine and have quite a zoo on their property also, it seems. Anyway, Kelli and Alex produced a video I'll call "Raising Goats for Idiots 101" (Happy Hobbit: Goat Basics—Episode 11) that was cute, funny, and educational. I was so enthralled and excited that I bought a breeding pair two days later from the local goat lady, baby Nubians. Fili lasted a year thankfully before she got pregnant (does go into heat or estrus every three weeks for goat's sake!) but was never healthy looking; her baby died the night she was born as I tried to bottle-feed her, to no avail. Fili died shortly thereafter of her illness or a mother's broken heart. Once again, my intuitive psychic connection to my animals instructed my spirit guide to be present, and I was there each time so neither of them died alone. For reasons far beyond explanation now, I feel no one should die alone. A loving hand, a tender caress can make all the difference during the last seconds of life. That's just me. I tried to never let my patients die alone. I would hold their hands and touch their upper chakras while I watched the monitor that showed flat-line, asystole. There are no words to describe the sensation of energy being transferred to a higher frequency during literally thousands of deaths I've experienced.

In the summer of 2016 we purchased a set of beautiful year-old *identical twin* brown Nubian does with white ears. Minnie wore a purple collar and Daisy a red collar for easy recognition at a distance. Mother Nature worked her magic, and Minnie birthed on New Year's Eve, December 31, just after dark (1700 hours in December). It just so happened I walked into the barn when the umbilical cords were still attached. It was raining cats and dogs, and apparently goats tonight, the temperature was dropping and getting cold very quickly, and the babies were still wet with amniotic fluid and blood. I towel dried a doe and a kid, Jules and Frodo, and added a large pile of straw for their manger, then found my two incubator heat lamps and hung them over their makeshift manger to keep them extra warm as they both cuddled with each other between nursing. I was wet and cold, and Papa Ron had serious frostbite, but Jules and Frodo survived that wintry New Year's Eve night. Happy New Year!

About a month later on February 7, my animal spirits summoned me to the barn again after feeding time. Daisy was birthing and had a doe and a kid I named after the enduring love affair in LOTR (*Lord of the Rings* for you, clueless geeks), Arwen and Strider. I was there for their births as well in an almost déjà vu kinda way. It was right at dusk, freezing cold, blowing winds, and raining heavily. Little rivulets of water followed gravity and trickled into parts of the barn stalls. I had to towel dry the babies and get them under the heat lamp, but left the placenta cleanup to momma Daisy.

Both moms were great and nursed without any problems, and both let their babies climb all over them when they started eating hay from the wall feeders. Now I had seven goats, four of them does. I started doing the math and realized they come into heat every three weeks; they could breed like rabbits (bad animal metaphor!) and

I could have thirty goats in a few years. Daisy again appeared to have been impregnated by Kili while she was still isolated with her babies when she was let out of her manger for a break. Turns out she wasn't pregnant; she was just bigger postpartum than her twin sister Minnie. That is how we tell them apart now: Docile Daisy and Skinny Minnie.

Kili was moved to another paddock, separated and alone. His horns turned a darker green each day as he butted the green-painted wooden fence, fortunately reinforced with metal no-climb fence wire. He still managed to knock several eight-foot sections of two-by-six wood fencing from their posts. That option certainly did not work out well; more fence repairs for me. He was finally transferred to another property, and now I had to learn how to neuter (wether) Frodo and Strider, both of whom could impregnate a doe at sixteen weeks of age. Most sites recommended you should take your goat to the vet and have "the doctor" do it, our closest being almost fifty miles away. After watching a few videos on YouTube, including a nine-year-old perform the procedure, I went out and spent about fifteen dollars for the hand tool castrator and some very small rubber cots at the local feed store.

At fifteen weeks of age, I gave each of them an adult aspirin dissolved in milk and waited thirty minutes. Karen and I easily applied the bands in less than two minutes, isolating both testicles and ensuring the two nipples were outside the band, released the band, and let them loose. They both acted as if nothing happened and ran with the rest of the herd, frolicking like baby goats frolic. About a month later, their scrotums fell off with the band, and suddenly Frodo and Strider became wethers.

Now with six goats, four does and two wethers, we decided to watch the four goatlings grow up and observe what six goats can do to our fourteen acres of forest and brush. Being the social herding creatures they are, all six of them are never far from each other. They enjoy human company, so every day if we peer out the windows in the kitchen or great room toward the backyard, we are usually met by all six of them staring in and bleating at us with tilted heads and blank expressions like Jar Jar Binks, the Gungan outcast on Naboo in the Star Wars saga, just on the other side of the fence. They also like interacting with the chickens and the dogs that are all nearby. They have not disappointed in their brush-clearing skills, starting near their exit gates from their one-acre corral. They moved on clearing trails to our backyard fence, kindly eating grasses (soon to be tall dry weeds) next to the fences so I don't have to weed eat there, eating all the tender leaves of invasive baby scrub oaks, and stripping brushy plants to spindly branches. That makes it much easier for me to see when I cut the branches in the fall for burning in brush piles. It costs me less than two dollars a day in hay costs in exchange for their love, entertainment, and brush-clearing skills. Goats are lovable, friendly, and don't leave huge poop piles like horses and cows. It's like owning a herd of deer with floppy ears. You just gotta love 'em!

With the exception of boarding horses when the occasion arose, this about rounded out the animal inventory at the Flying Monkey Ranch, not counting the reclusive flying monkeys. I preferred boarding to owning horses because of the expensive maintenance required and would prefer the owners intervene when they need a farrier or have to drive them fifty miles to the large animal vet for care. I did provide boarding and nursing care to two quarter horses that required daily wound care and other special needs at no extra charge since their owner is a dear friend and I learned from Julie "Jules" Diane about horses, so it was an even exchange of talents. I live vicariously through Julie now as she is a warm-hearted die-hard *Patriot* and a die-hard New England Patriot *fan* who loves Tom Brady.

I was an avid NFL fan (Packers!) but have disavowed the existence of "professional" football since the first player whose name will not tarnish these pages took a knee during the national anthem and denigrated me, our flag, our country, and the veterans and honored dead who made the ultimate sacrifice to overcome evil and protect our country. Also because the (NFL) "Non Football League" tried to bury the issue and denied the correlation between head injuries and CTE as Dr. Bennet Omalu brought to their attention years ago. If you want the digital version, just watch the movie *Concussion* with Will Smith portraying Dr. Omalu.

Over a period of less than four years, Karen and I had transformed an abandoned, run-down, overgrown, varmint-infested house into an updated, warm, comfortable redwood ranch home in the Sierra foothills, our dream home for retirement with privacy, co-ed naked gardening, lots of property, plenty of water, backup power source, and a lifetime supply of firewood. Now if we can only get rid of Jerry Brown-now-Gavin Newsome (nephew of Nancy Pelosi), Barbara Boxer, Diane Feinstein, and Frankenstein's daughter, Nancy Pelosi, along with several more political dinosaurs, we can truly experience "California Dreamin'!"

CHAPTER 22

Cold Turkey

O true apothecary! Thy drugs are quick.

—William Shakespeare

In order to broach this subject, I need to hop in the WayBack Machine with young carrot-top Sherman and his most accomplished dog mentor, the bespectacled canine genius Peabody, and go back to October 2011 when I went to see Dr. Gibson, my doctor in West Bend, Wisconsin.

Prior to my ER assault, I took an occasional Vicoprofen for my really bad HCV attack days. Motrin 800 mg kept me moving for many years running on cement floors in the ER and climbing in and out of cramped helicopters. Many days it did not work at all, and over the many years of almost daily use, it is likely my kidneys have suffered as a result. My post-assault headaches came on without aura or warning, and they were not relieved at all by Vicoprofen. My blood pressure was still sky high and uncontrolled, and the "which came first, the chicken or the egg" questions came up. Is the head injury causing hypertension, or is the hypertension triggering my headaches? Personally, I voted for option 1, a fifty-fifty guess.

Dr. Gibson suggested something stronger than Vicoprofen and instead prescribed oxycodone 5 mg tablets, one to two every four hours, and said I could get as many refills every month as long as I picked up the "Triplicate" prescription, required by federal law for most opiates, at his office. Thus began my "madventure" on my long fall down the rabbit hole.

I continued taking the oxycodone for the next sixteen months more and more frequently to dull the pain until we moved to California, and not waiting two months for our new health insurance, I secured a doctor who could prescribe all my meds, including oxycodone. Unfortunately, my doctor only worked two days a week and was frequently absent with her own serious illness, so there were blank periods when I ran out of my pain meds for a few days. Sadly, she died about a year later from her disease at a young age.

To further investigate the root cause of my chronic headaches, I was referred to and scheduled an appointment with a neurologist in Fresno, who interestingly was awarded the Bronze Star for bravery under fire as an Army doctor defending wounded soldiers at the same time I was in Viet Nam. He ran several in-office tests, some with electrodes that measured nerve conduction time, as well as a CT scan of my neck but not my head because he had recent head CT scans and reports in my medical record. At our follow-up visit, he vaguely mentioned all the chronic abnormalities in my neck but seemed fixated on my nerve conduction tests.

"I'm concerned because you have severe carpal tunnel syndrome in your left wrist. You will need surgery immediately, or you could lose function of your left hand," the doctor emphasized.

"But I'm right handed and have absolutely no pain or symptoms in my left hand, and I came to see you about my uncontrolled headaches from my head injury!" I declared, my PTSD buttons pushed, and suddenly Wolfman Jack was in my head on retro station KWTF spinning a vinyl release of David Bowie's *Space Oddity* released in November 1969, a few months after I returned from the jungles of East Asia. Major Tom and I both were listening to ground control's countdown in the space capsule before we both blasted off.

> *Ground Control to Major Tom*
> *(Ten, nine, eight, seven, six)*
> *Commencing countdown, engines on*
> *(Five, four, three)*

Check ignition and may God's
Love be with you
(Two, one, liftoff)

"I don't have any idea what is causing your headaches, Mr. Martin."

"Then I guess we're done here. Thank you for trying and informing me about carpal tunnel syndrome. I'll keep an eye on it and see someone if it gets worse." And I walked out his office none the wiser and thankful for good insurance. *Just keep on taking the oxycodone and numb the pain. It's actually still there, you just don't care about it being there,* I thought to myself.

Another follow-up with my PMD, and at my request, she referred me to a neurologist and pain specialist in Fresno. We chatted and discussed my extensive history of head, neck, and spine trauma. I explained to him that my goal was to get off opiates with his help. He prescribed me 120 tablets of oxycodone 10 mg every four to six hours and sent me on my way. A phone call to their office was required to request refills. Once again, the drive each month to his office thirty miles away to pick up my "Triplicate" prescription was a minor inconvenience, but any trip to Fresno we try to complete more than just one chore, so I stopped afterward and picked up dog food that is five to ten dollars cheaper for the big dog bags.

This went on for several months. Finally he switched me to Butrans (buprenorphine) transdermal system where one adhesive medicated patch is applied weekly. Unfortunately, he prescribed it during the very hot early fall firewood season, and despite my best efforts, with all the muscle movement and drenching sweat from cutting and brushing my oak trees, the patch refused to adhere and they were rendered useless. At our next visit the doctor discussed Botox injections and/or methadone alternatives that I quickly rejected, so he switched me back to oxycodone 10 mg every four hours.

The American Society of Addiction Medicine (ASAM) and the National Institute of Drug Abuse (NIDA) have stated that *drug overdose is now the leading cause of accidental death in America,* surpassing motor vehicle accidents as the leading killer of our young with 52,404 lethal drug overdoses in 2015; 20,101 were related to prescription opiates and 12,900 ODs from heroin.

That's pretty scary, and the numbers keep climbing. I was now taking 10 mg of oxycodone four to six times daily, or *more*. One of the weird paradoxical side effects of oxycodone is that it can cause rebound headaches when you are taking them for headache pain. The fog was getting thicker, and I began to feel like I was not totally in control. A veil of darkness began to surround me, and it became closer, cold, and lifeless. I was scared shitless. I felt like I had lost the ability to feel.

I'm stepping through the door
And I'm floating in a most peculiar way
And the stars look very different today

My doctors were all well-intentioned in prescribing opiates to control the pain I've experienced, and it helped me endure the pain for five years. ASAM defined *addiction* as "a primary, chronic and relapsing brain disease characterized by an individual pathologically pursuing reward and/or relief by substance use and other behaviors." I felt like I was reaching or had reached that plateau and felt helplessness and despair once again. Add a large dose of stubbornness and Marine never-say-die attitude, and I was looking for a miracle or divine intervention. Karma did come at the opportune time.

Prior to my karmic intervention, however, I experienced another life-altering experience six months earlier. After at least five years of drought and mammoth forest fires, California finally was rewarded and inundated with a river of storm after storm, raining for days on end. Our home has three fast-running seasonal creeks running through it, and the rain produced one two-hundred-foot-wide pond all the way through May, which is highly unusual for this area for decades. Suddenly, our property was inundated with frogs and toads; the croaking at night was almost deafening in the backyard facing most of the creeks and pond, and I have a serious documented hearing loss from the Marines (VA claim of course *denied!*).

The snowpack was 200 percent of "normal," and we had not seen "normal" in many years. This interpreted into great snowpack at the ski areas. Karen was anxious to go skiing more than me one morning since I had another of my headaches, but I accommodated her zeal by going against my better judgment. Talk about not listening to your gut instinct!

We are both excellent skiers who have skied for over forty years and don't take chances like we used to, following our know-no-fear kids when they would take us down double-black diamond runs making it look easy while we side-slipped down the moguls. We're not mogul fans anymore, preferring groomed steep slopes or really fresh powder. The days before the infamous February 12, 2016, incident unfortunately were warm with the occasional rain on top of the snow, with clear bitter cold nights that make for very icy morning ski conditions.

Karen and I took the lift at China Peak to the summit, surveyed the beautiful snowcapped mountains, and decided to traverse to the left and ski the blue intermediate runs. We had not skied since around 2010 in Wisconsin, and I do not consider their bumps on the surrounding flat landscape "ski mountains" (three-hundred-foot vertical drop!), so it had really been way back in 2007 when we skied Big Sky Montana while living in Livingston, Montana.

Karen liked me to lead, and she would follow my path of descent. The slopes were groomed the evening before, and hiding under the thin veneer of snow was one solid slab of ice. I decided to traverse the mountain laterally, almost with my skis in a wedge position to slow my speed. On the second right turn, my skis slipped on the ice and I went down hard, falling face-first on the steep slope. My body had suddenly become the Coors Light Love Train, racing downhill face-first and gaining speed with every passing second. I tried every maneuver I knew to try and release my skis and stop, to no avail; I was sliding too fast. Karen didn't even see me fall until after the crash landing.

Directly ahead in my path looking forward, I saw a very large dense stand of mature fir trees in my path a few hundred feet away. If I had hit one of those trees, I know I would have died for sure traveling at my speed head-first. My headlong slide was punctuated by a few bumps that sent me airborne, sending shock waves of pain to various parts of my body on landing, but I had traveled over two hundred yards before I finally got my ski bindings to release and was finally able to twist my body and flip again, landing face-first, feet facing downhill, right arm pinned under my body. Everything suddenly went dark on that sunny frosty beautiful day at seven thousand feet.

The first thing I remembered was a strange voice of a young woman repeating, "Are you okay? Are you okay?" followed by excruciating pain in my upper neck. I don't know how long I lay there before someone came along. Karen arrived a few minutes after the strange female voice I heard, and someone went looking for the ski patrol. As I started coming around and the stars were supplanted by the harsh reality of the bright sun shining in my eyes, I began my personal nursing self-assessment. The trauma of the event had put me in a mild state of shock, and it was too fresh to feel all my aches and pains, but one thing I was certain of: I broke my neck! The good news was that I was breathing and I could, so far, move all my extremities.

It took the ski patrol over thirty minutes to arrive; I guess they needed extra help when they heard "serious head and neck injury." So Ron lay in the snow not moving a muscle, the pain increasing with each passing minute, and hypothermia and cryoglobulinemia quickly setting in.

I vaguely recall six to eight people lifting me onto the backboard and securing me tightly in the ski patrol's snow sled, a most uncomfortable ride with attributes similar to a toboggan flying straight down the fall line of the mountain with no control, my life truly in the hands of one strange man in a red jacket.

They loaded me head-first with my head facing downhill (not my idea, but I was a patient now), adding more pressure to my head and neck. The whole ride down the mountain reinforced my awareness that my neck was broken as I felt every single pebble of snow we glided over like flaming ice crystals crashing into each other in my neck. When we reached a navigable area, the ski patroller was replaced by a snowmobile for the remainder of the ride to the first aid station.

On arrival an IV was placed and 100 mg of Fentanyl was given to me for the pain. Life was a little easier for a while. I suggested to the staff that with my type of injury, they should consider air ambulance transport rather than a three-hour drive bouncing in the back of an ambulance on a one-ton pickup chassis, a ride I did not desire to experience.

"You've got to be kidding me," one of the EMT's stated. "How did you know that? We always call for an air ambulance for serious neck injuries."

"I was chief flight nurse for a helicopter program for many years, and we always flew patients like me from outlying hospitals or from accident scenes. I've landed here several times over the years."

"Well, you're right. We already dispatched Sky Life out of Fresno. The helipad is a few miles away, so a ground ambulance will drive you there. Sky Life will take you directly to Community Medical Center (CMC), a level I trauma center."

"I used to work there years ago when it was called Valley Medical Center. I doubt their ER has changed much since then. At least they will call a trauma alert, so I won't have to wait for hours to even see a doctor."

Even the short ride to the heliport in the ambulance for ten minutes was very painful. Thank dog for clear skies and perfect flying conditions. The ambulance crew advised me I was lucky because I was going to fly in their Bell 222, a very classy helicopter. Fortunately, I had seen it up close before, because I now got the trauma patient's view, backboarded and C-spined just like the hundreds of patients I had personally flown in this same condition. Since the head and neck are immobilized, one can only look at the sky and then the ceiling of the inside of the helicopter. One of the nurses started a second IV of 0.9% normal saline and gave me an unsolicited dose of IV Fentanyl and an antiemetic, both of which helped my pain immensely.

> *For here am I sitting in a tin can*
> *Far above the world*
> *Planet earth is blue*
> *And there's nothing I can do*

There are not many things worse than a large C-spined patient lying on his back and strapped to the gurney suddenly start blowing chunks in a cramped cockpit. Besides the odor and mess, it could be potentially very serious or fatal to the patient. I used to fly with one particular flight paramedic, and every time one of our patients would puke, he would lose it and start hurling as well, so now I was stuck with two vomiting patients. My pilots would just look back at me, smile, and shake their heads at me in pitiful acknowledgment.

The amazing and expectedly smooth ride to CMC took about thirty minutes. In a matter of seconds after arrival in the ER, I was surrounded by multiple medical disciplines that all had assigned tasks and performed a full trauma assessment, removed me from the wooden backboard (aaaah!), cut off all my pricey ski clothes, and told me not to move anything. *As if!* I thought to myself. Trauma panel labs, x-rays, and multiple CT scans were performed over the next several hours. My pain was addressed once, but then as it got later into the shift, it became much busier and the nursing visits became less frequent. Been there, done that!

Finally the attending physician showed up with all the residents, interns, nurses, and whoever else was involved in my care (I could still only stare at the ceiling).

"Well, Mr. Martin, you have broken your neck. The lamina on both sides of C-2 have nondisplaced fractures. You are lucky to be alive. I have a call in to the neurosurgeon and he will determine whether the fracture is stable enough for you to go home or if you will need to be admitted and placed in halo-traction for several months. Oh, by the way, you broke your right ninth rib also. Tomorrow you will feel a lot sorer in spots you don't feel pain in now."

> *Tell my wife I love her very much, she knows*
> *Ground Control to Major Tom*
> *Your circuit's dead, there's something wrong*
> *Can you hear me Major Tom?*
> *Can you hear me Major Tom?*

Doom and gloom. The next several hours it took for the neurosurgeon to respond were arduous and stressful. Wearing halo-traction with a metal ring around your head with screws made of stainless steel screwed into your skull with bars attached to a shoulder apparatus would drive me mad. It would require lots and lots of sedation and amnesic drugs. You kind of look like Mr. Freeze (Otto Preminger) on the old Batman TV series spoof with it on. But I get ahead of myself. As it turned out, I did not require halo-traction and hospitalization. Instead I was fitted with a rigid cervical collar that was discomforting but functional. It kept my neck rigidly aligned and immobile. I went home with a neurosurgical follow-up; I already had pain meds, so I didn't even ask. The neck spasms were intense, and in retrospect I should have asked for muscle relaxer meds, but they were offered to me when I saw the neurosurgical PA the next week.

For twelve weeks I religiously wore the cervical collar 24-7, taking it off only to shower. It was nearly impossible for me to lie in bed and sleep. My leather recliner (Archie's chair) became my bed for the next four months. The ranch suffered greatly. All I could do was water and keep my plants alive. Weeds grew tall and became a fire hazard, and no outside work was undertaken until the middle of June when the cervical collar was finally removed after a repeat neck CT scan. My main priority was cutting the weeds on the property to reduce the fire hazard. Beyond that, it was slow going, because without mechanical support of my neck muscles, the pain persisted and my range of motion took a long time to regain. Thanks to Tammy Lee Anderson, my Rolfer and healer in Clovis for helping heal my body and for fixing things that had been out of kilter for decades!

My karmic intervention came only six weeks after my neck had healed sufficiently to remove my rigid neck brace and I painfully learned how to move my head and neck again. My chronic pains continued, and adding the strain of a serious neck fracture just compounded the problem. I was amply supplied with oxycodone up until the end of July. Since I was content and understanding of the reasons for being under contract to get opiate prescriptions only from my pain specialist, I needed to call his office when I needed a refill and

I was due to run out very soon. When I called my pain physician, I was informed he was out of town for the week and no one was available to prescribe my oxycodone until next week. Oxycodone is often referred to as "legal heroin" because chemically they are almost identical, just as addictive, as deadly, and as hard to kick.

The day was Monday, August 1, 2016.

Suddenly, another sudden intuitive leap of understanding occurred. It was time for me to take control of my life again, and five years of oxycodone usage had certainly changed my life. Without hesitation or feelings of regret, I made the decision that very moment I got off the phone with the doctor's office that I would stop taking oxycodone beginning that Monday in August. It's an easy date to remember and no time like now to get started.

Fortunately I am "retired" and only answerable to my loving wife and my many animals, so most of my days were spent on our Flying Monkey Ranch Rehab Center. This was a deliberate, self-imposed, home-managed cold turkey *withdrawal from opiate addiction with no medical intervention or rehab center!* Let me say this here and now to make all the medical community happy: *It is not recommended to stop taking oxycodone "cold turkey" without the help of a qualified medical professional.* I was well-informed of what symptoms to expect, plus I had the benefit of a critical care nurse to intervene if things went south, and undying resolve and fortitude. Only thing is, I didn't tell Karen I had stopped cold turkey until a couple of weeks had elapsed so I didn't have to worry about her trying to talk me out of it. Oh, what a stubborn fucking nurse I am. I experienced all the symptoms any other opiate addict felt; only I was armed with education and fierce determination. This was not how I was going to die!

Besides, I have survived worse things in my life and the sentence for abrupt withdrawal should usually not last more than a month. And most of the withdrawal symptoms I expected to experience, my body was already experiencing to some degree with TBI (and possibly CTE, I'll let you know *after* I have died), HCV, and PTSD. Acute withdrawal from opiates is not for the weak of heart and mind, as your physical, psychological, and emotional limits are constantly challenged every moment of your existence. It is similar to but much worse than having the flu; worse the first seventy-two hours, then very slowly improving over the next week to month. For me, it took over a month to feel "normal" again. What does normal mean?

Some of the physical symptoms included muscle and bone pain, headaches, hypertension, rhinorrhea (runny nose), night sweats, chills, fever, diarrhea, abdominal cramping, muscle spasms, tearing eyes, cardiac arrhythmia, tachycardia, nausea, vomiting, rapid breathing, yawning, goose bumps, dilated pupils, and uncontrollable shaking.

The psychological symptoms were more complex to deal with, because the brain is confused and conflicted with all the rapid biochemical changes taking place within its realm. They included, but were not limited to, anxiety, insomnia, restlessness, irritability, anorexia (loss of appetite), agitation, and depression. Just try sleeping or even sitting still with most of those symptoms occurring simultaneously, every day for a month. Like I stated above, it is recommended that one seek assistance from a qualified medical professional, so I took my advice as a professional RN and proceeded onward. Stubborn nurse! Bad nurse!

One major caveat to discontinuing my pain meds was that I still experienced pain almost daily. The withdrawal symptoms only exacerbated my preexisting symptoms, and there was no relief from pain except Advil, yoga, meditation, and breath control.

After much coaxing from Karen and many others, I finally took advantage of California Proposition 215, the Compassionate Use Act of 1996, and saw a physician who issued my recommendation for medical use of marijuana. It has become a panacea drug for a myriad of my complex symptomology of overlapping symptoms from my incongruous diagnoses.

I have since discovered and learned about a few of the 113 cannabinoids identified in the cannabis (marijuana) plant. Like the differences between sativa, indica, and cannabidiol (CBD), edibles, and oils. CBD has no psychogenic effects and therefore produces no "high" but works specifically for pain, PTSD, sleep disorders, and anxiety. I enjoyed the edibles and topical creams and smoke indica.

CBD is fast becoming my favorite, and it is actually legal in all fifty states (commercially made with hemp, not THC, so the effects are much less). I disagree however with the claims that it relieves pain as much as oxycodone and its opiate relatives. It never makes my pain go away, but does help reduce the severity.

And another really cool thing is, you can't overdose or die from smoking pot; the only way it can kill you is if a bale of it falls on your head (with my thanks to Willie Nelson)! And this is only my personal opinion, so do not take my word for it, but marijuana has never been addictive in my experiences. Yes, I have seen the propaganda movie *Reefer Madness* made in 1936, and I don't think I've laughed so much since watching *Animal House* and the *Austin Powers* movies for the first time. I personally have smoked marijuana and stopped for months, for years, and even for decades while I was a nurse, and experienced no withdrawal symptoms or cravings for more. I am probably just not an addictive type despite my iatrogenic bout with oxycodone. I can take it or leave it. No longer do I seek its inebriant qualities, but rather relief of my symptoms.

On July 4, 1970, I quit smoking cigarettes cold turkey just two months after my discharge from the Marine Corps. The same applied to alcohol. I quit for years with no cravings or desire to have a drink on numerous occasions. Alcohol has become taboo for me now for the rest of my life now because of hepatitis C and a severely damaged, cirrhotic liver. I don't miss alcohol, but if I see a salty margarita in a restaurant, I salivate like one of Russian physiologist Ivan Pavlov's experimental dogs. Hell, if I see a salty senorita in a restaurant, I salivate. I can't apologize for my extra Y chromosome; I'm a man with needs for dog's sake!

It's been well over three years now with no desire for opiates, and the carpal tunnel syndrome in my left hand doesn't hurt and it works just fine, thank you very much.

CHAPTER 23

Making Jell-O

I'd much rather be a woman than a man. Women can cry, they can wear cute clothes, and they're the first to be rescued off sinking ships.

—Gilda Radner

Karen still continues to work twelve-hour night shifts full-time at Fresno Heart and Surgical Hospital. She runs our two dogs, Blue and Molly, over a mile every day she has off work and does cardio training and thirty to sixty minutes of yoga as part of her daily routine. She loves to cook with wine, and sometimes she even adds it to the food. Despite her humble denial, she's a gourmet cook who loves to cook and eat great food.

We buy and grow our own organic food; avoid fast-food restaurants like Hillary avoids press conferences; take a fistful of vitamins and herbs daily; and drink ayurvedic "green shakes" with spirulina (icky tasting/smelling), coconut oil, almond milk, aloe vera juice, ashwagandha powder, turmeric, tulsi, yogarag guggulu, triphat, diatomaceous earth, beet root powder, and nutritional yeast flakes with bananas, blueberries, or strawberries to help make it palatable, while the Brits are having their afternoon tea and scones. She is a hardworking dynamo with unfathomable beauty, compassion, more energy than the Energizer bunny, always predictably in a good mood, almost never gets sick, and chose me as her soul mate. How can a man be any happier.

Our Flying Monkey Ranch is healthy and revived again after five years of hard work. Flowers bloom year-round, all our animals are loving creatures of God, and are healthy, happy, and full of life. All the different animals intermingle and get along with each other. The organic raised gardens and fruit trees are now prolific and are gopher- and squirrel-free, providing plenty of vittles to last us through the winter and freeze more apple pies, crisps, and applesauce than we can eat and give more away than we keep.

The twenty-four-foot diameter Sioux tipi is still standing; we just have to wait until it rains to have a fire inside, watching the wispy smoke linger upward through the open smoke flaps while lying on oversize dog pillows, gazing up at the stars. The firebreaks and trails I'm building are nearly completed, and the goatlings are providing even more weed clearing; I just need to catch up on burning my brush piles. We installed two oscillating water sprinklers and mounted them on the roof; they provide a combined 180-foot diameter water shower on our home and surrounding area in case of fire. We always have our "go bag" packed and a posted evacuation list.

Cal Fire has not yet visited our home to inspect our home for fire safety; however, an old friend visited recently, a retired fire chief from the rural Fresno area I have known for over thirty years. He stated that on large fires, one of his jobs was to assess which homes were defensible from an oncoming fire and those homes that were lost causes due to overgrowth of vegetation, etc. Our home passed his inspection with flying colors.

He even determined the probable direction of fire spread on our property based upon location and terrain. Amazingly, the same area that he pointed out has been one of my major priorities in property clearing since we bought our home because I sensed the same thing. A raging fire could race up a hilly overgrown area in minutes.

When we moved in, I began clearing brush and large dead branches as well as cutting down several hundred oak trees, mostly dead from the drought or diseased and infested with mistletoe. Lots more brush piles to burn, but also lots of free oak firewood to keep us warm in the winter! The land in question is on the north side of our home that slowly descends into what is now a grassy vale, but was once so thick with undergrowth, manzanita, and brush that it was nearly impassable and one could not see through all the green growth. A few old black oak trees that were about sixty feet tall and nearly as wide with three-foot diameter bases we had removed by a professional tree company. They dropped those huge trees right on the mark, not damaging any other surrounding landscaping.

We are truly blessed for all we have and give our thanks through prayer, yoga, meditation, healing essential oils, and smudging herbs. Smudging is a deeply spiritual meditation; each herb has its own unique energy and power, and breathing in their unique scents is intoxicating to the mind when sitting and meditating on the ground cross-legged in a circle of friends.

Our oldest son, Eric, lives just "over the hill" in Oakhurst ten miles north. His daughter Princess Ellery Rose is our first grand-child and is the happiest, most beautiful, funny, entertaining four-year-old. Absolute purity and innocence, growing independence, vigilance, fierce determination, unbridled energy, limitless creativity, and a proclivity toward defiance; the last trait is not from my bloodlines!

Karen and I decided early on that we wanted to play a big role in her life since she lives so close, so we negotiated with Eric and Heather one day a week that we could watch her. So every Monday is our play day with Ellery. Tuesday through Friday she attends day care the rest of the week. We don't even call it babysitting because she is so entertaining; we laugh and play and sing and dance and learn all day.

Ellery was dubbed at birth by me as the "Fifth Element." Mila Jovovich played Leeloo, a beautiful human/alien who, along with the other four elements Earth, Water, Air, and Fire, became the fifth element required to save Earth from total annihilation from overwhelming alien forces, along with the assistance and finally love confession of Korben Dallas, played by Bruce Willis. It is my belief, even though I probably will not live long enough to see it happen, but Ellery will someday do something that will change or alter the course of the world. Maybe a little far-fetched, but somehow I know she will one way or another play a major role on Mother Earth.

Middle child Katy Rose has spent years in college getting her proper teaching credentials to work with children with multiple mental and physical disabilities and currently teaches classes in Lewiston, Idaho, located on the beautiful Snake River. She calls her mom almost every day to check in and talk. Her husband, Adrian, is a master welder of anything metal and creates metal masterpieces as well as gates and fences for businesses. He currently fabricates large custom boats with conservative sticker prices starting in six figures. Many dogs and cats adorn their furniture. They are still working on becoming parents, and we're waiting to become grandparents again. Right now, the more grandkids I live to see, the merrier.

Youngest of our three combined children is Forrest; remember the skinny eleven-year-old kid who told his dad he was going to be a Navy SEAL when he grew up and is now six feet, four inches and 220 pounds of solid muscle? When he graduated from high school, he weighed 160 pounds! He got out of the Navy intact, bought a Harley Davidson, and landed a job with the US Forest Service "Hot Shot" crew fighting wildland fires in the national forests. From there he started working for Cal Fire and finally got hired full-time with them, currently working as an engineer. He was on the two largest fires in California history last year, one of them located in their backyard, the Sonoma County / Santa Rosa fire. He left from there to assist with the Thomas fire south of Santa Barbara, the largest fire ever recorded in California history, and worked all the way past Christmas with nary a day off. In the off-season, he graduated as an engineer finishing third academically and breaking several Cal Fire physical fitness standards records. His lovely wife, Margot Brown, just recently graduated from her doctor's residency program in June 2017 and had secured her first real job as an MD after taking several well-deserved months off. Margot had to evacuate her home alone that smoky night before her first day at work with their cat because Forrest was already on the fire lines and their home was under "mandatory evacuation" orders. Every one of our kids' homes was spared from fires despite being in the fires' paths and all of them having evacuation orders for their homes. It was quite a summer out West, not to mention several catastrophic hurricanes down South!

I suddenly realized I have no idea why I named this chapter "Making Jell-O!" Maybe "Nailing Jell-O to the Wall" would be more appropriate? That's what it seems like as a parent raising children, anyway. Really, don't sweat the small stuff and get over it.

CHAPTER 24

65 Minutes

The rush of battle is often a potent and lethal
Addiction, for war is a drug.

—Chris Hedges

Sixty-five minutes. Three thousand nine hundred seconds. One hour and five minutes. About the time it takes to cook and eat a home-cooked meal. Or barbecue a tri-tip steak on the grill. Or solve a cross-word puzzle. Unfortunately, sixty-five minutes is also the average amount of time each day that a United States Marine, Army, Navy, Air Force, or Coast Guard military veteran commits suicide.

It is an ongoing phenomenon comparing the high suicide rate of veterans to the general population. And that is the latest study published in 2013 by the United States Department of Veterans Affairs with other sources suggesting the rate is likely higher. And that data is nearly a decade old, from 1999 to 2010. There are more and more severely injured returning vets who would not have survived their injuries of previous wars, and a scandal in the VA health care system that impeded their deserved treatment so long that some vets died before treatment could be scheduled.

That amounts to *twenty-two soldiers a day, nearly seven hundred soldiers per month, and over eight thousand soldiers per year* who made the ultimate sacrifice to honor and defend their country, only to come home to America with horrendous memories and unfathomable traumatic experiences. Debilitating injuries, feelings of grief, anxiety, depression, hopelessness, isolation, trepidation, impulse control issues, anger, guilt, loss, rage, introversion, and loss of the ability to *feel alive*. The *annual* average of veteran suicide exceeded the total number of combat-related deaths in the Gulf War (383) and the Iraq and Afghanistan conflicts (6,773) spanning nearly two decades. *So sad!*

In 2007, the VA and the secretary of the US Department of Veterans Affairs implemented a comprehensive suicide prevention program (JOVSPA), the Joshua Omvig Veterans Suicide Prevention Act. These agencies contracted with NIMH (National Institute of Mental Health) to investigate possible reasons for the higher-than-normal veteran suicide rate and monitor the efficacy of the interventions and progress. The government is aware of the problem, but obviously too many slip through the cracks of bureaucracy, and many wait months for appointments or die first! Some are totally distrustful of the government, many deny any help, and some simply have experienced inexplicable horror and hurt too much, and suicide frees them from a life of pain and anguish, recurring nightmares… unforgettable memories.

JOVSPA was named obviously after Joshua Omvig, a twenty-two-year-old army specialist from Gillette, Wyoming, who had just returned from Iraq after a tour of duty with the 339th Military Police. He confided his feelings that he may have PTSD to his family upon returning from his eleven-month stint but did not seek treatment, fearing it would deleteriously affect his military career. The pain was too much for him to endure; in December 2005 Joshua killed himself with a gun in his parents' driveway shortly after returning home for the holidays.

Veterans (and others) with PTSD and concomitant depression are more likely to take their own lives. For all the veterans who die of suicide, 65% are over the age of fifty. Suicide risk for veterans is 22% higher than the rest of the population; 30 suicides per 100,000 population versus 14 suicides per 100,000 of the general population. The Department of Veterans Affairs stated that vets from the Vietnam War have the highest percentage (31%) of PTSD (that "police action" involved over 2.7 *million* troops!) than all US conflicts later combined. The cards were definitely stacked against me!

Over 30% of veterans returning from Afghanistan and Iraq have experienced a traumatic brain injury or have PTSD; sadly, only about half of them seek medical treatment. Many of them are prime candidates for PTSD and suicide.

These statistics have loomed in my subconscious and have always bothered me. When I was self-injecting my abdomen with a needle every other day with the outrageously expensive antiviral (BigPharma) interferon alfa-2a and anemia-inducing antiviral ribavirin to try to cure my hepatitis C in 1999, the physical side effects and pain were beyond description but were amplified even more psychologically. The sight of food caused me to vomit and thirty pounds were shed in the first two months of treatment. I thought often of suicide; the pain was unbearable, and I even felt homicidal. These invading thoughts occurred during the months I had to take off from my job as a flight nurse and I stayed home almost every day, thankfully. It was hard living with myself at the time, let alone what my wife and kids had to endure, and I prepared my family before starting therapy that with all the unknown side effects, I might say and do things I would regret. I became a real pain in the ass for months, and I knew it but seemed powerless to its control over me. The biochemical changes of those poisons had turned me into a curmudgeon and changed my personality into an evil Dr. Evil. My inner strength was definitely challenged, but my commitment to practice yoga and meditation daily with my wife, and my knowledge that Mr. Hyde would soon return to Dr. Jekyll, kept me marginally sane. I knew it was the horrible side effects of the interferon injections that had temporarily changed my personality into someone even I did not know and couldn't stand being around. I rarely looked in the mirror because I did not like the reflection of what I saw on the other side.

Fortunately, I was able to climb out of Alice's rabbit hole by the big tree and return with my sanity intact, despite nearly dying from the drug's side effects, and I have never felt the same physically since taking interferon alfa-2a. Good news: my pharmacologically induced psychosis stopped abruptly when I stopped the drug therapy. Bad news: the chemotherapy did not work after a year of self-imposed hell.

Why is the author writing about such morbid subjects? you wonder. A few years ago I went to see my private physician during the Christmas holidays. Predictably, he made more pharmaceutical changes, increasing my med doses.

Then one day in late December I looked at my clock and it read *sixty-four minutes.*

CHAPTER 25

George Bailey

There's no place like home!
There's no place like home!
There's no place like home!

—Dorothy Gale, *The Wizard of Oz*

The VA and other studies state that there are over 270,000 living Vietnam veterans with PTSD and other comorbidities. One could argue that number would more accurately be 270,001 because I was denied VA disability benefits for PTSD despite it being verified and confirmed by three social workers and three independent psychologists. In addition, my VA claims for documented hearing loss and a strong case for contracting hepatitis C were *denied*, so not much exists in their data banks. When Karen retires, I will be forced to enter the VA health care system. Our local VA facilities have received favorable reports from veterans, mostly from older vets in my age group.

Over the last 18,250 nights (that's equal to fifty years), I have languished and endured as I continue to see clear horrific images of a VC whose throat I cut; killing two seemingly innocent children (carrying enemy rifles); napalmed children running on fire reduced to black charred corpses; felonious psycho meth addict/dealer Sam Montalvo, who tried to kill me with a 12-gauge shotgun in the ER. And let's not forget the career-ending asshole, the psychotic, drunken, blood- and urine-soaked James A. Carvelli, who kicked me in the head and chest causing serious injury, and the patient whom I nearly killed in the ER!

Each day with PTSD is a challenge for me, but it is also a blessing to see the sunrise each day. There are a finite number of sunrises for all of us, and my sunrises are shrinking in number, as all our lives do. I still have days when people "push my PTSD button," and I've usually responded honestly and bluntly and expressed my true feelings rather than keeping quiet during those situations I usually walked away from quietly fuming. I've pissed off a lot of people. It's not healthy to sandbag and keep that shit inside anymore.

Computerized marketing phone calls, lying, stealing, abusing humans or animals, cheating, circuitous robotic phone trees that lead one in circles while never speaking to a human, trespassing, school shootings, and a long list of other nefarious and despicable acts could *potentially* push "the button." Fortunately, I am a Vietnam veteran who has been medicated for your safety. Well, most of the time.

Many frequent tall challenges were met head-on over and over and over and over. In February, I broke my second cervical vertebra and wore a rigid neck splint for four months. Shortly after that in August, I self-detoxed at home from oxycodone after five years of taking daily large doses freely prescribed by compassionate, well-meaning doctors for my headaches, and later for my broken neck that hurt like a red-hot poker in my brain stem.

Three months later in the late fall of 2016, almost constant mid-abdominal pain started, accompanied by nausea, anorexia, lost work time on the ranch, and a progressive 25 percent weight loss. It took five months to see a GI doctor who never examined my abdomen but convinced me, with the urging of Karen, to try the relatively new drug Harvoni that boasted 96–99 percent cure rate for patients never treated prior for HCV. Those who had prior treatment had lesser success rates, and must take the drug longer. After a battery of baseline blood tests, twelve weeks of Harvoni treatment began on June 6, 2017, and caused a host of horrible but not unexpected side effects, not including my headaches and constant abdominal pain. My only alternatives for treating the pain was Motrin and a combination of meditation, breath control, indica, and CBD oil.

Fortunately, after a three-month waiting period after finishing the therapy on August 28, I was declared clear of the virus on December 1, 2017. I was cured, or at least in remission. But the constant unrelenting abdominal pain that began over a year ago continued unabated. I still felt lousy every day and was shedding pounds without trying to lose weight. The pain precluded my desire to challenge my now-defiant GI tract. If it told me, "Don't you dare eat that or you will see it again real soon," I heeded my stomach's advice, and sometimes it took a few inhalations to stimulate my appetite enough to allow me to eat a few bites of cottage cheese, toast, or oatmeal. By year's end I had lost sixty pounds! This weight loss method is not recommended. I would not advocate Slim Fast either after looking at Whoopi Goldberg.

I changed GI doctors and found a real doctor who explained things, asked pertinent questions, suggested a plan, asked for my input, listened intently, *and* performed a full complete abdominal assessment like I was trained as a nurse to do, and performed same to my patients in the ER for over three decades. We developed a good rapport and shared by ruling out what the causes for the weight loss and pain was *not* (not a diabetic) first and then talked about possible causes, cancer in my colon or exocrine cancer of the pancreas.

Based upon my reported symptomology, Dr. Singh suspected my pancreas could be the cause. The location and function of the pancreas can make it hard to diagnose, especially in the early stages, taking sometimes a year to discover it. He ordered a slew of lab tests, an oral (barium) and IV contrast of the abdomen and pancreas, a colonoscopy, and upper endoscopy with biopsies. I discussed with my doctor and the CRNA (certified registered nurse anesthetist) that I only wanted light sedation with Versed, *no* opiates, and if I could not handle the pain, he had propofol as backup. Propofol, nicknamed "milk of amnesia" because of its white milky appearance and extraordinary clinical effects, has a rapid onset and very short half-life in the bloodstream. The effects can be dramatic, but it is quickly metabolized and the patient is amnesic to the events occurring during their pharmacologic dream state. Jocko took just a little bit too much, so sad to lose such a talented superstar.

After 3 mg of Versed, I told my doctor I was ready to proceed. At my request, the image of my colon on the color monitor screen was situated so I could view the Hershey Highway in high-def and ask questions along the route. During the procedure, the doctor maneuvering the northbound six-foot black snake asked me if the pain was tolerable or if I wanted anything for the pain. I told him that I was indeed having pain from the colonoscope but had been experiencing a similar but worse type of pain constantly for the past year and declined his opiate offer. A few precancerous polyps were removed, but otherwise it was unremarkable. Once again, the bowel prep preceding the actual procedure was the most uncomfortable.

During the waning months of the year, I had multiple repeated blood tests, an MRI of the head and abdomen, and all the aforementioned GI exams. The constant pain and weight loss continued, I still could not eat a normal meal, and my depression was escalating. Not surprisingly, of course, my doctor doubled the dose of the SSRI escitalopram (Lexapro). My suicidal thoughts were never discussed; Dr. Manjal never asked, and I didn't offer.

The holiday season was upon us, and dreary skies loomed on the horizon. Interesting paradox: the Christmas season is a festive time celebrating the birth of Jesus, yet statistics reflects an increase in suicides during this period. The added stressors we allow ourselves to affect our behaviors only compound the threat. From a family perspective, this Christmas would be spent in relative isolation. Karen was scheduled to work her regular F-T shifts plus extra night shifts on December 13–16, 19–20, and 23–27. So it was just me and the Flying Monkey Ranch critters to entertain each other.

Family turmoil erupted in November when Eric and Heather permanently split up with our fifth element Ellery stuck in the middle and left a grandpa and grandma with broken hearts. Due to situational constraints, we were not allowed to see Ellery on her second birthday, which occurred on Thanksgiving Day, and as it turned out later, Christmas as well. Katy and husband Adrian did visit the week before Christmas for a few days. Forrest was working straight through the holidays sans days off, fighting the Thomas Fire in So-Cal, and Margot was in her first months working as a physician.

The intolerable and constant abdominal pain, anorexia, dysphagia, headaches, myalgias, unsteady erratic gait, confusion, irritability, sleep disturbances with night sweats and frequent nightmares, family strife, uncertainty, and not knowing what was making me so sick was even more depressing than if the doctor would have found some serious, life-threatening disease. I had dug myself an emotional abyss of helplessness, despair, and depression, and the only way to look was up. The clock counting down to sixty-five minutes was tick-tick-ticking away, and nothing stood in its way.

Friday, December 22, 2017

El Sol Amarillo rose in the East with the cool refreshing crispness of a fresh-picked apple from our orchard. The full supermoon on December 3 was in perigee closest to Earth, and tonight it would be but a silver waxing crescent as it approached the first quarter anticipating the next blue supermoon on December 31. It was Karen's only day off before working five straight 1900–0700 shifts caring for open-heart surgical patients in the CICU, so we spent a lazy day at home. Coincidentally, today was Festivus Eve.

Festivus, is a noncommercial secular annual holiday popularized by the "it's a show about nothing" hit series *Seinfeld* in the 1997 episode "The Strike." In the parody spoof, Festivus is created by Frank Costanza (Jerry Stiller), neurotic George Costanza's (Jason Alexander) hot-tempered red-haired father. It celebrates an alternative to the pressures of commercialization of the Christmas holiday that now, sadly, begins before Halloween in early October. The pagans dance around an unadorned aluminum pole, supplanting the tinseled tree, while celebrating the "Airing of Grievances," followed by Festivus Dinner, Festivus Miracles, and later Feats of Strength. Officially, Festivus was not over until the head of the household is wrestled to the floor and submits. This is Festivus for the Rest of Us! With that in mind, I suggested that since she would essentially be gone the next five days (work all night; sleep during the day; yoga, shower, shared "green shake," then back to work, total awake time at home two and one-half hours. Repeat × 5!), we should celebrate Festivus together on her last night off.

With the winter solstice and shortest day of the year only a mere twenty-four hours past, the sun set at 1645 (4:45 p.m.). Would this be my last sunset? The last supper? All the animals were fed and settled; the solar and low-voltage lights on the property emitted a soft glow of light that allowed outside navigation with less fear of stumbling in the darkness. It was time for some serious pole dancing.

We both held hands as we navigated our way down the driveway in sustained rainfall to our aluminum Festivus pole, an illuminated twenty-foot aluminum flagpole. We were both in our natural state, with only the American Flag and Marine Corps Flag as passive silent witnesses to this spontaneous bizarre event, waving in the faint wind from high above, questioning what pagan ritual was about to take place. We danced naked like faeries in the night, laughing and giggling with total abandon. Instead of Airing of Grievances, we both blessed our good fortune, health, family, love, serenity. The festivities outdoors concluded when the fingers and toes started getting numb, so it was inside for Festivus Dinner and a warm fire in the woodstove to thaw out.

Dinner was a delectable delight from the get-go. Home-made baked stuffed portobella mushroom appetizers followed by the entrée: baked lobster with butter sauce, organic veggies from our garden, and sliced sourdough bread dipped in Sciabica's rosemary-infused EVOO with complimentary balsamic vinegar. A nice cold bottle of champagne to tease the palate was opened with one in reserve, just in case. After a tasty dessert consisting of French vanilla ice cream topped with fresh strawberries, cocoa powder, and sliced walnuts with a dash of Bailey's Irish Cream, we settled on the floor next to our dogs Molly and Blue warming themselves by the woodstove. We laid out a special altar cloth and placed a tripod-mounted abalone shell filled with sand in its center, then lit a few small charcoal tablets, and prepared for the ancient native American Indian tradition of smudging herbs.

This is a great hour-long meditation that stimulates all six senses and helps forge the strong bonds between the participants on a metaphysical plane. One can smudge many herbs, plants, minerals, and crystals in any particular order and number; it's up to the individual's personal preference. Following is the orderly sequence that I developed years ago, and we have followed the same ritualistic path experiencing the multitude of feelings and sensations from their distinct aromatic emanations.

The first herb is desert sage for purification and cleansing. Mayan white copal crystals remove negative spirits and are intoxicatingly stimulating to cranial nerve V, the trigeminal nerve. To clear the light body and further enhance relaxation, lavender flowers are smudged next. In order to summon one's animal totem, cedar shavings are then burned. Frankincense crystals, representing consecration and purity, come next, followed by myrrh crystals for healing, peace, and protection. By now, the senses are in a state of calm hyperawareness and peaceful homeostasis, effects of the combination of six potent herbs smoldering and swirling slowly in unison and harmony. Kashmiri and sandalwood follow those same two precious gifts presented by the magi to Jesus in Bethlehem under Caesar Augustus's reign over two thousand years ago, both promoting spirituality and enhancing the meditation. As the meditation continues, sweetgrass helps clear and prevent the return of any remaining negative spirits. Lastly, as one slowly begins to become aware of their immediate surroundings and return from their spiritual meditative journey, patchouli, a bushy herbal plant from the *Lamiaceae*, or "mint" family, concludes the meditation with spiritual fulfillment and grounding.

Participants usually sit on the floor in a small circle on a zabuton with beaded (faux) eagle feathers to help fan and circulate the smoke. Others (like me!) hold "shaman stones," or moqui marbles, in a clasped palm mudra with thumb and forefinger forming a circle, wrists resting just above the knees, while comfortably sitting in the half (me) or full (Karen) lotus position, experiencing the distant memories and pulse of these magical, mystical stones. Discovered at the base of Navajo sandstone formations, roughly the size of a walnut with a sandstone center surrounded with iron, phosphorus, and lime, these heavy, dense stones are estimated to be between 130 and 150 million years old, eons before some dinosaurs roamed what is now North America. Their powers are alleged to include spiritual protection, healing powers, absorbing negativity and replacing with positive energy, and increasing the upward flow through the seven chakras. They also connect with Mother Earth's energies and contact animal spirits, totems, spirit guides, and shape-shifting.

Upon rising from the floor, and totally disregarding the incoming, distressing sensory impulses from the cartilage, bones, and muscles of my knees, my now erect and temporarily vertically challenged position was greeted with the cumulative smoke cloud of ten herbs and crystals hovering throughout our home about five feet AGL. Their collective aromatic mixture reignited primal memories and allowed a temporary hiatus from my perceived insurmountable problems.

Karen and I exchanged a small gift to each other, then we settled on our couch with red fox blanket and a bowl of popcorn to watch *It's a Wonderful Life*, the 1946 quintessential Christmas classic directed by Frank Capra. George Bailey (Jimmy Stewart) a small-town banker from Bedford Falls, was experiencing despair, ruin, and serious financial problems and was contemplating suicide on Christmas Eve. Just before plunging himself into the icy river from the bridge above, George Bailey chooses instead to jump in to save another jumper, his guardian angel. When he discovers what life would have been without him, how wonderful life really is despite one's woes, he is ultimately redeemed. All is well in Bedford Falls, and his guardian angel gets his wings. I have watched this movie many times over the years but never had it had such a profound influence on my being. While watching the movie, I was feeling the same feelings of helplessness, despair, and depression. Outwardly, I projected a serene persona, but inside I felt like I was going to melt down quicker than the Wicked Witch of the West at a Water Park.

Sleep evaded me that night like a bipartisan congressional vote. The physical pain holding my body hostage had carried on longer and more relentlessly than Robert Mueller seeking Russian collusion in the White House. Desperation. Frustration. Exasperation. I had reached my nadir and was ready to tumble down the abyss into darkness, never to return...

The sun shone brightly the next morning, and a quick surprise visit from middle daughter Katy Rose and husband Adrian and their three dogs Otis, Gaia, and Half-Pint brightened the day despite my perceived gathering of dark storm clouds approaching with frightening intensity. Then we received the phone call everyone retrospectively hates answering. Karen's close cousin Colleen called to inform us that her husband, Jim, an electrical engineer who had just retired, died of an acute myocardial infarction (AMI, heart attack) in his living room chair while playing fantasy football on his sixtieth birthday. Death had darkened our door from afar, yet it felt so near I could touch it, taste it, smell it. We four humans, five dogs, two cats, and six goats walked the mile-long trail around the perimeter of our property, enjoying each other's company and sharing moments in reflective silence. Even my troupe of flying monkeys quietly hummed an elegy from the treetops above.

Suddenly, out of nowhere I was stuck by yet another epiphany, a sudden intuitive realization that all my pain, suffering, and dark feelings come from within and nobody but me could change me but me. It all felt so insignificant. In this life-altering moment, I stopped hating myself and forgave myself, and all thoughts of selfish suicidal thoughts vanished and have yet to return. My life suddenly had value and meaning again. A new beginning. I had just experienced a George Bailey moment. Only one more variable in my medical equation required serious consideration that had been completely overlooked by the medical community, but the one that I was always most paranoid and most suspicious of. It would require even more sacrifice, and it would not be without its inherent risks, but at this point in my life, I was desperate and willing to try almost anything to feel better. Something drastic had to change.

My guardian angel had just received his new pair of wings.

CHAPTER 26

White Rabbit

Suicide rates have not slumped under the onslaught of antidepressants, mood-stabilizers, anxiolytic and anti-psychotic drugs; the jump in suicide rates suggests that the opposite is true. In some cases, suicide risk skyrockets once treatment begins (the patient may feel not only penalized for a justifiable reaction, but permanently stigmatized as malfunctioning). Studies show that self-loathing sharply decreases only in the course of cognitive-behavioral treatment.

—Antonella Gambotto-Burke, *The Eclipse: A Memoir of Suicide*

Thus far, my esteemed Eastern (Indian) Western medicine physicians had emptied their collective bag of magic tricks much like one of my childhood cartoon heroes Felix the Cat, though without interference from the Professor and Poindexter, and they still offered no solace or even a remote hint of a diagnosis. Intractable abdominal pain, weakness, and fatigue with severe 25 percent weight loss are all symptoms, not diagnoses. Despite working as a nurse for decades, I always possessed the knowledge and recognition of the multiple alternative modalities of healing that has superseded Western medicine for centuries. Ingesting synthetic pharmaceuticals approved by the most corrupt federal agency, my personal albeit shared opinion by many, the Food and Drug Administration, had always been of the lowest priority for me. Many drugs are beneficial and oftentimes necessary for survival, like insulin and epinephrine; I've utilized these drugs uncountable times to help save lives including my own. I do not dispute the medical necessity of the myriad of lifesaving drugs. It's the overprescribing and insane costs driven by greed and profit. Unfortunately for me, however, I fell into the trap of Big Pharma by dutifully following my physicians' well-intentioned instructions, expecting improvement but receiving progressive deterioration instead.

If not for the hospital assault of October 2, 2011, I quite possibly could have achieved my goal of independence from prescription drugs. Since that infamous day, a myriad of doctors have had a field day prescribing multiple combinations of antihypertensives, antidepressants, benzodiazepines for PTSD, opiates for pain, and hypnotics for sleep, sometimes as many as nine different drugs several times a day. It was time once again to take control of my life, much like my unforgettable experience the year prior detoxifying from oxycodone.

Two long painful months passed while I pondered my course of action while still feeling blessed to view each consecutive sunrise. All my diagnostic tests were indeterminate, "consistent with senescent changes" as one of the radiologists who had never met me dictated in his notes, further dictating and subsequently charging for incorrect medications during the conscious sedation procedure based upon a computer software "template" designed for expediency, rather than taking the time to peruse the medication record or the supposed nurses notes. That snafu created quite a stir when I received the bill for medications I refused to take (Fentanyl) and never did receive. No, I'll never going back to that place again! My temple is not a *template*.

Armed with knowledge of the human body and blessed with discriminating diagnostic abilities and a keen sensitivity and intimate connection with my own body, I knew instinctively that there were exogenous causes for my continued debilitating condition. Hours were spent re-researching my medications, short- and long-term side effects, drug interactions, and dependency issues. After six years of taking daily medications and tricking the body to act in discordance with its natural homeostatic condition, on Monday, March 5, 2018, Baron Ron Von Martinstein once again locked himself in the la-*bor*-atory at the Flying Monkey Ranch and made the long-considered and much-anticipated decision to discover if my suspicions would be confirmed. The long and winding road lay ahead, with a steep incline, I might add. Never did I consider the path would be easy; rather, quite the opposite.

The AM radio tuner mysteriously turned on inside my head again to the all-too-familiar station KWTF. The Wolfman had the night off. The Jefferson Airplane with San Francisco vocalist/lyricist and rock goddess Grace Slick slowly pulsated to the enchanting "White Rabbit"...

> *One pill makes you larger,*
> *And one pill makes you small*
> *And the ones that mother gives you*
> *Don't do anything at all.*
> *Go ask Alice, when she's ten feet tall.*

That Monday morning a resolute decision was made to take the steep high road. My mind was prepared for battle again with Sauron and the evil dark forces of the pharmaceutical world, but now I was a veteran in the arena of acute toxic drug withdrawal symptoms. The steep ascent would include many of the same aforementioned side effects of oxycodone withdrawal plus some I had yet to experience because I was withdrawing from four completely different classes of drugs.

The benzodiazepine clonazepam (Klonopin) was prescribed by my PMD/psychologist for PTSD symptoms after "the incident" back in 2011, and I took them as prescribed three times daily for over six years. Benzodiazepine withdrawal symptoms can be extremely harsh, oftentimes harder to exorcise than opiates and with a longer duration of deleterious side effects.

Escitalopram (Lexapro) is a serum serotonin reuptake inhibitor (SSRI) drug for depression and anxiety and an approved drug for PTSD. It was the most recent replacement drug for a regimen of others that I reluctantly tried and found to be ineffective, deleterious, or sensitive to.

The sedative/hypnotic zolpidem (Ambien) was prescribed for sleep, and I found them to be relatively ineffective more times than not; however, it was sometimes the only bridge between sleep and insanity in desperate times when sleep eluded me for hours or days on end, tossing and turning while my mind was in hyperdrive or my body screamed in painful silence. Interestingly, Ambien can also cause drug dependence and can paradoxically *impede* sleep patterns.

Lastly and most critical was propranolol ER, a beta-adrenergic blocking agent with multiple applications, but in my case it was for high blood pressure that took my collective of doctors five years to get under control. My sixty-plus-pound weight loss over the last year had a positive effect on lowering my blood pressure, and I still methodically check it three to four times daily. The propranolol has remained on my required list for my BP control.

The first few weeks of March were reminiscent of my August 2016 confrontation with oxycodone withdrawal. Worsening abdominal pain, anorexia, tachycardia, night sweats, myalgias, arthralgias, neuralgias, cramping. Anxiety, restlessness, agitation, "crawling" skin, worsening insomnia.

> *And if you go chasing rabbits*
> *And you know you're going to fall*
> *Tell them a hookah-smoking caterpillar*
> *Has given you the call*
> *And call Alice, when she was just small.*

The days passed slowly and painfully, and the days turned into weeks, weeks into months. The lingering symptoms progressed longer than I had anticipated, but I remained ever vigilant and hopeful that my hypothesis would be proven correct.

Another severe concussion and neck hyperextension on Saturday, May 12, 2018, Mother's Day Eve, dealt a serious blow, both literally and figuratively to my recovery efforts. While trying to capture one of my younger ~80 kilo wether goats to replace his collar he had outgrown, Strider escaped my leaping effort and my body became a flying projectile, striking my left frontal lobe on the edge of one of the vertical four-by-four wood support beams inside the barn, snapping my head and neck backward, landing supine on my back in straw and goat poop, immovable for twenty minutes.

Karen witnessed the incident and was at my side in a heartbeat while my goatlings all gathered 'round and stared quizzically with feigned interest at my agonizing cries of pain. The frontal hematoma with expansive abrasions continued to grow in size to that of a walnut while I lay there unable to move. I would have put my pain level at 10 out of 10, and I rarely quantify my pain score that high. At that same moment, I was feeling blessed that I was not unconscious. The intense sensations felt just like the pain I experienced after breaking both sides of C-2 in my neck two years prior but accompanied with intractable head pain as well.

After twenty minutes I finally regained my composure and was tired of lying on the poopy manger floor. Karen helped me up perpendicular to Mother Earth and held on to me for a few minutes until I regained control of my upright status. I looked Strider in the eye and the chase was on once again; only this time I negotiated a successful quick takedown, and I placed a larger collar around his neck while Karen removed the old tight one. Improvise, adapt, and overcome! Oohrah, mission accomplished! Time for ice packs and Advil to diminish the intense pain I was experiencing.

The unwelcomed return of a familiar sensation from the past was disconcerting. Coldness and paresthesia in my left arm radiated down to my thumb and middle fingers, reminiscent of a previous injury decades earlier that resulted in a herniated left cervical disc at C4-C5 and successful cervical laminotomy as the final outcome. Another possible MRI loomed in my future. I was conscious, breathing, lucid, and could again move all my extremities. The situation and outcome could have been much worse. Blessed be! And no, I did not call an ambulance or go to the hospital. Stubborn nurse, bad nurse!

As the month of May wound down, my withdrawal symptoms began to wane, and I began to feel alive again. My HCV had now been in remission for six months. My neck pain now became the primary distraction as the rest of my body began to heal, and my internal biochemical composition began normalizing after being betrayed and deceived for six years by pharmaceuticals. With each passing day my energy levels began to increase exponentially.

Unfortunately, my head and spine were exempt from this new-found power surge. Postconcussion hyperextension injury (PCHI) number 1 occurred only a week after Mother's Day. While working on the corral fence behind our barn, I opened a gate and ducked under the near-invisible electric fence wire mounted at about eye level surrounding the four-foot-tall goat fence instead of temporarily disconnecting it. Sadly, I forgot about the near-invisible wire upon re-entry to the corral and struck the taut wire at forehead level full-stride! My hard hat prevented further head injury, but my neck snapped back harder than "Devil in the Blue Dress" Monika Lewinsky's under the Oval Office's resolute desk. My Bad!

PCHI number 2 was realized on the following Monday with the innocent assistance of our then two-and-a-half-year-old granddaughter Princess Ellery Rose. While sitting on the floor leaning back against a firm leather sofa, Ellery climbed up my torso and unexpectedly plopped the full weight of her twenty-eight-pound body on my face, forcing my unsupported neck rapidly backward nearly ninety degrees against the sofa seat. The tension and pain in the stretched muscles and ligaments forced my shoulders to rise up to meet my ears, and my neck remained fixed in neutral position, the slightest movement sending shock waves of pain throughout my spine.

Knowing that SHIT (shit happens in threes!) happens in threes, I became even more cautious but also felt like, "Doom on you, Ronbo." The inevitable is, well, inevitable. It's only a matter of how, where, and when. PCHI number 3 was simmering on the back burner, patiently waiting for its opportunity to fulfill its predetermined destiny.

It takes about two full eight-to-twelve-hour workdays of tractor work to cut the weeds on the intricate matrix of trails, fire-breaks, roads, meadows, and forest I've created on our property. The process needs to be repeated every few weeks during the early spring until it stops raining and the green wildflowers of spring become the dry weeds of summer and a severe fire danger. The last major cutting usually occurs sometime in June. I was on my last half hour of cutting on day two on what I hoped would be the final major cutting until next spring.

An ancient large mature black oak tree lives just outside the main gate to "the back fifteen," comprising most of our fenced property where the animals graze. The trunk is thirty inches in diameter, providing a shady canopy for the swing that dangles from a sixteen-inch branch extending horizontally about six feet AGL. Cutting the weeds around this special mammoth tree was the "coup de gras(s)" before heading through the gate to the house and calling it a day.

While I was paying close attention to not tangling my tractor in the swing ropes, the inexorable PCHI number 3 struck with unmatched intensity as my head with firmly attached hard hat with hearing protection and eye shield struck the horizontal branch obliquely yet firmly. My neck stretched backward and to the left, knocked the helmet off my head, and my body tumbled off the left side of the tractor, landing hard on the dry powdery dirt and prickly stubble of now-dried weeds. Thankfully, the safety features on the John Deere immediately shut off the engine and stopped the three spinning mower blades, preventing potential further injury.

I lay on the scorched dry earth feeling like I had just been tased after getting struck by a telephone pole, or maybe a telephone truck. Sweaty, hot, dusty, dry mouth, tired, pained, stunned, and alone I lay on Mother Earth, praying for her warm embrace and the ability to still achieve an erection. My legs first began to move under autonomic control. My arms moved but there was a painful, burning, electrical shock feeling from the skull, neck, shoulders, and arms. Called a "burner" or "neck stinger," it feels like being struck by one of Thor's lightning bolts. Thor was kind enough today to give me a free firm hammer stroke to my forehead as well. This stinger was a much more intense pulsing than the shock delivered by the goat corral electric fence that I personally test for power on occasion sans gloves. *Zzzzztttt!*

During my extended supine trauma self-assessment, my field of vision looking directly up at the bright midday sky was suddenly filled with six inquisitive, horny, floppy-eared ruminants. Minnie and her kids Frodo and Jules and Minnie's identical twin sister Daisy and her two kids Strider and Arwen all surrounded me and bleated their collective caprine concerns with heads slightly atilt, which caused me to break out laughing. Thankfully, innervation to the bladder was still functioning because I hadn't peed on myself. My Nubian goatlings came to my rescue!

Recovery from these repetitive injuries will likely take months to heal. Neck pain and a cold, numb left arm are now a persistent distraction. Multiple holistic modalities have been employed with minimal yet gradual improvement. What a pain in the neck!

Despite the daily pain distraction in my neck, my chronic daily abdominal pain *disappeared*. My appetite improved and I actually gained almost ten pounds after losing sixty. Strength, coordination, stamina, energy, proprioception, mentation, memory, balance, creativity, attitude, insomnia, anxiety, depression, activity, spirituality, health, and love of self *all* improved since *stopping* the recommended, prescribed, safe, and approved by the FDA pharmaceuticals!

The individual, synergistic, and anti-symbiotic side effects of all the synthetic chemicals coursing through my blood for years had in reality intensified and exacerbated the very symptoms their manufacturer proclaimed were supposedly beneficial in treating. My prescribed medications were paradoxically responsible for making me sicker! Thank you, Dr. Von Martinstein, your hypothesis was correct. You may take your seat.

> *When the men on the checkerboard get up*
> *And tell you where to go*
> *And you've just had some kind of mushroom,*
> *And your mind is moving low.*
> *Go ask Alice, I think she'll know.*

My trinity knot of life began to prosper and blossom with my returning health, resurging energy, and spiritual rebirth. Though still limited in the amount of hours I choose to work outdoors, I can still easily cut down four of my dead oak trees; limb and stack the slash in brush piles; cut the wood into logs, load the wood in my trailer, and haul it back up to the house; then restack it all neatly in the woodpile near the house before calling it a day.

The Summer Scorch Trials of California sequel repeated this summer with a vengeance as well, with zero rain for eight months and sustained temperatures over 100 degrees for over thirty days straight, combined with a ninety-eight-thousand-acre forest fire just to our north that closed Yosemite National Park for weeks, devastated the local tourism at peak season, and covered our skies, hills, and homes with toxic dense smoke and ash for six straight weeks.

Many days the air quality was so unhealthy it was ill-advised to go outdoors without wearing at least an N95 mask or respirator. Even with slightly improved breathing while working outside with my N95, the eyes burned and teared, visibility was severely impaired, and the Flying Monkey Ranch was covered with gray ash that took on the appearance of the monochromatic landscape of Pepperland after the Blue Meanies, Apple Droppers, Snapping Turks, and the Glove invaded, destroying beauty and music and freezing its inhabitants in the Beatles classic movie *Yellow Submarine*. It was a very long, hot, arid, smoky, scary, toxic summer for the second year in a row for our mountain community.

It was a sad day for us in July when our grown bonny bairn Katy Rose and her wonderful husband Adrian moved from Paradise, California, to live in Lewiston, Idaho, on the Snake River to be nearer Adrian's parents. As it turned out, we could not have been happier for their move. At 0630 on Thursday, November 8, a brush fire started on Camp Creek Road in the Feather River Canyon. Within twenty-four hours, over thirty-one square miles or twenty thousand acres were blackened by fire and the town or Paradise was completely destroyed, reduced to smoldering ash, tragedy, and death. Not until desperately needed rain fell for several days beginning on the twenty-first was the deadly Camp fire in Butte County declared officially 100 percent contained on November 25. It was responsible for over eighty-five deaths with hundreds initially missing or unaccounted for; 153,336 acres scorched, 13,696 residences and nearly 19,000 structures destroyed; every school and the only hospital gone. The

Camp fire has become the most destructive wildfire in California history and the nation's deadliest in over one hundred years.

The month of November was once again spent mostly indoors or outdoors with an N95 mask. San Francisco, 150 miles southwest of Paradise, even instituted poor air quality measures by closing the famous Cable Cars, universities canceled classes, while paradoxically the Mad Baron busied himself cutting brush, downing dead oak trees, clearing more fire trails, and stacking more oak firewood.

The comparatively cooler temperatures of the morning as compared to 106 degrees at 1500 prompted me to work early and quit early, reserving the heat of the afternoons to perform less arduous physical activities. Nevertheless, the last two years of near-cataclysmic forest fires in our own physicality and the entire western US was more than adequate incentive for creating more fire access roads and hard protection for our home and property in the wee hours and eschewing the oppressive omnipresent midday heat.

During the Summer Scorch Trials of 2018, nearly one hundred of my trees were cut into firewood, creating over sixty brush piles that continued to sprout and grow in numbers, most the size of a midsize car. They quickly became havens for the plentiful coveys of quail and rabbits that live on our property, and of course the ubiquitous rattlesnake in search of prey. When the first rain in eight months finally arrived on Thanksgiving Eve and continued intermittently for several days, fire restrictions were finally rescinded and the San Joaquin Valley Air Pollution Control District Hazard Fuel Reduction Program phone recording finally stated, "For the foothills and mountains of Madera County, today, Friday, November 30, it is a permissive burn day at all elevations between the hours of 9:00 a.m. and 4:00 p.m. Please contact your local fire department if your permit requires you to do so."

NCIS Special Agent Leroy Jethro Gibbs's rule 29 states, as I recall, "There are no coincidences." Mountain Roofing from Oakhurst arrived on Wednesday, November 21, with trailers, equipment, supplies, scaffolding, and forklift to begin removal of our old roof before installing a new metal roof just as it started to rain after eight continuous months of zero precipitation. We had signed our contract in early July but were on a lengthy waiting list. The assembled scaffolding, forklift, and trailer with roofing materials did not deter the shaky Christmas Eve landing of Kris Kringle and his nine reindeer (it was raining *and* foggy!) on our half-metal, half-plastic covered unfinished roof during a heavy rainstorm. The roof was finally completed in mid-January between the frequent drenching rain days that continued until mid-May.

The quail and rabbits quickly sought other lodging as the eager pyromaniac Baron Von Brush, armed with large propane tank and homeowner-designed flame thrower, chainsaws, shovels, rake, and trusty green JD, adroitly addressed the ever-growing population of piles, and by year's end, thirty-six brush piles were reduced to small mounds of ash in the ten allotted days of legal burning by the SJVAPCDHFRP. The remaining thirty piles were gone by March.

It amazes me that at age seventy, despite all the recent and long-term traumas in my life, I am leaner and meaner and a hell of a lot wiser than my early years as a US Marine! Maybe a little bit slower and clumsier, though. I still do the same stupid shit; it just takes me longer. And I've independently and systematically discontinued taking opiates for pain, benzodiazepines for anxiety and PTSD, SSRIs, ARBs, ACE inhibitors, diuretics, antidepressants, hypnotics for sleep, and I would be pharmaceutical-free if not for my continued labile hypertensive episodes.

> *When logic and proportion*
> *Have fallen sloppy dead*
> *And the white knight is talking backwards*
> *And the red queen's off with her head*
> *Remember what the dormouse said.*
>
> *Feed your head.*
> *Feed your head!*
> *Feed your HEAD!*

Sounds like good advice to me. I'm following the White Rabbit.

CHAPTER 27

Mitakuye Oyasin

*The whole course of human history may depend on a change
of heart in one solitary and even humble individual. For it is
in the solitary mind and soul of the individual that the battle
between good and evil is waged and ultimately won or lost.*

—M. Scott Peck

So, for the last 37,000,000 minutes God has granted me the opportunity to walk the earth in this carbon-based shell, I have learned to live within the company of my fellow humans and abide by the established laws that govern our actions and behavior, with a few minor inconsistencies in the established social norms.

It is truly a blessing and a privilege to live for so many years, as so many people do not experience the joys and heartaches of living so long. Each gray hair, or *chrome* in my case, represents fond memories and experiences of great times from the past. The varicose veins in my legs are the roadmaps to wisdom and understanding of oneself and represent the many happy roads traveled on adventures. The knowledge and wisdom that is assimilated in one's life is directly proportional to the efforts one puts forth to grow and achieve in their lifetime.

Armed with the awareness that my special gift as a caregiver made a positive impact in so many people's lives has provided abundant compensation and given me the strength to embrace every morning the sun greets me in the east to carry on and to humbly seek passive permission to extend my visit on Mother Earth and enjoy my short time here practicing patience, perseverance, tolerance, love, and acceptance.

My Southern Baptist, Midwestern, sheltered youth, complimented with a strong nuclear family, better than average intelligence, great education, *and* uncommonly good looks, laid the foundation for my successful transition into young adulthood. I still question to this day how and why I was chosen to survive Viet Nam, in spite of my youthful capricious belief that I was immortal and indestructible. And believe me, my tour of duty was *gravy* compared to most who served. I worked in a building surrounded by huge temperamental room-filling-sized computers. Aircraft from the First Marine Air Wing (First MAW) didn't get bombs, fuel, or parts until data was programmed, entered, verified, processed, and printed out on sofa-sized cacophonous dot-matrix printers. It was my personal choice to spend my free time off base applying the philosophy of Vietnamization, strongly endorsed by Marine Generals Walt, Krulak, and Green, to explore the surrounding dangerous countryside and place myself in danger engaging in risky behavior.

Everyone observes, experiences, catalogs, interprets, and stores traumatic occurrences in their lives differently on the conscious and the subconscious levels. Our impulsive unconscious mind drives our desires and emotions while instinctively learning through the experience, becoming a very powerful force in controlling conscious behavior. Many thousands encountered much more death and destruction than me; some acquired a taste for it, many "state" it did not affect them, while others still recall those unshakable life-altering incidents with laser clarity and acknowledge their awesome significance. It was not until many years later before I discovered I was not alone in my unexplained feelings. Why some veterans were hauntingly and deeply affected and others were not is beyond the scope of my knowledge; perhaps, maybe if someone asked me when I was much younger and still knew it all.

And I still regularly wonder what my lifetime batting average with the New York Yankees would have been.

Capricorns are astrologically endowed with leadership, integrity, honesty, ambition, fierce loyalty, determination, pragmatism, sensuality, stubbornness, and love for all things living. Everything that surrounds our perceived consciousness, I believe, is alive and has a vibrational and spiritual energy: plants, animals, rocks, trees, water, earth, wind, and fire. We are all related! They should all be revered with grace and humility. I had no interest in the study of astrology, nor did I take classes to discover the innate traits of Capricornicus, the horned goat, to map out my life. Nay, I was closer to 280 dog years old when I first discovered astrology second-hand from Karen, and only then realized I was a horny goat as well, and shared several similar attributes of Capricornicus. Jesus was a Capricorn. So was Richard Nixon. Go figure.

Along the long and winding road of life I've learned that air goes in and out, blood goes 'round and 'round, and saving lives is much more preferable to taking them. Forgiveness is absolutely essential to healing. Healing is an ongoing ordeal that helps define pain much like darkness defines light. They must both coexist; you cannot have one without the other. Somatic pain is a constant visitor whom I have grown accustomed to yet refuse to embrace, and rejoice in each moment when it leaves my body. Psychological pain is the eternal flame that invades the quietest moments and darkest recesses, completely uninvited and at the most inopportune times. Sleep offers no escape from its cold fingers; oftentimes though less frequently I am awakened by my own screams in a cold sweat, unable to fall back to sleep. Again, the darkest memories help draw a clearer distinction between the great moments that far surpass the bad.

The saddest thing about betrayal is that it never comes from your enemies. It's a very difficult precept for me, the fiercely loyal Capricorn, to wrap my head around. Malcolm X once said, "To me, the only thing that is worse than death is betrayal. You see, I could conceive death, but I could not conceive betrayal!" Each lifelong memory of betrayal left behind a trail of enmity and lack of closure that was not easily forgotten nor erased from the memory banks, nor from my soul. Forgiveness now has successfully supplanted my anger and resentment that, left unchecked, would have eroded my highest, strongest walls of defense and created lasting dis-ease. Forgive but do not forget.

My life has truly been blessed beyond my wildest expectations. Karen and I spent New Year's Eve, after being stuck in traffic for hours in a snowstorm due to a jackknifed semi blocking both lanes of traffic, in the spiritual electromagnetic vortex town of Sedona, Arizona. We stayed in an upscale hotel on a hilltop with 360-degree views of the snowcapped red sandstone formations.

After an elegant dinner, we returned to our room and walked about one hundred feet in deep snow to the outdoor hot tub. We were fortunate to be the only humans braving the eight inches of fresh snow and unexpectedly freezing cold weather that night, so we were fortunate to have the whole area to ourselves, sitting in a huge outdoor bubbling cauldron that could easily accommodate twenty, under a mostly starry night with a waning sliver of the moon providing a reverential glow to the surrounding red sandstone buttes and snow-covered landscape, interspersed with snow showers.

After a long soak and a long toke, we returned to our room. Each room shared a large partly covered landscaped patio that extended twenty feet beyond the rooms with tables, chairs, and comfortable cushioned seating areas with oversize elevated firepits, except tonight everything was blanketed in eight inches of progressives snowflakes. There were four firepits on each of the three levels of our hotel, and only one was lit when we returned, the one right outside our room on the third level. I believe we made a good impression at the registration desk. Gracious tips pay dividends.

We brought plenty of winter clothes for this short vacation, so we were able to sit outside around a wonderful warm fire on frozen cushions, just the two of us, counting our blessings as we rang in the New Year under the watchful eyes of Orion, Canis Major, Taurus, and the Pleiades high in the midnight sky.

Three days later we arrived in Gilbert, Arizona, east of Phoenix, at my older brother's beautiful southwestern home to visit Rich and his wife, Sally. My seventieth birthweek wish was for Karen and me to visit my older brother, whom we have not seen in over ten years. I've known this human longer than anyone on the planet, like my whole life, and in spite of our philosophic differences, we are both Marines and share many traits similar to De Vito and Schwarzenegger in the classic movie *Twins.* Subtleties and nuances in mannerisms and behavior that are evident to me and unseen by others. We have both cheated and postponed death despite many attempts by disease and trauma to hasten our early departures into the next dimension.

The night of January 3, 2019, family and friends met for my seventieth birthday and shared dinner and libation at a wonderful steak house. A dear friend and long-time Harley motorcycle companion, Fred Pascarelli, gave me his personal sage advice twenty years ago on my birthday when I turned fifty. "Never trust a fart and never waste a hard-on," he said. That same advice applies at age seventy, I might add, and Fred and Jane were there to share in more fond memories twenty years later.

While looking in the mirror when I awoke to brush my teeth the following morning, I noticed my heretofore brown conforming eyebrows had both metamorphosed overnight into twisted, gnarly, spiky white bristles that took on the sinister appearance of J. R. Ewing's menacing brows on *Dallas.* If only the hair on my head grew half as fast as nare-hair and otic-hair, the chrome hair on my head would be tied back in a ponytail by now!

Life at the Flying Monkey Ranch goes on, unfettered by the divisiveness, hatred, and insanity infecting our state, our country, and the volatile world at large. The hypocrisy, hatred, vitriol, fear-mongering, and social disease and moral decay afflicting our beloved Mother Earth has created a planetary sphenopalatine ganglioneuralgia—global brain freeze! Critical mass has been reached! My more-than-subtle dislike of all things Clinton and Obama is evident in my "liberal" use of metaphorical references. The political climate of our republic has not been this derisive, contemptuous, divisive, and disdainfully disgusting since the Viet Nam era of the late '60s and early '70s. The protests of the '70s helped to shorten the war and hasten the departure of President Nixon, Tricky Dick, who also was not on my speed dialer despite his many positive accomplishments, so I do not play party favorites; I just find objectionable those who are amoral, depraved, corrupt, and dishonorable. The list is long.

Fast-forward fifty years, and once again it's time we stop children, what's that sound? Everybody look what's goin' round.

Many times on life's pleasant journey have I tumbled down the rabbit hole facing a complex matrix of challenges from the deplorable Red Queen of Hearts. And, fortunately for me, each time I have prevailed. Confronting one's demons is just as essential as forgiveness for healing to occur. I am fortunate to have been blessed with strong self-determination (stubbornness) and have been able to individually conquer my iatrogenically induced addiction to oxycodone, benzodiazepines, hypnotics, antidepressants, and a host of other "diagnosis-related" dangerous pharmaceuticals in the comfort of my own home with no *unexpected* undesirable consequences. Enduring the anguish of acute drug withdrawal two times was a short-term investment with long-term gains and simply a matter of having the time, support, positive outlook, and the lush surroundings of the Flying Monkey Ranch to recover in my personal mountain spa resort, complete with six emotional support goats. Mental illness and hepatitis C linger like the apparitions of unexpected house guests that refuse to leave. My PTSD, anxiety, and depression symptoms are less frequent yet persistent visitors, and my HCV is in remission for now. The good days now incrementally outnumber the bad days. I'm still holding on to the ace of spades and my Uno "draw four" card for my inevitable final encounter with the Jabberwocky. It's always better to lose the last deal with a good hand.

Alcohol!

From the earliest exposure in a child's life, the brain is constantly bombarded with images that mentally condition the unconscious mind to teach us that alcohol is pleasurable, sophisticated, and a panacea for almost any occasion. Alcohol is almost sacrosanct, an expectation and perceived necessity in most social intercourse. So why do we as a species promote ingesting an extremely addictive, distasteful (methanol), sweetened, lethal poison that is responsible for more pain, heartache, suffering, death, and destruction than any other drug on the planet?

Everyone is consequentially influenced by alcohol and its effects at some time in their lives; it's how we as individuals decide to effectively confront and conduct ourselves while still completely surrounded by alcohol's subliminal lifelong universal social acceptance that holds meaning. Cirrhosis and decades of living with symptomatic HCV are two very significant reasons for total abstinence. However, it required relearning what I had learned, that which may not be true, much like Yoda's sage advice to young Jedi Luke Skywalker: "No. No different. Only different in your mind. You must *unlearn* what you have *learned*." Beyond the overt reasons for quitting (i.e., drinking toxic addictive poison), what potential benefits have I received from humans drinking alcohol recently? Not crazy Coarsegold Jack! Certainly not James A. Carvelli! And absolutely not the countless hundreds of lives lost who have needlessly died in vehicle crashes on my watch.

No need to cue the balloons or throw confetti or strike up the band or uncork the champagne. In inimitable fashion, I have *forever* individually forsaken the ingestion of the impure, infamous, insidious, injurious instrument of iniquity—alcohol. Karen has also made that same conscious decision to quit for her own raison d'être, and a collaborative mindset and approach to maintaining complete sobriety is the preferred method for us. Well, isn't that special! Church Lady would be so proud. Eliminating alcohol required special acquiescence only because of its unfortunate universal social acceptance. I do not advocate for either abstinence or indulgence; the decision to quit is a deeply personal one that everyone must decide for themselves and not taken on without seriousness and sincerity, honesty, conviction, and self-discipline. My life, my choice. However, I would advise extreme caution and suggest maintaining a twenty-foot perimeter from me if you are drunk and out of control. It could get ugly.

In her best-selling book, Annie Grace's *This Naked Mind*, I was profoundly moved and inspired by her insightfulness concerning drinking alcohol and how to control it, because we have all shared similar experiences. Her thesis is "to reverse the conditioning in your unconscious mind by educating your conscious mind. By changing your unconscious mind, you eliminate your desire to drink. Without desire, there is no temptation. Without temptation, there is no addiction." We have both closed that long and interesting chapter of our lives and made the conscious decision to abstain forever and have successfully made that transitional adjustment on the wheel of life. It is positively transformational in ways that cannot be properly explained in the confines of these pages.

Protest marches are now a daily occurrence in every corner of the globe as humans openly display their oft-misplaced anger, ignorance, and total dissatisfaction with whatever narrative is on the day's agenda, many with violent outcomes and/or violations of other innocent people's rights. If an individual or a group of people do not get their way, or feel that others do not share their extremist views exactly as them, these reprehensible, intolerant, fearful people are more than ready to restrict and usurp your right to free speech oftentimes with extreme violence (Antifa!) if you do not concede to their radical doctrine and share their beliefs. These same objectionable groups take great pleasure in hurling unfounded hate-filled epithets like racist, Nazi, nihilist, xenophobe, Islamophobe, intolerant, deplorable, misogynist, misanthrope, and terrorist, often without even a faint comprehension of the meanings of their own hate speech that the Socialist protest sponsors neatly printed on their expensive protest signs.

Social order, obedience of laws, decency, honesty, integrity, and respect for our fellow man are summarily dismissed and have spun out of control. It is *inspired* and *conspired* by the radical left socialist-progressive movement that perversely criticize, demonize, politicize, and weaponize any event, person, or topic of public interest into their ultraradical narrative of left-wing dogma. The weirder and farther from logic and reason, the better the optics will appear on the MSM networks that no longer report objective impartial news; rather, they spew opinionated, malicious, hateful vitriol. Objective journalism sadly is now an American anachronism. That is why we now have "quiet spaces" on college campuses for fear-inspired progressive snowflakes to escape from perceived racist red baseball caps; gender-neutral bathrooms for all twenty-four subcategories; scantily clad transgenders and nonbinaries (WTF!) dancing erotically for grade-school children in elementary schools; and emotional support peacocks flying business class. I will always defend their right to (peacefully) protest, but I also respect their right to be stupid! The behavior of our elected representatives on both sides of the aisle is reprehensible, and I am sad for my country because of their selfish, sophomoric behavior. The opposite of *progress* is *Congress*. Case in point: the recent character assassination of Chief Justice Brett Kavanaugh by the usual suspects. Nuf said!

All the above actions signal a disturbing paradigm shift in planetary social behavior, values, morals, religion, and thinking, which pose serious threats to our cultural, educational, legal, and political institutions. Gandalf in the Third Age of Arda said, "Sauron believes that it is only great power that can hold evil in check. But that isn't what I've found. I have found it is the small things, everyday deeds of ordinary folk that keep the darkness at bay. Simple acts of kindness and love. Why Bilbo Baggins? Perhaps it is because I'm afraid… and he gives me courage." Truer words were never spoken. That will always be my ethos as long as my heart continues to beat, and beyond.

Breathe, meditate, pray. Exercise and eat organic food; it's medicine. Laugh, and frolic in the grass with your dog each day. Do yoga; it is your spiritual guide to becoming who you are. Treat every person you meet with the dignity and respect that they deserve. Be responsible and accountable for your own actions. Improvise, adapt, and overcome. Call your mom! Love yourself and you will find it easy to love others.

Mitakuye Oyasin!

Go ask Alice. I think she'll know.

APPENDIX

THIRTEEN LAWS OF THE HOUSE OF GOD
Dr. Samuel Shem

1. GOMERs don't die.
2. GOMERs go to ground.
3. At a cardiac arrest, the first procedure is to take your own pulse.
4. The patient is the one with the disease.
5. Placement comes first.
6. There is no body cavity that cannot be reached with a 14-gauge needle and a good strong arm.
7. Age + BUN = Lasix dose.
8. They can always hurt you more.
9. The only good admission is a dead one.
10. If you don't take a temperature, you can't find a fever.
11. Show me a medical student who only triples my work and I will kiss his feet.
12. If the radiology resident and the medical student both see a lesion on the chest x-ray, there can be no lesion.
13. The delivery of medical care is to do as much nothing as possible.

AUTHOR'S NOTES

In chapter 9, "On Death and Dying," some of the characterizations of the more remote prehospital personnel mentioned in this tragic event were overstated, but they personify the volunteer's daily reality and by no means was there any intent to misrepresent the tremendous sacrifices made by volunteer fire agencies. This heartrending event exemplified those brave, selfless acts performed with dedication and without thought of remuneration or reward.

The same applies to the patient Mr. Romanov in chapter 11, "Dream Catcher." His character was a permutation, depicting him from a medley of analogous patients typifying the intense challenges we routinely faced, and an exemplary instance of the good fortune we were blessed with as a critical care flight crew, pursuing our passion while performing nearly flawless lifesaving maneuvers under the most challenging circumstances.

ABOUT THE AUTHOR

Born in the postwar era of WWII and raised in the Midwest surrounded by a close nuclear family with strong Christian values strongly influenced Mr. Martin's life. The experiences of horror and death during young adulthood while serving with the Marines in Viet Nam both troubled and inspired him to pursue his greater passion to fly in helicopters while helping others. The classic rock songs of the '60s—spawned by the political turbulence, social upheaval, and global transformation brought on by the free speech movement, demonstrations, riots, assassinations, racial injustice, and an unjust war—were inspirational catalysts in him achieving personal self-awareness, searching for replies to unanswered questions, and seeking sanity in an insane world, while maintaining his unconventional wit.

Mr. Martin worked for nearly forty years in the field of emergency medicine as an EMT, ER nurse, paramedic, flight nurse and educator, attributing his luminous accomplishments and career longevity to his satirical sense of humor.

Mr. Martin and his wife Karen currently live in Coarsegold, California and share their magical seventeen-acre Flying Monkey Ranch in the foothills of the Sierra Nevada range just south of Yosemite National Park with their menagerie of four-legged critters.